Cases in Cardiac Resynchronization Therapy

Cases in Cardiac Resynchronization Therapy

Cheuk-Man Yu, MD, FRCP (London/Edin), FRACP, FHKAM (Medicine), FHKCP, FACC, MBChB
Division of Cardiology
Department of Medicine and Therapeutics
Prince of Wales Hospital
The Chinese University of Hong Kong
Hong Kong SAR

David L. Hayes, MD, FACC, FHRS
Professor of Medicine
Mayo Clinic College of Medicine
Rochester, Minnesota

Angelo Auricchio, MD, PhD
Director, Clinical Electrophysiology Unit
Fondazione Cardiocentro Ticino
Lugano, Switzerland;
Professor of Cardiology
University of Magdeburg
Magdeburg, Germany

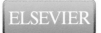

1600 John F. Kennedy Blvd.
Ste 1800
Philadephia, PA 19103-2899

Notices

Knowledge and best practice in this field are constantly changing. As new research and experience broaden our understanding, changes in research methods, professional practices, or medical treatment may become necessary.

Practitioners and researchers must always rely on their own experience and knowledge in evaluating and using any information, methods, compounds, or experiments described herein. In using such information or methods they should be mindful of their own safety and the safety of others, including parties for whom they have a professional responsibility.

With respect to any drug or pharmaceutical products identified, readers are advised to check the most current information provided (i) on procedures featured or (ii) by the manufacturer of each product to be administered, to verify the recommended dose or formula, the method and duration of administration, and contraindications. It is the responsibility of practitioners, relying on their own experience and knowledge of their patients, to make diagnoses, to determine dosages and the best treatment for each individual patient, and to take all appropriate safety precautions.

To the fullest extent of the law, neither the Publisher nor the authors, contributors, or editors, assume any liability for any injury and/or damage to persons or property as a matter of products liability, negligence or otherwise, or from any use or operation of any methods, products, instructions, or ideas contained in the material herein.

Library of Congress Cataloging-in-Publication Data

Cases in cardiac resynchronization therapy / [edited by] Cheuk-Man Yu, David
L. Hayes, Angelo Auricchio.
    p. ; cm.
 Includes bibliographical references and index.
 ISBN 978-1-4557-4237-0 (hardcover : alk. paper)
 I. Yu, Cheuk-Man, editor of compilation. II. Hayes, David L., editor of compilation. III. Auricchio, Angelo, editor of compilation.
 [DNLM: 1. Cardiac Resynchronization Therapy. WG 168]
 RC685.C6
 616.1'2306--dc23   2013041661

Executive Content Strategist: Delores Meloni
Senior Content Development Specialist: Taylor Ball
Publishing Services Manager: Jeff Patterson
Senior Project Manager: Anne Konopka
Design Direction: Ellen Zanolle

Printed in China

Last digit is the print number: 9 8 7 6 5 4 3 2 1

To Joan, Yannick, Ryan, and our extended families for the love and support.
Cheuk-Man Yu

To Sharonne, Sarah, and Drew.
David L. Hayes

To Heike, Luisa, Francesco, and Marta for always being there.
Angelo Auricchio

Contributors

Marta Acena, MD
Attending Physician
Division of Cardiology
Fondazione Cardiocentro Ticino
Lugano, Switzerland
Novel Wireless Technologies for Endocardial Cardiac
  Resynchronization Therapy
Guide Wire Fracture During Cardiac Resynchronization
  Therapy Implantation and Subsequent Management
Significant Residual or Worsening Mitral Regurgitation
  (MitraClip)

Samuel J. Asirvatham, MD
Professor of Medicine and Pediatrics
Division of Cardiovascular Diseases and Internal
  Medicine
Department of Pediatrics and Adolescent Medicine
Mayo Clinic
Rochester, Minnesota
Right Ventricular Pacing–Related Cardiomyopathy
Successful Cardiac Resynchronization Therapy Implantation:
  When to Consider the Middle Cardiac Vein
Management of Frequent Ventricular Extrasystoles

Angelo Auricchio, MD, PhD
Director, Clinical Electrophysiology Unit
Fondazione Cardiocentro Ticino
Lugano, Switzerland
Professor of Cardiology
University Magdeburg
Magdeburg, Germany
Novel Wireless Technologies for Endocardial Cardiac
  Resynchronization Therapy
Guide Wire Fracture During Cardiac Resynchronization
  Therapy Implantation and Subsequent Management
Significant Residual or Worsening Mitral Regurgitation
  (MitraClip)

Matthew T. Bennett, MD, FRCPC
Division of Cardiology
University of British Columbia
Vancouver, British Columbia, Canada
Efficacy of Cardiac Resynchronization Therapy in Right
  Bundle Branch Block
Efficacy of Cardiac Resynchronization Therapy in New York
  Heart Association II

Pierre Bordachar, MD, PhD
Département de Rythmologie du Pr Haïssaguerre
Hôpital Haut-Lévêque
Centre Hospitalier Universitaire de Bordeaux
Pessac, France
Endocardial Left Ventricular Lead: High Approach

Martin Borggrefe, MD, PhD
Director of the Department of Cardiology
University Medical Centre Mannheim
First Department of Medicine
Mannheim, Germany
Cardiac Contractility Modulation in a Nonresponder to
  Cardiac Resynchronization Therapy

Frieder Braunschweig, MD, PhD, FESC
Associate Professor of Cardiology
Karolinska Institutet
Department of Cardiology
Karolinska University Hospital
Stockholm, Sweden
Intrathoracic Impedance (Dietary Incompliance)

Haran Burri, MD
Associate Professor
Cardiology Service
University Hospital of Geneva
Geneva, Switzerland
Persistent Left Superior Vena Cava: Utility of Right-Sided
  Venous Access for Coronary Sinus Lead Implantation
Persistent Left Superior Vena Cava: Cardiac
  Resynchronization Therapy with Left-Sided Venous Access

David Cesario, MD, FACC, FHRS
Associate Professor of Clinical Medicine
Director of Cardiac Electrophysiology
University of Southern California
Los Angeles, California,
Role of Cardiac Computed Tomography Before Implant:
  Diagnosis of a Prominent Thebesian Valve as an
  Obstacle to Left Ventricular Lead Deployment in Cardiac
  Resynchronization Therapy

Chin Pang, Chan, MBChB, FHRS
Division of Cardiology
Department of Medicine and Therapeutics
Prince of Wales Hospital
The Chinese University of Hong Kong
Hong Kong SAR
Role of Optimal Medical Therapy
Pacemaker Indication

Joseph Y. S. Chan, MBBS, MSC
Consultant, Division of Cardiology
Department of Medicine and Therapeutics
Prince of Wales Hospital
Shatin, Hong Kong
Recognition of Anodal Stimulation

Wandy Chan, MB ChB, PhD, FRACP
Christchurch Heart Institute
University of Otago, Christchurch
Christchurch, New Zealand
Pulmonary Hypertension and Cardiac Resynchronization
*   Therapy: Evaluation Prior to Implantation and Response*
*   to Therapy*

Yat-Sun Chan, FHKAM
Division of Cardiology
Department of Medicine and Therapeutics
Prince of Wales Hospital
The Chinese University of Hong Kong
Hong Kong SAR
Atrioventricular Optimization by Transthoracic
*   Echocardiography in a Patient with Interatrial Delay*

Vishnu M. Chandra
Carnegie Mellon University
Pittsburgh, Pennsylvania
Successful Cardiac Resynchronization Therapy Implantation:
*   When to Consider the Middle Cardiac Vein*

Maria Rosa Costanzo, MD, FACC, FAHA
Medical Director
Midwest Heart Specialists–Advocate Medical Group
    Heart Failure and Pulmonary Arterial Hypertension
    Programs
Medical Director
Edward Hospital Center for Advanced Heart Failure
Naperville, Illinois
Cardiac Resynchronization Therapy in Patients with Right
*   Heart Failure Resulting from Pulmolnary Arterial*
*   Hypertension*

Jean-Claude Daubert, MD
Service de Cardiologie
Centre cardio-pneumologique
Rennes, France
Cardiac Resynchronization Therapy in a Patient with QRS
*   Duration Between 120 and 150 Milliseconds*

Kenneth Dickstein, MD, PhD, FESC
Department of Cardiology
Stavanger University Hospital
Stavanger, Norway
University of Bergen
Bergen, Norway
Cardiac Resynchronization Therapy Defibrillator
*   Implantation in Atrial Fibrillation*

Erwan Donal, MD, PhD
Service de Cardiologie
Centre cardio-pneumologique
Rennes, France
Cardiac Resynchronization Therapy in a Patient with QRS
*   Duration Between 120 and 150 Milliseconds*

Fang Fang, PhD
Division of Cardiology
Department of Medicine and Therapeutics
Prince of Wales Hospital
The Chinese University of Hong Kong
Hong Kong SAR
Atrioventricular Optimization by Transthoracic
*   Echocardiography in a Patient with Interatrial Delay*

Edoardo Gandolfi, MD
Electrophysiology and Pacing Unit
Department of Cardiology
Humanitas Clinical and Research Center
Rozzano, Milano, Italy
Atrial Fibrillation Therapy in Refractory Heart Failure

Joseph J. Gard, MD
Electrophysiology Fellow
Division of Cardiovascular Diseases and Internal
    Medicine
Mayo Clinic
Rochester, Minnesota
Right Ventricular Pacing–Related Cardiomyopathy
Successful Cardiac Resynchronization Therapy Implantation:
*   When to Consider the Middle Cardiac Vein*

Maurizio Gasparini, MD
Head of Electrophysiology and Pacing Unit
Department of Cardiology
Humanitas Clinical and Research Center
Rozzano, Milano, Italy
Atrial Fibrillation Therapy in Refractory Heart Failure
Resumption to Sinus Rhythm After Cardiac
*   Resynchronization Therapy in a Patient with Long-*
*   Lasting Persistent Atrial Fibrillation*

Stefano Ghio, MD
Department of Cardiology
Fondazione IRCCS Policlinico San Matteo
University of Pavia
Pavia, Italy
*Difficulties in Prediction of Response to Cardiac
Resynchronization Therapy*

John Gorcsan III, MD
Professor of Medicine
University of Pittsburgh School of Medicine
Pittsburgh, Pennsylvania
*Cardiac Resynchronization Therapy in Non–Left Bundle
Branch Block Morphology*

Juan B. Grau, MD, FACS, FACC
Associate Professor of Surgery at
Columbia University Medical Center
Columbia University College of Physicians and Surgeons
The Valley Columbia Heart Center
Director of Minimally Invasive and Robotic Cardiac
Surgery
Director of Translational Cardiovascular Research
New York, New York
Adjunct Assistant Professor of Surgery
The University of Pennsylvania School of Medicine
Philadelphia, Pennsylvania
*Video-Assisted Thoracotomy Surgery for Implantation of an
Epicardial Left Ventricular Lead*
*Robotically Assisted Lead Implantation for Cardiac
Resynchronization Therapy in a Reoperative Patient*

David L. Hayes, MD, FACC, FHRS
Professor of Medicine
Mayo Clinic College of Medicine
Rochester, Minnesota
Management of Frequent Ventricular Extrasystoles

Antereas Hindoyan, PhD
Cardiovascular Medicine Fellow
Division of Cardiovascular Medicine
Department of Medicine
Cardiovascular Thoracic Institute
Keck School of Medicine
University of Southern California
Los Angeles, California
*Role of Cardiac Computed Tomography Before Implant:
Diagnosis of a Prominent Thebesian Valve as an
Obstacle to Left Ventricular Lead Deployment in Cardiac
Resynchronization Therapy*

Gerhard Hindricks, MD
Head of the Department of Electrophysiology
University of Leipzig Heart Center
Leipzig, Germany
*Implantation of a Biventricular Implantable Cardioverter-
Defibrillator Followed by Catheter Ablation in a Patient with
Dilated Cardiomyopathy and Permanent Atrial Fibrillation*

Azlan Hussin, MD
Consultant Cardiologist and Electrophysiologist
Electrophysiology Unit
Department of Cardiology
National Heart Institute
Kuala Lumpur, Malaysia
*Mapping the Coronary Sinus Veins Using an Active Fixation
Lead to Overcome Phrenic Nerve Stimulation*
*Utility of Active Fixation Lead in Unstable Left Ventricular
Lead Positions in the Coronary Sinus for Left Ventricular
Stimulation*

Pierre Jaïs, MD, PhD
Département de Rythmologie du Pr Haïssaguerre
Hôpital Haut-Lévêque
Centre Hospitalier Universitaire de Bordeaux
Pessac, France
Endocardial Left Ventricular Lead: High Approach

Christopher K. Johnson, BS
The Valley Columbia Heart Center
Columbia University College of Physicians and
Surgeons
Ridgewood, New Jersey
*Video-Assisted Thoracotomy Surgery for Implantation of an
Epicardial Left Ventricular Lead*
*Robotically Assisted Lead Implantation for Cardiac
Resynchronization Therapy in a Reoperative Patient*

Jagdesh Kandala, MD, MPH
Research Fellow in Medicine
Harvard Medical School
Massachusetts General Hospital
Boston, Massachusetts
*Role of Scar Burden Versus Distribution Assessment by
Cardiovascular Magnetic Resynchronization in Ischemia*

Paul Khairy, MD
Associate Professor of Medicine
University of Montreal
Electrophysiologist
Department of Cardiology
Montreal Heart Institute
Montreal, Canada
A Difficult Case of Diaphragmatic Stimulation

Simon Kircher, MD
University of Leipzig, Heart Center
Department of Electrophysiology
Leipzig, Germany
*Implantation of a Biventricular Implantable Cardioverter-
Defibrillator Followed by Catheter Ablation in a Patient with
Dilated Cardiomyopathy and Permanent Atrial Fibrillation*

Karl-Heinz Kuck, MD
Asklepios Hospital St. Georg
Department of Cardiology
Hamburg, Germany
*Paroxysmal Atrial Fibrillation in Patients Undergoing
    Cardiac Resynchronization Therapy: Challenge or Routine?*

Jürgen Kuschyk, MD
Head of Device Therapy
University Medical Centre Mannheim
First Department of Medicine
Mannheim, Germany
*Cardiac Contractility Modulation in a Nonresponder to
    Cardiac Resynchronization Therapy*

Emanuele Lebrun, PhD
Department of Heart and Vessels
University of Florence
Florence, Italy
Medtronic Italia
Sesto San Giovanni, Italy
*Loss of Left Ventricular Pacing Capture Detected by Remote
    Monitoring*

Christophe Leclercq, MD, PhD, FESC
Professor, Service de Cardiologie et Maladies Vasculaires
Centre Hospitalier Universitaire de Rennes
Rennes University
CIT-IT 804 Rennes
France
*Left Ventricular Quadripolar Lead in Phrenic Nerve
    Stimulation: It Is Better to Prevent Than to Treat*

Francisco Leyva, MD, FRCP, FACC
Consultant Cardiologist
Reader in Cardiology
President, British Society of Cardiovascular Magnetic
    Resonance
Queen Elizabeth Hospital
Birmingham, United Kingdom
*Use of Cardiovascular Magnetic Resonance to Guide
    Left Ventricular Lead Deployment in Cardiac
    Resynchronization Therapy*

Josef J. Marek, MD
Postdoctoral Fellow
University of Pittsburgh School of Medicine
Pittsburgh, Pennsylvania
*Cardiac Resynchronization Therapy in Non–Left Bundle
    Branch Block Morphology*

Raphaël P. Martins, MD
Service de Cardiologie
Centre cardio-pneumologique
Rennes, France
*Cardiac Resynchronization Therapy in a Patient with QRS
    Duration Between 120 and 150 Milliseconds*

Christopher J. McLeod, MBChB, PhD
Assistant Professor of Medicine
Division of Cardiovascular Diseases and Internal
    Medicine
Mayo Clinic
Rochester, Minnesota
*Intercommissural Lead Placement into a Right Ventricular
    Coronary Sinus*
*The Importance of Maintaining a High Percentage of
    Biventricular Pacing*

Theofanie Mela, MD
Director, Pacemaker and Implantable Cardioverter-
    Defibrillator Clinic
Massachusetts General Hospital
Assistant Professor of Medicine, Harvard Medical
    School
Boston, Massachusetts
*Role of Scar Burden Versus Distribution Assessment by
    Cardiovascular Magnetic Resynchronization in Ischemia*

Andreas Metzner, MD
Asklepios Hospital St. Georg
Department of Cardiology
Hamburg, Germany
*Paroxysmal Atrial Fibrillation in Patients Undergoing
    Cardiac Resynchronization Therapy: Challenge or
    Routine?*

Tiziano Moccetti, MD
Medical Director and Head of Cardiology
Division of Cardiology
Fondazione Cardiocentro Ticino
Lugano, Switzerland
*Novel Wireless Technologies for Endocardial Cardiac
    Resynchronization Therapy*
*Significant Residual or Worsening Mitral Regurgitation
    (MitraClip)*

John Mark Morgan, MA, MD, FRCP
Professor, School of Medicine
University of Southampton
Southampton, United Kingdom
*Left Ventricular Endocardial Pacing in a Patient with an
    Anomalous Left-Sided Superior Vena Cava*

Dan Musat, MD
The Valley Columbia Heart Center
Columbia University College of Physicians and
    Surgeons
Ridgewood, New Jersey
*Video-Assisted Thoracotomy Surgery for Implantation of an
    Epicardial Left Ventricular Lead*

Avish Nagpal, MBBS
Division of Infectious Diseases
Mayo Clinic
Rochester, Minnesota
Complications of Cardiac Resynchronization Therapy:
Infection

Razali Omar, MD, FACC, FHRS
Director, Electrophysiology Unit
National Heart Institute
Kuala Lumpur, Malaysia
Mapping the Coronary Sinus Veins Using an Active Fixation
Lead to Overcome Phrenic Nerve Stimulation
Utility of Active Fixation Lead in Unstable Left Ventricular
Lead Positions in the Coronary Sinus for Left Ventricular
Stimulation

Mary P. Orencole, MS, ANP-BC
Nurse Practitioner
Resynchronization and Advanced Cardiac Therapeutics
Program
Massachusetts General Hospital
Boston, Massachusetts
Role of Remote Monitoring in Managing a Patient on
Cardiac Resynchronization Therapy: Medical Therapy
and Device Optimization

Luigi Padeletti, MD
Department of Heart and Vessels
University of Florence
Florence, Italy
Gavazzeni Hospital
Bergamo, Italy
Loss of Left Ventricular Pacing Capture Detected by Remote
Monitoring

Kimberly A. Parks, DO, FACC
Advanced Heart Failure and Cardiac Transplantation
Massachusetts General Hospital
Instructor in Medicine
Harvard Medical School
Boston, Massachusetts
Role of Left Atrial Pressure Monitoring in the Management
of Heart Failure

Laura Perrotta, MD
Department of Heart and Vessels
University of Florence
Florence, Italy
Loss of Left Ventricular Pacing Capture Detected by Remote
Monitoring

Silvia Pica, MD
Cardiomyopathies, Heart Failure and Cardiac
Transplant Unit
Department of Cardiology
San Matteo Hospital
University of Pavia
Pavia, Italy
Difficulties in Prediction of Response to Cardiac
Resynchronization Therapy

Paolo Pieragnoli, MD
Department of Heart and Vessels
University of Florence
Florence, Italy
Loss of Left Ventricular Pacing Capture Detected by Remote
Monitoring

Sebastiaan R.D. Piers, MD
Fellow, Cardiac Electrophysiology
Department of Cardiology
Leiden University Medical Centre
Leiden, The Netherlands
Managing Ventricular Tachycardia: Total Atrioventricular
Block After Ablation in a Patient with Nonischemic
Dilated Cardiomyopathy
Prevention of Effective Cardiac Resynchronization Therapy
by Frequent Premature Ventricular Contractions in a
Patient with Nonischemic Cardiomyopathy

Luca Poggio, MD
Electrophysiology and Pacing Unit
Department of Cardiology
IRCCS Istituto Clinico Humanitas
Rozzano, Milano, Italy
Resumption to Sinus Rhythm After Cardiac
Resynchronization Therapy in a Patient with Long-Lasting
Persistent Atrial Fibrillation

Claudia Raineri, MD
Cardiomyopathies, Heart Failure and Cardiac
Transplant Unit
Department of Cardiology
San Matteo Hospital
University of Pavia
Pavia, Italy
Difficulties in Prediction of Response to Cardiac
Resynchronization Therapy

François Regoli, MD, PhD
Attending Physician
Division of Cardiology
Fondazione Cardiocentro Ticino
Lugano, Switzerland
*Novel Wireless Technologies for Endocardial Cardiac
    Resynchronization Therapy*
*Guide Wire Fracture During Cardiac Resynchronization
    Therapy Implantation and Subsequent Management*
*Significant Residual or Worsening Mitral Regurgitation
    (MitraClip)*

Giuseppe Ricciardi, MD
Department of Heart and Vessels
University of Florence
Florence, Italy
*Loss of Left Ventricular Pacing Capture Detected by Remote
    Monitoring*

John Rickard, MD
Electrophsyiology Fellow
Cleveland Clinic
Cleveland, Ohio
*Extraction of a Biventricular Defibrillator with a Starfix
    4195 Coronary Venous Lead*

Philippe Ritter, MD
Département de Rythmologie du Pr Haïssaguerre
Hôpital Haut-Lévêque
Centre Hospitalier Universitaire
de Bordeaux
Pessac, France
Endocardial Left Ventricular Lead: High Approach

Gregory Rivas, MD
Cardiac Electrophysiology Fellow
Division of Cardiovascular Medicine
Department of Medicine
Cardiovascular Thoracic Institute
Keck School of Medicine
University of Southern California
Los Angeles, California
*Role of Cardiac Computed Tomography Before Implant:
    Diagnosis of a Prominent Thebesian Valve as an
    Obstacle to Left Ventricular Lead Deployment in Cardiac
    Resynchronization Therapy*

Susanne Roeger, MD
Heart Failure Specialist
University Medical Centre Mannheim
First Department of Medicine
Mannheim, Germany
*Cardiac Contractility Modulation in a Nonresponder to
    Cardiac Resynchronization Therapy*

Matteo Santamaria, MD, PhD
Attending Physician
Division of Cardiology
Fondazione Cardiocentro Ticino
Lugano, Switzerland
*Guide Wire Fracture During Cardiac Resynchronization
    Therapy Implantation and Subsequent Management*

Farhood Saremi, MD
Professor of Radiology
University of Southern California
Keck Hospital
Los Angeles, California
*Role of Cardiac Computed Tomography Before Implant:
    Diagnosis of a Prominent Thebesian Valve as an
    Obstacle to Left Ventricular Lead Deployment in Cardiac
    Resynchronization Therapy*

Beat Andreas Schaer, MD
Assistant Professor, Departement of Cardiology
University of Basel Hospital
Basel, Switzerland
Up and Down in Device Therapy

Mark H. Schoenfeld, MD, FACC, FAHA, FHRS
Clinical Professor of Medicine
Yale University School of Medicine
Director, Cardiac Electrophysiology and Pacemaker
    Laboratory
Hospital of Saint Raphael
New Haven, Connecticut
*Nonresponders to Cardiac Resynchronization Therapy:
    Switch-Off If Worsening*

Jerold S. Shinbane, MD, FACC, FHRS, FSCCT
Associate Professor of Clinical Medicine
Director, USC Arrhythmia Center
Director, Cardiovascular Computed Tomography
Division of Cardiovascular Medicine
Department of Medicine
Cardiovascular Thoracic Institute
Keck School of Medicine
University of Southern California
Los Angeles, California
*Role of Cardiac Computed Tomography Before Implant:
    Diagnosis of a Prominent Thebesian Valve as an
    Obstacle to Left Ventricular Lead Deployment in Cardiac
    Resynchronization Therapy*

Jagmeet P. Singh, MD, DPhil
Director, Resynchronization and Advanced Cardiac
    Therapeutics Program
Director of the Holter and Non-invasive
    Electrophysiology Laboratory
Massachusetts General Hospital
Associate Professor of Medicine
Harvard Medical School
Boston, Massachusetts,
*Role of Left Atrial Pressure Monitoring in the Management
    of Heart Failure*
*Role of Remote Monitoring in Managing a Patient on
    Cardiac Resynchronization Therapy: Medical Therapy
    and Device Optimization*

Erlend G. Singsaas, MD
Department of Cardiology
Stavanger University Hospital
Stavanger, Norway
*Cardiac Resynchronization Therapy Defibrillator
    Implantation in Atrial Fibrillation*

M. Rizwan Sohail, MD
Assistant Professor of Medicine
Divisions of Infectious Diseases and Cardiovascular
    Diseases
Mayo Clinic College of Medicine
Rochester, Minnesota
Complications of Cardiac Resynchronization Therapy: Infection

Jonathan S. Steinberg, MD
Director, Arrhythmia Institute
Valley Health Center
Professor of Medicine
Columbia University College of Physicians and Surgeons
New York, New York and Ridgewood, New Jersey
*Video-Assisted Thoracotomy Surgery for Implantation of an
    Epicardial Left Ventricular Lead*
*Robotically Assisted Lead Implantation for Cardiac
    Resynchronization Therapy in a Reoperative Patient*

Christian Sticherling, MD, FESC
Professor of Cardiology
Departement of Cardiology
University of Basel Hospital
Basel, Switzerland
Up and Down in Device Therapy

Anthony S. L. Tang, MD, FRCPC
University of Ottawa
Ottawa, Ontario, Canada
Royal Jubilee Hospital
Victoria, British Columbia, Canada
*Efficacy of Cardiac Resynchronization Therapy in Right
    Bundle Branch Block*
*Efficacy of Cardiac Resynchronization Therapy in New York
    Heart Association II*

Robin J. Taylor, MRCP
Clinical Research Fellow
University of Birmingham and Queen Elizabeth
    Hospital Birmingham,
United Kingdom
*Use of Cardiovascular Magnetic Resonance to Guide
    Left Ventricular Lead Deployment in Cardiac
    Resynchronization Therapy*

Bernard Thibault, MD
Professor of Medicine
University of Montreal
Electrophysiologist
Department of Cardiology
Montreal Heart Institute
Montreal, Canada
A Difficult Case of Diaphragmatic Stimulation

Tobias Toennis, MD
Asklepios Hospital St. Georg
Department of Cardiology
Hamburg, Germany
*Paroxysmal Atrial Fibrillation in Patients Undergoing
    Cardiac Resynchronization Therapy: Challenge or
    Routine?*

*Skand Kumar Trivedi, MBBS, MD (Gen Medicine),
DM (Cardiology), FACC, FESC, MNAMS*
Professor and Head
Department of Cardiology
Bhopal Memorial Hospital and Research Centre
Bhopal, India
*Persistent Left Superior Vena Cava: Cardiac
    Resynchronization Therapy with Left-Sided Venous Access*

Richard Troughton, MB ChB, PhD, FRACP
Christchurch Heart Institute
University of Otago, Christchurch
Christchurch, New Zealand
*Pulmonary Hypertension and Cardiac Resynchronization
    Therapy: Evaluation Prior to Implantation and Response
    to Therapy*

Fraz Umar, MRCP
Clinical Research Fellow
University of Birmingham and Queen Elizabeth
    Hospital Birmingham,
United Kingdom
*Use of Cardiovascular Magnetic Resonance to Guide
    Left Ventricular Lead Deployment in Cardiac
    Resynchronization Therapy*

Niraj Varma, MA, DM, FRCP
Section of Electrophysiology and Pacing
Heart and Vascular Institute
Cleveland Clinic
Cleveland, Ohio
Role of Remote Monitoring in Managing a Patient on Cardiac Resynchronization Therapy: Atrial Fibrillation

Bruce L. Wilkoff, MD
Director of Cardiac Pacing and Tachyarrhythmia Devices
Department of Cardiovascular Medicine
Professor of Medicine
Cleveland Clinic Lerner College of Medicine of Case Western Reserve University
Cleveland, Ohio
Extraction of a Biventricular Defibrillator with a Starfix 4195 Coronary Venous Lead

Erik Wissner, MD
Director, Magnetic Navigation Laboratory
Asklepios Hospital St. Georg
Department of Cardiology
Hamburg, Germany
Paroxysmal Atrial Fibrillation in Patients Undergoing Cardiac Resynchronization Therapy: Challenge or Routine?

John A. Yeung-Lai-Wah, MB, ChB, FRCPC
Division of Cardiology
University of British Columbia
Vancouver, British Columbia, Canada
Efficacy of Cardiac Resynchronization Therapy in Right Bundle Branch Block

Cheuk-Man Yu, MD, FRCP (London/Edin), FRACP, FHKAM (Medicine), FHKCP, FACC, MBChB
Division of Cardiology
Department of Medicine and Therapeutics
Prince of Wales Hospital
The Chinese University of Hong Kong
Hong Kong SAR
Role of Optimal Medical Therapy
Pacemaker Indication

Katja Zeppenfeld, MD, PhD, FESC
Director of Cardiac Electrophysiology
Professor of Cardiology
Leiden University Medical Centre
Leiden, The Netherlands
Managing Ventricular Tachycardia: Total Atrioventricular Block After Ablation in a Patient with Nonischemic Dilated Cardiomyopathy
Prevention of Effective Cardiac Resynchronization Therapy by Frequent Premature Ventricular Contractions in a Patient with Nonischemic Cardiomyopathy

Foreword

With over 500,000 new cases of heart failure per year and 300,000 deaths per year, heart failure is a major public health problem. Cardiac resynchronization therapy has become a cornerstone for the treatment for patients with congestive heart failure and conduction system disease. It is an important therapy and demands knowledge about heart failure management, hemodynamics, cardiac imaging, and device management. This textbook from three leading authorities in this field is the perfect combination of all these disciplines.

This textbook represents a major contribution to this important and evolving field. It provides much valuable information to clinicians that is indispensable to anyone who cares for these patients. Through an impressive array of cases that span virtually every aspect of this field, cardiologists will find reading and reviewing these cases to be a spectacular learning experience. Each case is written from a different perspective by an expert in the field and provides valuable insight into how a heart failure specialist might approach a patient with right ventricular dysfunction and an implanted cardiac resynchronization device who has not responded optimally. In other chapters, approaches to patients with a wide variety of other simple or complex problems are discussed in detail and in a clinically meaningful fashion. Each discussion is clinically oriented, and specific patient-related problems are analyzed. This outstanding text will appeal to clinicians from widely varying backgrounds, and each will learn something valuable. The editors are to be congratulated on providing what is truly a practical and essential guide to best practices of cardiac resynchronization therapy that will improve the care of these patients on a daily basis. This is a remarkable book and provides a truly unique perspective on this important clinical practice.

Kenneth A. Ellenbogen, MD
Kontos Professor of Cardiology
Chairman, Division of Cardiology
Virginia Commonwealth
University School of Medicine
Richmond, Virginia

Preface

Cardiac resynchronization therapy has transformed the practice of heart failure treatment. Since the first human cases conducted in 1989 by a Dutch cardiac surgeon, Dr. Patricia Bakker, and by Dr. Morton Mower, the inventor of biventricular pacing, the therapy has evolved significantly. Armed with the knowledge acquired from more than two decades of research on the effect of cardiac pacing and resynchronization on cardiac mechanics, with lead placement technologies that tackle the complex coronary vein anatomy considered inaccessible just a short time ago, and with the results of large-scale clinical trials involving progressively less ill patients, we are confidently treating a large variety of patients today.

Naturally it is expected that cardiac resynchronization therapy will continue to change rapidly. It is challenging for the practitioner to stay current on these developments, and publications attempting to teach electrophysiologists risk becoming antiquated just as they are being published. Nevertheless, many underlying concepts and principles endure through the years and require proficiency by competent practitioners.

Currently, several outstanding books in cardiac electrophysiology provide comprehensive information in conventional textbook format. *Cases in Cardiac Resynchronization Therapy* differs from these traditional books by focusing on a case-based approach to teach the core principles of patient selection, therapy delivery, patient follow-up, and outcome assessment. Each case illustrates one or more important and enduring concepts that competent cardiac device specialists should be expected to master. Careful study of numerous individual cases helps the practitioner appreciate the many nuances of cardiac resynchronization therapy.

Each case presentation is formatted to include the relevant clinical background and representative images necessary to understand the problem addressed. Still-frame images appear within the text, and when necessary, angiograms, ultrasound images, cardiac magnetic resonance images, or computed tomography images are provided. The outcomes of the cases and management strategies are discussed, along with supportive didactic information and the most important and relevant literature. Key concepts are summarized at the end of the discussion.

Cases in Cardiac Resynchronization Therapy is designed principally for fellows enrolled in cardiac electrophysiology training programs and for practicing electrophysiologists and cardiac device implanters preparing for board examination or recertification. In addition, general cardiology fellows, nurses and technicians, cardiology nurse practitioners, and physician assistants will find this information highly relevant and of interest.

Cheuk-Man Yu

David L. Hayes

Angelo Auricchio

Contents

SECTION 9

Device-Based Diagnostics for Heart Failure Monitoring and Remote Monitoring

Video Table of Contents

SECTION I

Current Indications

CASE 1

Paroxysmal Atrial Fibrillation in Patients Undergoing Cardiac Resynchronization Therapy: Challenge or Routine?

Tobias Toennis, Andreas Metzner, Erik Wissner, and Karl-Heinz Kuck

Age	Gender	Occupation	Working Diagnosis
58 Years	Female	Housewife	Dilated Cardiomyopathy

HISTORY

The patient has had a known cardiomyopathy for 3 years. She had coronary artery disease, with implantation of a bare metal stent (BMS) in the proximal circumflex artery in 2006. The left ventricular ejection fraction was 32% at the last visit to the cardiologist. The patient reported a rhythm disorder, but an electrocardiogram (ECG) has not been performed. She had peripheral artery disease class IIb, with a percutaneous transluminal angioplasty of the femoral artery on the left side in 2007.

Comments

The etiology of cardiomyopathy was unknown. She had cytomegalovirus-related hepatitis in the history, a myocardial biopsy revealed no active inflammation and no bacterial or viral burden, and magnetic resonance imaging did not show signs of inflammation or other structural heart disease.

CURRENT MEDICATIONS

The patient's current medications are acetylsalicylate 100 mg/day, enalapril 5 mg/day, metoprolol succinate 95 mg/day, spironolactone 25 mg/day, torasemide 5 mg/day, and atorvastatin 20 mg/day.

Comments

The medication dosage for congestive heart failure was reduced by the cardiologist because of recurrent hypotensive episodes.

CURRENT SYMPTOMS

In June 2008, the patient was admitted to the hospital because of recurrent chest pain unrelated to exercise. In addition, she reported shortness of breath during minimal physical efforts.

PHYSICAL EXAMINATION

BP/HR: 110/70 mm Hg/68 bpm
Height/weight: 160 cm/53 kg
Neck veins: No elevation of jugular venous pressure
Lungs/chest: Breath sounds clear bilaterally without crackles, rhonchi, or wheezing
Heart: Regular rate and rhythm with systolic murmur radiating to axilla
Abdomen: Soft, nontender, nondistended in all quadrants; positive bowel sounds; no palpable masses
Extremities: Warm, without clubbing or cyanosis; slight edema at the ankles

Comments

No actual signs of cardiac decompensation are present and only slight peripheral edema as a sign of congestion.

LABORATORY DATA

Hemoglobin: 12.7 g/dL
Hematocrit/packed cell volume: 0.37%
Mean corpuscular volume: 92 fL
Platelet count: 237/nL
Sodium: 134 mmol/L

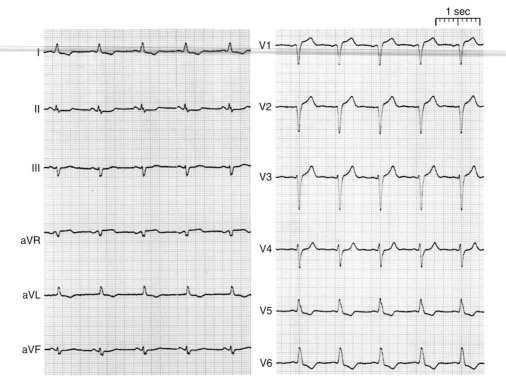

FIGURE 1-1 12 Lead ECG at admission showing sinus rhythm with a heart rate of 68 bpm and LBBB.

Potassium: 4.61 mmol/L
Creatinine: 0.9 mg/dL
Blood urea nitrogen: 51 mg/dL
Troponin T: <0.01 µg/L (normal, <0.04 µg/L)
Creatinine kinase: 44 units/L
Creatinine kinase–myocardial bound: 13 units/L

Comments

No relevant abnormalities were reported in the laboratory results. The myocardial markers remained normal in following tests.

ELECTROCARDIOGRAM

Findings

The ECG recorded a sinus rhythm, heart rate of 68 bpm, left axis deviation, left bundle branch block (LBBB), PQ interval 160 ms, QRS 160 ms, and QT 480 ms (Figure 1-1).

Comments

The ECG identified complete LBBB, with QRS greater than 150 ms, which had been described previously.

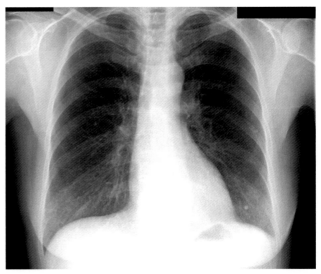

FIGURE 1-2 Chest radiograph at admission.

CHEST RADIOGRAPH

Findings

Radiography findings were no infiltrates, no congestion, no pleural effusion, normal heart/thorax ratio, and normal heart size. A small calcified, circular formation was seen in the lower left lobe, consistent with a granuloma (Figure 1-2).

Comments

The chest radiograph was normal.

ECHOCARDIOGRAM

Findings

The patient's left atrial diameter (LAD) was 35 mm, left ventricular end-diastolic diameter (LVEDD) was 62 mm, and left ventricular end-systolic diameter (LVESD) was 54 mm. She had a severely reduced left ventricular ejection fraction (30%), global hypokinesia of the left ventricle, akinesia of posterior wall, septal-to-posterior wall motion delay of 140 ms, aortic preejection time of 150 ms, moderate mitral regurgitation, slight aortic and tricuspid regurgitation, and no pericardial effusion, The inferior vena cava (IVC) and hepatic veins were not dilated (Figure 1-3).

Comments

Highly reduced left ventricular function with significant dyssynchrony was found, with no relevant signs of right heart failure.

CATHETERIZATION

Hemodynamics

Hemodynamic monitoring found highly reduced left ventricular function at 28%, moderate mitral regurgitation, no aortic stenosis, left ventricular end-systolic pressure of 128 mm Hg, left ventricular end-diastolic pressure of 20 mm Hg, pulmonary capillary wedge pressure of 34 mm Hg, pulmonary artery pressure of 64/26/44 mm Hg, right ventricular pressure of 60/0/9 mm Hg, right atrial pressure of 6 mm Hg, and cardiac output of 2.8 L/min.

Findings

The left main artery, the left anterior descending artery, and the right coronary artery showed no significant stenosis. A nonsignificant in-stent restenosis of the circumflex artery was found (Figure 1-4).

Comments

Coronary angiography revealed coronary disease in one vessel, without significant stenosis; severely reduced left ventricular function; and pulmonary hypertension.

FOCUSED CLINICAL QUESTIONS AND DISCUSSION POINTS

Question

What therapy options are available?

Discussion

The medical therapy of heart failure in this patient could not be intensified because of recurrent hypotensive episodes. No reversible reason for the reduced left ventricular function could be found. Based on the chronic, severely reduced left ventricular function (≤35%) under best possible medical treatment, the patient had an indication for implantable cardioverter-defibrillator for primary prevention of sudden cardiac death. In addition, because therapy for heart failure could not be intensified and the patient had an LBBB of more than 150 ms in New York Heart Association (NYHA) class II, she qualified for cardiac resynchronization therapy (CRT) according to the European guidelines.[1] The documented dyssynchrony on echocardiography is not part of the guidelines but supports the indication for the resynchronization therapy.

FINAL DIAGNOSIS

The final diagnosis was dilated cardiomyopathy with severe reduction of left ventricular function, NYHA III, LBBB, and coronary artery disease (single-vessel disease), with no need of intervention.

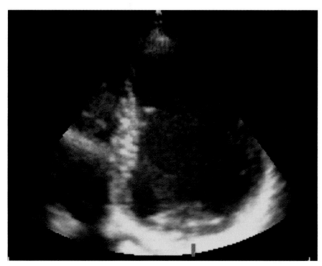

FIGURE 1-3 Echocardiography with an apical four-chamber view showing a severe dilatation of the left ventricle, highly reduced left ventricular function, and signs of dyssynchrony.

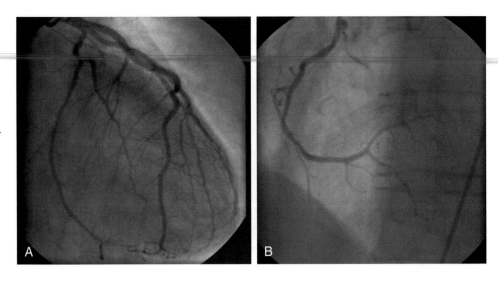

FIGURE 1-4 Coronary angiography of left **(A)** and right **(B)** coronary artery in a right anterior oblique 30-degree view **(A)** and a left anterior oblique 60-degree cranial 30-degree view **(B)**.

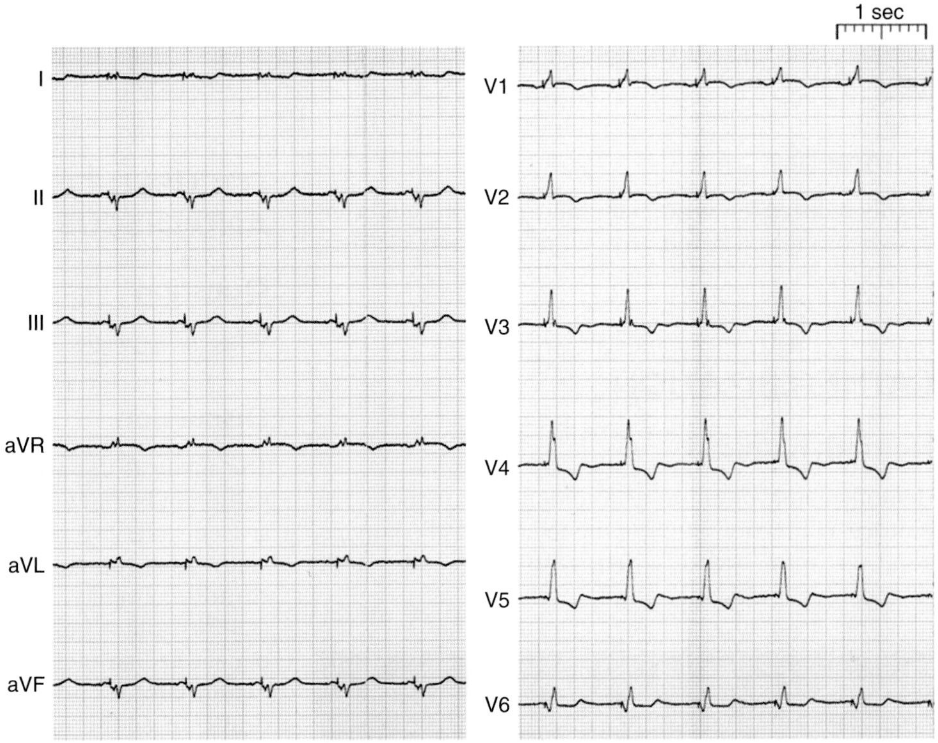

FIGURE 1-5 12-Lead electrocardiogram after implantation of a cardiac resynchronization therapy–implantable cardioverter-defibrillator device in sinus rhythm.

PLAN OF ACTION

The treatment plan consisted of resynchronization therapy for heart failure and primary prevention of sudden cardiac death by implantation of a CRT-ICD device.

INTERVENTION

The planned intervention was implantation of a CRT defibrillator device (the CRT-D system) with remote monitoring.

POSTIMPLANT ELECTROCARDIOGRAM

Findings

The postimplant ECG demonstrated atrial pacing and sequential atrio-biventricular pacing at a heart rate of 70 bpm, PQ interval of 110 ms, QRS of 115 ms, and QT of 470 ms (Figure 1-5).

Comments

The ECG identified paced rhythm with biventricular stimulation and significant reduction of QRS width.

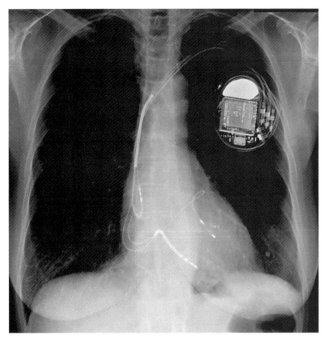

FIGURE 1-6   Chest radiograph after implantation of a CRT-ICD device showing the device, a bipolar atrial lead, a dual-coil right ventricular lead, and a bipolar left ventricular lead in a lateral branch of the great cardiac vein.

POSTIMPLANT CHEST RADIOGRAPH

Findings

The postimplant radiogram showed no infiltrates, no congestion, no pleural effusion, normal heart/thorax ratio, and a heart of normal size. A left-pectoral ICD with three leads—one in the right atrium, one in the apical right ventricle, and one in the lateral coronary sinus—was placed. The chest x-ray showed on the left side and ICD and 3 leads—one in the apex of the right ventricle, and one on the lateral wall of the left ventricle. A known small calcified, circular formation, consistent with a granuloma, was noted in the lower left lobe of the lung (Figure 1-6).

Comments

The postimplant chest radiograph was normal, with normal ICD findings and ICD lead positions.

ECHOCARDIOGRAM (8 WEEKS AFTER IMPLANTATION)

Findings

The 8-week echocardiogram showed left atrial diameter of 36 mm, LVEDD of 54 mm, LVESD of 45 mm, moderately reduced left ventricular ejection fraction

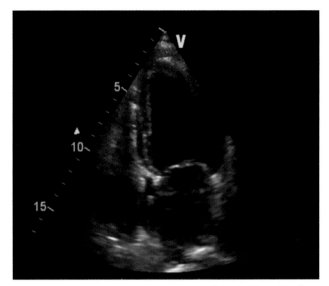

FIGURE 1-7   Echocardiography with apical four-chamber view 8 weeks after implantation with reduced left ventricular end-diastolic and end-systolic and slightly improved ejection fraction.

(32%), global hypokinesia of the left ventricle, septal-to-posterior wall motion delay of 80 ms, aortic preejection time of 105 ms, moderate mitral regurgitation, slight aortic and tricuspid regurgitation, right ventricular systolic pressure of 42 mm Hg, and no pericardial effusion, The IVC and hepatic veins were not dilated (Figure 1-7).

Comments

The echocardiogram showed remarkable reduction of left ventricular diameters and improvement of mechanical dyssynchrony. The left ventricular ejection fraction was moderately reduced, there was no sign of mechanical dyssynchrony, and there was no sign of right heart congestion.

Outcome

A few days after implantation the patient noticed remarkable improvement of exercise tolerance. She was discharged 2 days after implantation of the CRT-D system.

Course

Three months after implantation of the CRT-D, the patient developed paroxysmal atrial fibrillation with recurrent cardiac decompensation because of an intermittent loss of ventricular capture. Antiarrhythmic therapy of amiodarone 200 mg daily was initiated, as well as oral anticoagulation therapy with phenoprocoumon, based on a CHADS-VASC score of 3.

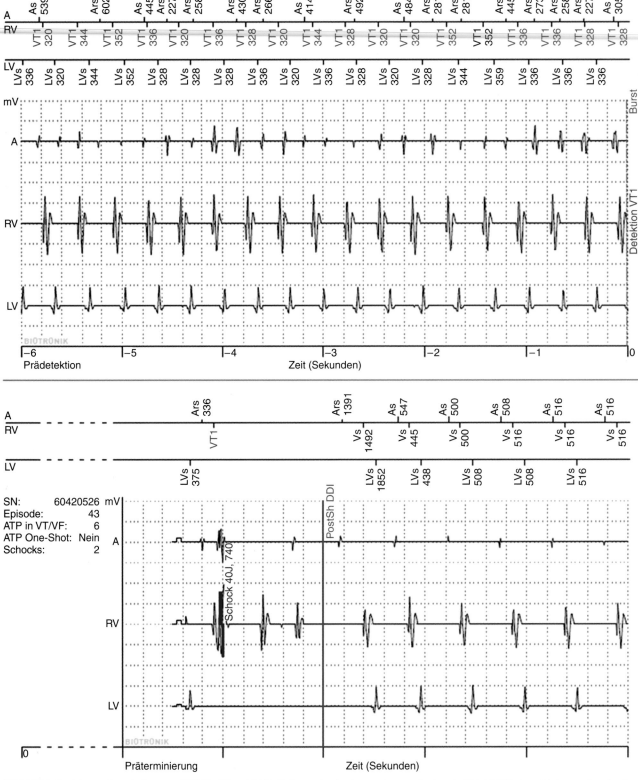

FIGURE 1-8 Intracardiac electrogram (EGM) of the atrial fibrillation episode via remote monitoring. *A,* Atrial EGM; *Ars,* atrial sense in refractory period; *AS,* atrial sense; *LV,* left ventricular EGM; *LVS,* left ventricular sense; *RV,* right ventricular EGM; *VT1,* right ventricular sense in *VT1*-zone; *Zeit,* time in seconds. After shock (40J) sinusrhythm was reestablished.

Twelve months after implantation, the patient experienced four ICD shocks. Investigation revealed episodes of atrial fibrillation to be the cause for inappropriate ICD intervention.

Findings

Recording of arrhythmia episodes by home monitoring with intracardiac electrogram documented atrial fibrillation with fast AV conduction, thus resulting in the detection of rapid ventricular rhythm. The episode terminated after six ineffective antitachycardia pacing therapies and two shocks. Sinus rhythm was reestablished at the end of the episode (Figure 1-8).

Comments

As a result of tachyarrhythmic episodes of atrial fibrillation, the patient experienced several inappropriate ICD interventions, even while on antiarrhythmic therapy with amiodarone.

FOCUSED CLINICAL QUESTIONS AND DISCUSSION POINTS

Question

What therapy options apart from the medical treatment are available?

Discussion

In patients with recurrent episodes of atrial fibrillation despite antiarrhythmic drug treatment, catheter-based ablation for complete electrical isolation of the pulmonary veins is another treatment option,[4] as implemented in the latest guidelines[5] for atrial fibrillation therapy. In contrast to application in patients with chronic persistent atrial fibrillation, AV node ablation is not a recommended treatment strategy in patients with paroxysmal atrial fibrillation. First, the absence of the hemodynamic effect of the physiologic atrial contraction can result in deterioration of the heart failure. Second, after AV node ablation, patients depend on the rate response function of the device, which does not sufficiently replicate physiologic sinus node function and will lead to worse exercise tolerance.

Question

When is the best moment to perform the pulmonary vein isolation in these patients?

Discussion

As could be seen in the current case, atrial fibrillation in patients with CRT-D devices may cause severe problems by two mechanisms. Rapidly conducted atrial fibrillation can lead to worsening of heart failure in patients who are CRT responders by loss of biventricular stimulation.[3] Furthermore, it can result in inadequate ICD therapies, which can be dangerous and traumatic to the patient and are of prognostic relevance.[2,6] Therefore early pulmonary vein isolation should be considered even after onset of atrial fibrillation. In addition remote monitoring is a very useful feature and should be recommended for early detection of atrial fibrillation in those patients.

PLAN OF ACTION

As a result of ineffective antiarrhythmic drug-based treatment, pulmonary vein isolation was indicated.

INTERVENTION

After three-dimensional reconstruction of the left atrium, pulmonary vein isolation was performed by

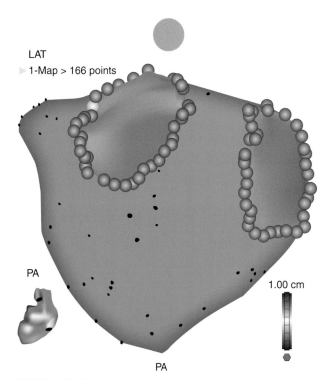

FIGURE 1-9 Posterior-anterior view of a three-dimensional CARTO reconstruction of the left atrium and circumferential ablation lines around the ipsilateral pulmonary veins.

circumferential radiofrequency catheter–based ablation. Electrical isolation was assessed based on spiral mapping catheter recordings (Figure 1-9).

OUTCOME

The patient remained in stable sinus rhythm. The symptoms of heart failure were reduced, resulting in much better exercise tolerance (NYHA I). Echocardiographic findings remained stable.

Selected References

1. Calkins H, Kuck KH, Cappato R, et al: 2012 HRS/EHRA/ECAS expert consensus statement on catheter and surgical ablation of atrial fibrillation: recommendations for patient selection, procedural techniques, patient management and follow-up, definitions, endpoints, and research trial design—a report of the Heart Rhythm Society (HRS) Task Force on Catheter and Surgical Ablation of Atrial Fibrillation, *Heart Rhythm* 9:632-696, 2012.

2. Dickstein K, Vardas PE, Auricchio A, et al: ESC Committee for Practice Guidelines: 2010 focused update of ESC guidelines on device therapy in heart failure: an update of the 2008 ESC guidelines for the diagnosis and treatment of acute and chronic heart failure and the 2007 ESC guidelines for cardiac and resynchronization therapy—developed with the special contribution of the Heart Failure Association and the European Heart Rhythm Association, *Europace* 12:1526-1536, 2010.

3. Ouyang F, Bänsch D, Ernst S, et al: Complete isolation of the left atrium surrounding the pulmonary veins: new insights from the double-lasso technique in paroxysmal atrial fibrillation, *Circulation* 110:2090-2096, 2004.

4. Poole JE, Johnson GW, Hellkamp AS, et al: Prognostic importance of defibrillator shocks in patients with heart failure, *N Engl J Med* 359:1009-1017, 2008.

5. Santini M, Gasparini M, Landolina M, et al: Device-detected atrial tachyarrhythmias predict adverse outcome in real-world patients with implantable biventricular defibrillators, *J Am Coll Cardiol* 7:167-172, 2011.

6. Wilton SB, Leung AA, Ghali WA, et al: Outcomes of cardiac resynchronization therapy in patients with versus those without atrial fibrillation: a systematic review and meta-analysis, *Heart Rhythm* 8:1088-1094, 2011.

Implantation of a Biventricular Implantable Cardioverter-Defibrillator Followed by Catheter Ablation in a Patient with Dilated Cardiomyopathy and Permanent Atrial Fibrillation

Simon Kircher and Gerhard Hindricks

Age	Gender	Occupation	Working Diagnosis
64 Years	Male	Teacher	Dilated Cardiomyopathy and Permanent Atrial Fibrillation

HISTORY

The patient has dilated cardiomyopathy with an initial left ventricular ejection fraction (LVEF) of 25%, permanent atrial fibrillation (AF), and the cardiovascular risk factors of obesity (body mass index 32 kg/m²) and arterial hypertension.

The diagnosis of nonischemic dilated cardiomyopathy was established 1 year previously after angiographic exclusion of significant coronary artery disease, and medical heart failure therapy was initiated. Additionally, an antiarrhythmic treatment with amiodarone and an oral anticoagulation with phenprocoumon were initiated because of highly symptomatic paroxysmal AF mainly manifesting as debilitating palpitations. The amiodarone therapy, however, had to be terminated as a result of drug-induced hyperthyroidism after 3 months of treatment. Over the past several months, paroxysmal AF progressed to less symptomatic persistent AF, and after recent electrical cardioversion had failed to restore sinus rhythm, AF was considered permanent because the decision was made to cease further attempts of rhythm control interventions and to continue with a rate control strategy with metoprolol and digitoxin.[2]

The patient arrived for treatment with slowly progressive breathlessness, fatigue, marked limitation of physical activity corresponding to New York Heart Association (NYHA) functional class III, and ankle swelling despite optimal medical heart failure treatment. He also reports recurrent episodes of irregular heart action.

CURRENT MEDICATIONS

The patient's current medications are metoprolol 95 mg twice daily; phenprocoumon with a target international normalized ratio of 2.5 (range 2.0 to 3.0); digitoxin 0.07 mg once daily; torasemide 10 mg twice daily; ramipril 10 mg once daily; and spironolactone 25 mg once daily.

CURRENT SYMPTOMS

The patient demonstrated progressive breathlessness, marked limitation of physical activity (NYHA functional class III), fatigue, severely reduced exercise capacity, mildly symptomatic irregular heart action, and recurrent ankle swelling. Anginal pain, dizziness, and syncopal events were denied.

PHYSICAL EXAMINATION

BP/HR: 110/70 mm Hg/70 bpm
Height/weight: 184 cm/107 kg
Neck veins: Not distended

Lungs/chest: Slight fine crackles over both lung bases during inspiration, no decrease in breath sounds, no dullness during percussion of the lungs

Heart: Irregular heart beat, heart rate about 60 bpm, no murmur, no third heart sound (S_3) or fourth heart sound (S_4)

Abdomen: Soft, adipose, nontender, nondistended, no hepatosplenomegaly, bowel sounds present in all four quadrants

Extremities: No cyanosis, mild peripheral edema

LABORATORY DATA

Hemoglobin: 9.4 mmol/L
Hematocrit/packed cell volume: 45%
Mean corpuscular volume: 90.6 fL
Platelet count: 254/nL
Sodium: 137 mmol/L
Potassium: 4.5 mmol/L
Creatinine: 101 μmol/L
Blood urea nitrogen: 7.5 mmol/L

ELECTROCARDIOGRAM

Findings

The electrocardiogram recorded atrial fibrillation with a heart rate of about 55 bpm, normal QRS axis, left bundle branch block with a QRS duration of 150 ms, QT interval duration of 440 ms, and secondary repolarization abnormalities (Figure 2-1).

CHEST RADIOGRAPH

Findings

The major radiograph findings on posteroanterior view were global cardiac enlargement, slight pleural effusions, and subtle pulmonary congestion (Figure 2-2).

ECHOCARDIOGRAM

Findings

Transthoracic 2-dimensional echocardiography revealed LV dilation (LV end-diastolic volume 222 mL, LV end-diastolic diameter 66 mm) and severe systolic dysfunction with a LVEF of 35% (Figure 2-3). Both the parasternal long-axis view and the 4-chamber view demonstrated a substantial dilation of the left atrium (50 mm in the parasternal long axis) (Figure 2-4). Clinically relevant valvular heart disease could be excluded.

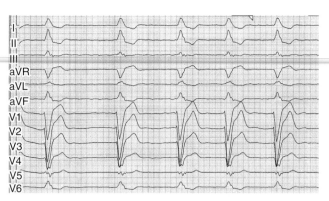

FIGURE 2-1   Surface 12-lead electrocardiogram, recording speed 50 mm/sec *(see text for interpretation).*

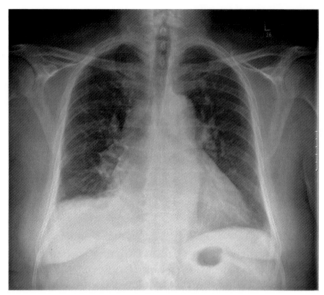

FIGURE 2-2   Chest radiograph, posteroanterior view *(see text for interpretation).*

FOCUSED CLINICAL QUESTIONS AND DISCUSSION POINTS

Question

Does evidence from clinical trials exist that supports cardiac resynchronization therapy (CRT) in patients with systolic heart failure, wide QRS complex, and permanent AF?

Discussion

Patients with AF are highly underrepresented in randomized trials of CRT. This is in contrast to routine practice because more than 20% of patients undergoing CRT have episodes of AF.[3] A meta-analysis of prospective cohort studies demonstrated that patients with persistent or permanent AF had a substantial benefit from CRT with respect to cardiac performance and functional outcomes.[11] Moreover, in the Multicentre Longitudinal Observational Study, mortality rates of patients with sinus rhythm or permanent AF who had undergone CRT were similar during a median

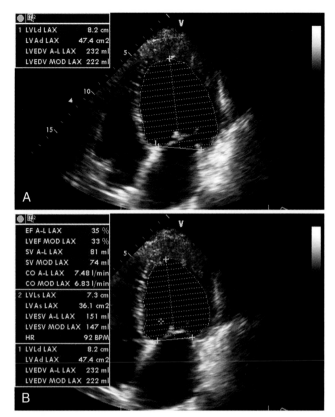

FIGURE 2-3 Two-dimensional transthoracic echocardiographic still-frame images from the 4-chamber view during diastole **(A)** and systole **(B)** *(see text for interpretation).*

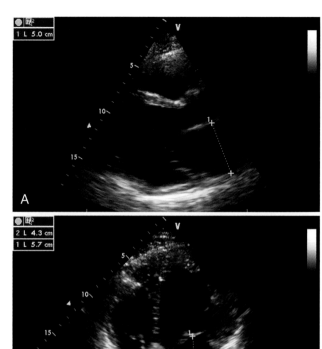

FIGURE 2-4 Two-dimensional transthoracic echocardiographic still-frame images from the parasternal long axis **(A)** and the 4-chamber view **(B)** *(see text for interpretation).*

follow-up period of 34 months.[6] Current guidelines of the European Society of Cardiology (ESC) recommend that implantation of a biventricular pacemaker or implantable cardioverter-defibrillator (ICD) should be considered to reduce morbidity in patients with permanent AF, NYHA functional class III/IV, a LVEF of 35% or less, an intrinsic QRS width of 130 ms or greater (120 ms or greater according to recently published 2013 ESC guidelines), and/or pacemaker dependency with frequent ventricular pacing (class IIa recommendation).[1,4]

Question

Should an atrial lead be implanted in patients with permanent AF undergoing CRT device implantation?

Discussion

AF is defined as permanent if cardioversion fails to restore sinus rhythm or if no rhythm control interventions are pursued.[2,7] It might be argued that an atrial lead is not required in these patients and that additional atrial lead placement would unnecessarily increase the risk for perioperative complications. In a multicenter, retrospective, longitudinal study, 330 patients with a CRT device and permanent AF were followed for a median of 42 months.[7] During the study period, spontaneous sinus rhythm

resumption occurred in approximately 10% of patients. A post-CRT QRS of 150 ms or less, a LV end-diastolic diameter of 65 mm or less, a left atrial diameter of 50 mm or less, and AV junction ablation were predictors of sinus rhythm resumption.

Question

Are ablative strategies, that is, AV node ablation or left atrial catheter ablation, able to improve outcome in patients with CRT and persistent or permanent AF?

Discussion

The rationale for AV node ablation in patients with CRT and permanent AF is to control ventricular rate to ensure a maximum biventricular pacing time and obtain a regular ventricular rhythm, because the benefit of CRT depends on a 100% biventricular pacing rate and RR-interval irregularity is associated with worsening of cardiac function.[9,10] In a study by Gasparini and colleagues including 673 patients with heart failure and CRT, patients with permanent AF demonstrated substantial and sustained long-term improvements in LV performance and functional capacity similar to those in patients with sinus rhythm only if ablation of the AV junction had been performed.[5] Additionally, it was demonstrated that AF patients with AV junction ablation had a significantly lower all-cause mortality rate in contrast to patients with AF with medical rate control only.[6] Current ESC guidelines state that AV nodal ablation may be required to ensure adequate pacing.[1,4] The role of AF catheter ablation in patients with no or moderate cardiac disease is well established, especially in those with paroxysmal AF.[2] Catheter ablation of patients with systolic heart failure, however, is less well established. In the Pulmonary Vein Antrum Isolation vs. AV Node Ablation with Biventricular Pacing for Treatment of Atrial Fibrillation in Patients with Congestive Heart Failure (PABA-CHF) trial, 81 patients with drug-refractory AF (~50% had persistent or long-standing persistent AF) and a LVEF of 40% or less were randomly assigned to pulmonary vein isolation (plus additional linear lesions) or AV node ablation with biventricular pacing.[8] After 6 months, 71% of patients in the catheter ablation group were free from AF without concomitant antiarrhythmic drug treatment. Catheter ablation was superior to AV node ablation and CRT with respect to an improvement in LVEF, functional capacity, and quality of life. The 2012 Heart Rhythm Society, European Heart Rhythm Association, and European Cardiac Arrhythmia Society Expert Consensus Statement on Catheter and Surgical Ablation of Atrial Fibrillation states that according to current studies, catheter ablation may be a reasonable treatment option in strictly selected patients with heart failure.[2]

FINAL DIAGNOSIS

The patient's final diagnoses were highly symptomatic dilated cardiomyopathy with a LVEF of 35% and a wide QRS complex, and permanent AF.

PLAN OF ACTION

The patient fulfilled the criteria for CRT according to current guidelines (LVEF of 35%, NYHA functional class III despite optimal medical treatment, and QRS width of 150 ms).[1,4] Therefore, implantation of a biventricular ICD device with an atrial lead was scheduled after cardiac recompensation.

INTERVENTION

A biventricular ICD was successfully implanted.

OUTCOME

Six months after CRT implantation, slight improvement of cardiac function was found on echocardiography. This improvement, however, did not translate into a clinical benefit because the patient remained highly symptomatic (NYHA functional class III) despite effective CRT (biventricular pacing rate approximately 98%). Therefore a rhythm control strategy was reconsidered and the patient was scheduled for left atrial catheter ablation. This decision was based on data from the PABA-CHF study showing that sinus rhythm could be restored in a considerable number of patients despite distinct dilation of the left atrium (mean left atrial diameter in the pulmonary isolation group measured 49 ± 5 mm).[8]

After transseptal access to the left atrium and registration of a CT-derived three-dimensional model of the left atrium in the electroanatomic mapping system (Figure 2-5), circumferential ablation lines were placed around the ipsilateral pulmonary vein pairs at the antral level to achieve complete pulmonary vein isolation (i.e., bidirectional conduction block). Subsequently, a bipolar voltage map of the left atrium was created to identify potential AF

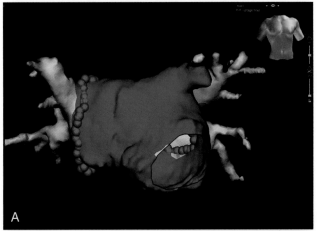

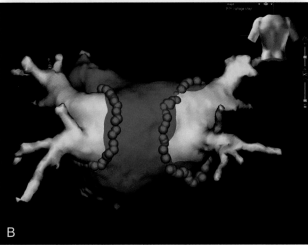

FIGURE 2-5 Anterior-posterior **(A)** and posterior-anterior **(B)** view of a three-dimensional model of the left atrium and the pulmonary veins acquired by preprocedural computed tomography and registered into the electroanatomic mapping system. *Red dots* indicate the circumferential ablation line, purple areas represent bipolar voltages with an amplitude greater than 0.5 mV (normal voltage by definition).

triggers or substrate for the perpetuation of AF. The voltage map, however, revealed exclusively voltages greater than 0.5 mV which by definition represent normal tissue. Thus no further substrate modification was performed. At the end of the procedure, sinus rhythm was restored and no sustained atrial arrhythmia could be induced by atrial burst pacing.

Findings

Up to 6 months after catheter ablation, no mode-switch episodes indicating AF recurrences or atrial tachycardias have been observed during routine interrogations. Functional status improved significantly by one NYHA functional class, and LVEF increased to 40%.

Selected References

1. Brignole M, Auricchio A, Baron-Esquivias G, et al: 2013 ESC guidelines on cardiac pacing and cardiac resynchronization therapy, *Eur Heart J* 34:2281-2329, 2013.
2. Calkins H, Kuck KH, Cappato R, et al: 2012 HRS/EHRA/ECAS Expert Consensus Statement on Catheter and Surgical Ablation of Atrial Fibrillation: recommendations for patient selection, procedural techniques, patient management and follow-up, definitions, endpoints, and research trial design, *Europace* 14:528-606, 2012.
3. Dickstein K, Bogale N, Priori S, et al: The European cardiac resynchronization therapy survey, *Eur Heart J* 30:2450-2460, 2009.
4. Dickstein K, Vardas PE, Auricchio A, et al: 2010 Focused Update of ESC Guidelines on device therapy in heart failure: an update of the 2008 ESC Guidelines for the diagnosis and treatment of acute and chronic heart failure and the 2007 ESC Guidelines for cardiac and resynchronization therapy. Developed with the special contribution of the Heart Failure Association and the European Heart Rhythm Association, *Europace* 12:1526-1536, 2010.
5. Gasparini M, Auricchio A, Regoli F, et al: Four-year efficacy of cardiac resynchronization therapy on exercise tolerance and disease progression: the importance of performing atrioventricular junction ablation in patients with atrial fibrillation, *J Am Coll Cardiol* 48:734-743, 2006.
6. Gasparini M, Auricchio A, Metra M, et al: Multicentre Longitudinal Observational Study (MILOS) Group: Long-term survival in patients undergoing cardiac resynchronization therapy: the importance of performing atrio-ventricular junction ablation in patients with permanent atrial fibrillation, *Eur Heart J* 29:1644-1652, 2008.
7. Gasparini M, Steinberg JS, Arshad A, et al: Resumption of sinus rhythm in patients with heart failure and permanent atrial fibrillation undergoing cardiac resynchronization therapy: a longitudinal observational study, *Eur Heart J* 31:976-983, 2010.
8. Khan MN, Jaïs P, Cummings J, et al: PABA-CHF Investigators. Pulmonary-vein isolation for atrial fibrillation in patients with heart failure, *N Engl J Med* 359:1778-1785, 2008.
9. Koplan BA, Kaplan AJ, Weiner S, et al: Heart failure decompensation and all-cause mortality in relation to percent biventricular pacing in patients with heart failure: is a goal of 100% biventricular pacing necessary? *J Am Coll Cardiol* 53:355-360, 2009.
10. Melenovsky V, Hay I, Fetics BJ, et al: Functional impact of rate irregularity in patients with heart failure and atrial fibrillation receiving cardiac resynchronization therapy, *Eur Heart J* 26:705-711, 2005.
11. Upadhyay GA, Choudhry NK, Auricchio A, et al: Cardiac resynchronization in patients with atrial fibrillation: a meta-analysis of prospective cohort studies, *J Am Coll Cardiol* 52:1239-1246, 2008.

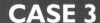

CASE 3

Efficacy of Cardiac Resynchronization Therapy in Right Bundle Branch Block

Matthew T. Bennett, John A. Yeung-Lai-Wah, and Anthony S. L. Tang

Age	Gender	Occupation	Working Diagnosis
71 Years	Male	Retired Electrician	Ischemic Heart Disease and Persistently Reduced Ejection Fraction

HISTORY

The patient is a 71-year-old man who has been followed for 20 years. He is a former smoker, having smoked from the age of 20, with 50 years of smoking at one pack per day. He formerly had hypertension. His mother had a myocardial infarction at the age of 60 years; no other family members had known premature vascular disease. He initially sought treatment at the age of 52 years with an anterior myocardial infarction. Thrombolysis was performed at that time, and he was placed on aspirin 325 mg daily.

The patient returned to medical attention 9 years ago with worsening angina (Canadian Cardiovascular Society [CCS] III). An exercise methoxyisobutylisonitrile (MIBI) test demonstrated ST depression in the anterior leads starting 6 minutes into exercise. He was able to exercise for 9 minutes. The maximal ST depression was 0.2 mV in amplitude and persisted 3 minutes into recovery. The nuclear images showed a large reversible defect occupying most of the anterior wall and anterior septum. A subsequent angiogram showed 90% stenosis in the proximal left anterior descending (LAD) artery, 40% stenosis of the left mainstem artery, 50% stenosis of the proximal and mid–right coronary artery, and 60% stenosis of the circumflex artery. Angioplasty was performed, and a bare metal stent was placed in the proximal LAD. He was then started on an angiotensin-converting enzyme (ACE) inhibitor, a statin, and a thienopyridine in addition to his aspirin and was enrolled in a cardiac rehabilitation program.

His echocardiogram at that time showed an ejection fraction of 50%, normal right ventricular function, mild-to-moderate mitral regurgitation, mild tricuspid regurgitation (no other valvulopathy), and right ventricular systolic pressure of 25 mm Hg.

One year ago the patient returned to medical attention with an acute inferior myocardial infarction. He had been on holiday camping and sought treatment 30 hours after the onset of pain. He underwent an angiogram, which revealed an occlusion of the proximal right coronary artery. Collaterals from the circumflex artery filled the distal right coronary artery. The stenosis of the circumflex artery was 75%. The stenosis of the left mainstem artery was 60%. The LAD artery now had a 70% stenosis in its midportion. The left ventricular angiogram showed an ejection fraction of 45% with severe mitral regurgitation.

A subsequent echocardiogram confirmed an ejection fraction of 45% and demonstrated severe mitral regurgitation. Akinesis of the inferior wall and hypokinesis of the anterior wall were noted. The mitral valve appeared morphologically normal. The mitral regurgitation jet was directed posteriorly, thought to be due to a tethered posterior leaflet resulting from the inferior wall motion abnormality.

Coronary artery bypass surgery and mitral valve repair or replacement was recommended. This was undertaken before discharge. He received the following grafts: left internal thoracic artery to mid-LAD with a skip graft to the second diagonal artery; saphenous vein graft from the aorta to a large first obtuse marginal artery with a skip graft to the second obtuse marginal artery; and saphenous vein graft from the aorta to the distal right coronary artery. On examining the mitral valve, the surgeon thought the best result would be obtained with a mechanical mitral valve replacement, which was implanted simultaneously.

The patient's immediate postprocedure echocardiogram showed no mitral regurgitation and an ejection fraction of 20%. Despite this, his hospital stay was complicated by pulmonary and peripheral edema. He was discharged to home 10 days after surgery on aspirin, an ACE inhibitor, a statin, a diuretic, and a low-dose beta blocker.

17

He has been attending the heart function and heart failure clinic weekly; his medications have been slowly increased to his target doses. He has had no hospital admissions for heart failure.

He is referred to a cardiac electrophysiologist 3 months after surgery for an opinion regarding device therapy.

Comments

In summary, this patient is a 71-year-old retired electrician with ischemic heart disease and persistently reduced ejection fraction despite revascularization and maximal medical therapy.

CURRENT MEDICATIONS

The patient's medications are ramipril 10 mg, aspirin 81 mg, and coumadin (dose titrated to achieve an international normalized ratio of 2.5-3.5) every morning and bisoprolol 10 mg, spironolactone 25 mg, and atorvastatin 80 mg every evening.

Comments

The patient appears to be on optimal medical therapy.

CURRENT SYMPTOMS

The patient currently denies orthopnea and paroxysmal nocturnal dyspnea. He is able to walk one block on a flat surface and has to stop because of shortness of breath.

Comments

He has New York Heart Association class III heart failure symptoms despite being revascularized and on optimal medical therapy.

PHYSICAL EXAMINATION

BP/HR: 98/60 mm Hg (left arm, seated position)/ 55 bpm at rest
Height/weight: 177.5 cm/82 kg
Neck veins: 3 cm above the sternal angle, positive abdominojugular reflux
Lungs/chest: Good breath sounds, no crepitations or wheezes
Heart: Normal mechanical first heart sound (S_1); wide split second heart sound (S_2), presence of a third heart sound (S_3), no fourth heart sound (S_4), and no audible murmurs
Abdomen: No hepatosplenomegaly, no aortomegaly
Extremities: Warm, well perfused; grade 2 pedal edema

Comments

The patient appears mildly volume overloaded.

LABORATORY DATA

Hemoglobin: 123 g/L
Hematocrit/packed cell volume: 38%
Mean corpuscular volume: 82 fL
Platelet count: 200 × 10^3/μL
Sodium: 141 mmol/L
Potassium: 4.1 mmol/L
Creatinine: 152 mmol/L
Blood urea nitrogen: 7 mmol/L

COMMENTS

The patient's renal insufficiency is long-standing. He has had three previous episodes of acute renal insufficiency resulting from prerenal azotemia. His creatinine has been at this level over the last 12 months.

ELECTROCARDIOGRAM

Findings

The 12-lead electrocardiogram (ECG) shows sinus bradycardia at a rate of 60 bpm, right bundle branch block (RBBB), and left and anterior hemiblock (Figure 3-1).

Comments

The important finding on ECG is that the RBBB is very wide, with a QRS duration of 220 msec.

ECHOCARDIOGRAM

Findings

The echocardiogram performed the week before the patient was referred for device therapy demonstrated an ejection fraction of 20%. The left ventricular end-diastolic and end-systolic dimensions are 66 and 52 mm, respectively. Mitral valve hemodynamics are normal, and paradoxical septal motion was noted. Left atrial diameter was 62 mm.

Comments

The parasternal long axis image shown in Figure 3-2 demonstrates the very dilated left ventricle with poor ejection fraction.

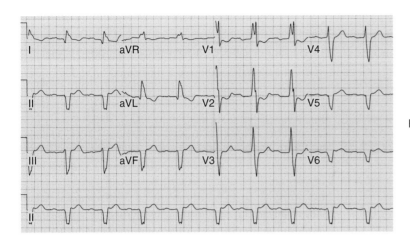

FIGURE 3-1

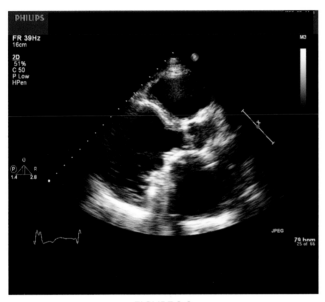

FIGURE 3-2

FOCUSED CLINICAL QUESTIONS AND DISCUSSION POINTS

Question

What is the benefit of a biventricular implantable cardioverter defibrillator (Bi-V ICD) over an implantable cardioverter-defibrillator (ICD)?

Discussion

Dyssynchrony is defined as the lack of synchronization between chambers or between the walls within the same chamber. This can refer to atrioventricular dyssynchrony, which is lack of synchronization between the atria and ventricles; V-V dyssynchrony (also known as interventricular dyssynchrony), which is lack of synchronization between the left and right ventricles; or intraventricular dyssynchrony, which is dyssychrony between the walls within one of the ventricles.

BBB creates V-V dyssynchrony by delaying the activation of the ipsilateral ventricle. This is one reason why investigators attempted to improve the symptoms of patients with heart failure and BBB by adding a left ventricular lead and resynchronizing the chambers.

Both randomized and nonrandomized trials have shown the efficacy of biventricular ICDs and pacing in patients with wide QRS duration and reduced ejection fraction. These trials included patients with left bundle branch block (LBBB) and RBBB. However, to date only four randomized trials have examined the efficacy of biventricular pacing on death or hospitalization for heart failure in subgroups stratified by QRS morphology.

The Comparison of Medical Therapy, Pacing and Defibrillation in Heart Failure (COMPANION) trial; the Cardiac Resynchronization in Heart Failure (CARE-HF) trial; the Multicenter Automatic Defibrillator Implantation with Cardiac Resynchronization Therapy (MADIT-CRT) study; and the Resynchronization–Defibrillation for Ambulatory Heart Failure Trial (RAFT) showed the benefit of biventricular pacing or ICD over medical therapy or a biventricular ICD over standard ICD therapy.[1,3,5,6] In each of these trials, patients with LBBB and RBBB were included and as a group had a significant reduction in the primary end points (usually mortality and hospitalization for heart failure or a cardiovascular event) (Table 3-1). In each of these trials, there was no benefit of biventricular pacing in the RBBB subgroup or the combined RBBB and intraventricular conduction delay subgroup.

It would appear that although patients with LBBB and RBBB have interventricular dyssynchrony, additional factors such as left ventricular intraventricular dyssynchrony must be present that confer a benefit from biventricular pacing. Are these factors and RBBB mutually exclusive or are there patients with RBBB who have these factors and thus will benefit from biventricular pacing?

In the RAFT trial the efficacy of biventricular pacing was further analyzed by QRS duration in the group of patients with RBBB. In the group of patients with a QRS duration of less than 160 msec, there was no benefit to biventricular ICD over ICD. However, in the patients with RBBB and a QRS duration of 160 msec or greater, benefit was seen of the cardiac resynchronization therapy device (CRT-D) over ICD in reducing mortality and heart failure hospitalizations.[1]

On further review of the patient's chart, it was noted that he previously had an LBBB (Figure 3-3). Presumably, the previous LBBB was actually very slow left bundle conduction and not complete LBBB. The left bundle actually conducted, but so slowly that it appeared to be 'blocked'. This was only apparent when there was right bundle branch block present. This demonstrates that patients with RBBB may have underlying left bundle disease.

Question

Would there be an expected improvement in mortality or morbidity with a Bi-V ICD if the QRS showed nonspecific interventricular conduction delay?

Discussion

Three of the trials described previously analyzed the efficacy of biventricular pacing in patients with nonspecific intraventricular conduction delay (IVCD). In the CARE-HF trial, only 10 patients randomized had IVCD. There appeared to be no difference in the event rates between the group randomized to biventricular pacing (2/4) and the group randomized to medical therapy (2/6).[4] In the 308 patients with IVCD in the MADIT-CRT trial no benefit was seen to biventricular pacing with respect to the end point of heart failure event or death.[7] In the RAFT trial, death and heart failure hospitalization event rates were similar in the 207 patients with IVCD who were randomized between biventricular ICDs and ICDs alone.[6]

TABLE 3-1   Trials That Analyzed the Efficacy of Biventricular Pacing Depending on QRS Morphology

Trial	No.	Control	Intervention	End Point	RRR Overall (%)	RRR in Non-LBBB
COMPANION	1520	Medical therapy	Biventricular pacemaker/ICD	Death from or hospitalization from heart failure	Biventricular pacemaker 34% Biventricular ICD 40%	No difference
CARE-HF	813	Medical therapy	Biventricular pacemaker	Death or hospitalization for a major cardiovascular event	37%	No difference
RAFT	1798	ICD	Biventricular ICD	Death or heart failure hospitalization	25%	No difference*
MADIT-CRT	1820	ICD	Biventricular ICD	Death or heart failure event	44%	No difference

*See text: Overall no difference was found in the RBBB group, but when analyzed by QRS width, patients with RBBB and a QRS >160 msec derived benefit from biventricular ICD therapy.

CARE-HF, Cardiac Resynchronization in Heart Failure trial; *COMPANION,* Comparison of Medical Therapy, Pacing and Defibrillation in Heart Failure trial; *ICD,* implantable cardioversion defibrillator; *LBBB,* left bundle branch block; *MADIT-CRT,* Multicenter Automatic Defibrillator Implantation with Cardiac Resynchronization Therapy study; *RAFT,* Resynchronization–Defibrillation for Ambulatory Heart Failure Trial; *RRR,* Relative Risk Reduction.

FIGURE 3-3

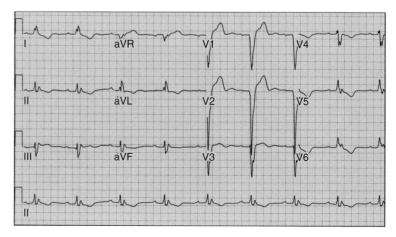

Question

What are the additional risks in implantation of a CRT-D over an ICD?

Discussion

Both the MADIT-CRT and RAFT trials randomized patients between CRT-Ds and ICDs alone.[5,6] Both trials enrolled patients during a time when currently available coronary sinus access tools and subselection sheaths were used and where left ventricular lead deployment techniques were well known. The risk for hemothorax and pneumothorax was higher in CRT-D than ICD implantation (RAFT, 1.2% vs. 0.9%; MADIT-CRT, 1.7% vs. 0.8%). The risk for pocket hematoma requiring intervention occurred more commonly in the CRT-D group than the ICD group (RAFT, 1.6% vs. 1.2%; MADIT-CRT, 3.3% vs. 2.5%). Device pocket infection occurred more commonly in the CRT-D group than the ICD group (RAFT, 2.4% vs. 1.8%; MADIT-CRT, 1.1% vs. 0.7%). An increased rate of lead dislodgement occurred, requiring intervention in the CRT-D group in contrast to the ICD group (RAFT, 6.9% vs. 2.2%; MADIT-CRT, 4% need for left ventricular lead repositioning). In addition, patients in the CRT-D group had a 0.7% to 1.2% risk for coronary sinus dissection.

FINAL DIAGNOSIS

The patient is a 71-year-old man with ischemic heart disease and mitral regurgitation. After mitral valve replacement, coronary artery bypass graft surgery, and optimal medical therapy, he had persistently low ejection fraction and NYHA III symptoms. His ECG shows a RBBB with a QRS duration of 220 msec.

PLAN OF ACTION

After a discussion with the patient regarding the risks and benefits of implantation of a CRT-D versus ICD, the patient wished to proceed with a CRT-D.

INTERVENTION

CRT-D was undertaken; the coronary sinus venogram identified a suitable posterolateral coronary sinus branch within which a left ventricular lead was inserted (Figure 3-4). At the time of the procedure a high-voltage ICD lead was inserted first, followed by a right atrial pace and sense lead. After this, a coronary sinus venogram was performed (Figures 3-5 and 3-6). The only suitable vein for a coronary sinus lead was a lateral

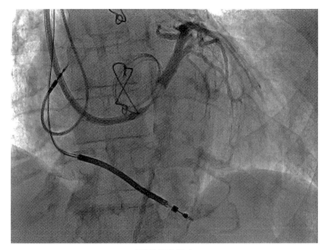

FIGURE 3-4

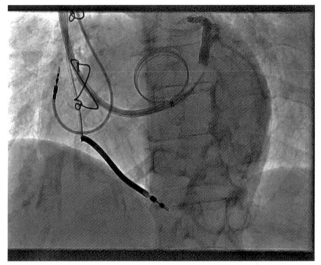

FIGURE 3-5

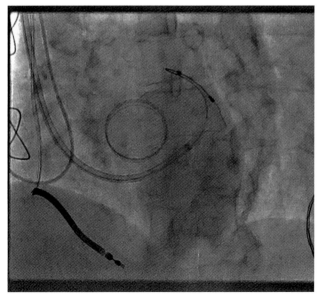

FIGURE 3-6

branch of the coronary sinus. An angioplasty wire was required to advance the wire to its final position (Figure 3-7).

The device was programmed DDDR to 50 to 120 bpm. The sensed atrioventricular delay was programmed to 180 msec, and the programmed atrioventricular delay was programmmed to 150 msec. The V-V delay was programmed so the left ventricular stimulus was delivered 20 msec before the right ventricular stimulus.

The patient's follow-up ECG shows sinus rhythm with biventricular pacing. The QRS is much more narrow than before the procedure.

His chest radiograph shows cardiomegaly (Figures 3-8 and 3-9). The position of both the right ventricular and right atrial leads are satisfactory. The left ventricular lead is in the lateral left ventricle (Figure 3-10).

OUTCOME

The patient returned to the clinic 1 month later. His symptoms had improved such that now he could walk seven blocks before stopping and overall felt an improvement in his energy. All of his medications remained the same.

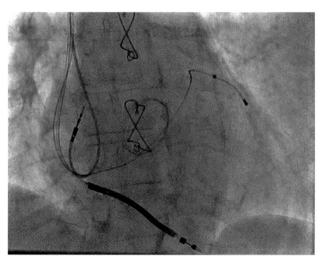

FIGURE 3-7

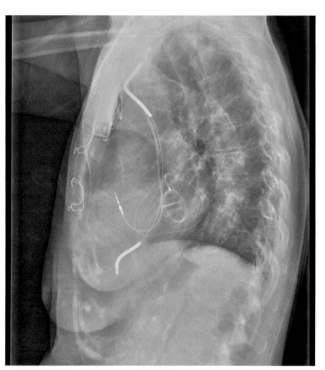

FIGURE 3-9

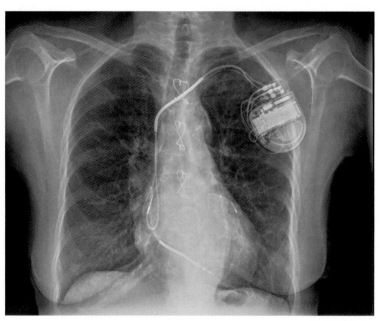

FIGURE 3-8

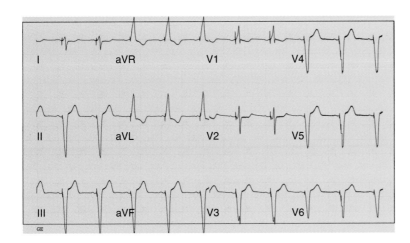

FIGURE 3-10

Selected References

1. Birnie DH, Ha A, Higginson L, et al: Importance of QRS duration and morphology in determining response to cardiac resynchronization therapy: results from the Resynchronization-Defibrillation for Ambulatory Heart Failure Trial (RAFT). *Heart Rhythm,* 9(Suppl 5): S295-S296, 2012.
2. Bristow MR, Saxon LA, Boehmer J, et al: Cardiac-resynchronization therapy with or without an implantable defibrillator in advanced chronic heart failure, *N Engl J Med* 350:2140-2150, 2004.
3. Cleland JG, Daubert JC, Erdmann E, et al: The effect of cardiac resynchronization on morbidity and mortality in heart failure, *N Engl J Med* 352:1539-1549, 2005.
4. Gervais R, Leclercq C, Shankar A, et al: Surface electrocardiogram to predict outcome in candidates for cardiac resynchronization therapy: a sub-analysis of the CARE-HF trial, *Eur J Heart Fail* 11:699-705, 2009.
5. Moss AJ, Hall WJ, Cannom DS, et al: Cardiac-resynchronization therapy for the prevention of heart-failure events, *N Engl J Med* 361:1329-1338, 2009.
6. Tang AS, Wells GA, Talajic M, et al: Cardiac-resynchronization therapy for mild-to-moderate heart failure, *N Engl J Med* 363:2385-2395, 2010.
7. Zareba W, Klein H, Cygankiewicz I, et al: Effectiveness of cardiac resynchronization Therapy by QRS Morphology in the Multi-center Automatic Defibrillator Implantation Trial-Cardiac Resynchronization Therapy (MADIT-CRT), *Circulation* 123: 1061-1072, 2011.

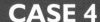

CASE 4

Cardiac Resynchronization Therapy in a Patient with QRS Duration Between 120 and 150 Milliseconds

Raphaël P. Martins, Erwan Donal, and Jean-Claude Daubert

Age	Gender	Occupation	Working Diagnosis
68 Years	Female	Retired	Congestive Heart Failure Leading to Diagnosis of Primary Left Ventricular Dysfunction with Severe Dyssynchrony, Moderately Prolonged QRS, and Lack of Left Ventricular Dilation

HISTORY

This patient had a history of lymph node tuberculosis during childhood, thyroid carcinoma (treated surgically and with radiotherapy), and depressive disorders.

A normal electrocardiogram (ECG) was recorded 20 years earlier at the time of the thyroidectomy. However, a progressive left bundle branch block (LBBB) pattern appeared with a QRS duration of 120 and 135 ms, 8 and 2 years earlier, respectively. Transthoracic echocardiography was performed 2 years earlier and showed normal left ventricular ejection fraction (LVEF) of 60%.

Comments

The patient's history demonstrated a progressive widening of QRS complex and appearance of LBBB with a normal left ventricular function.

CURRENT MEDICATIONS

The patient is currently taking levothyroxine 75 mcg daily.

CURRENT SYMPTOMS

Over a 1-year period, the patient progressively experienced exercise intolerance, weight gain related to lower extremity edema, and shortness of breath (New York Heart Association [NYHA] class III). Treatment by ramipril, bisoprolol, and furosemide was initiated without significant efficacy. She was then hospitalized for a first episode of congestive heart failure.

Comments

The patient's clinical history is suggestive of progressive congestive heart failure.

PHYSICAL EXAMINATION

BP/HR: 115/70 mm Hg/80 bpm
Height/weight: 165 cm/80 kg (+10 kg in contrast to weight)
Neck veins: Jugular veinous distention
Lungs/chest: Shortness of breath (NYHA class III), increased breathing rate, crackles throughout the lung field
Heart: Regular heart sounds, no murmurs detected
Abdomen: No ascites detected, hepatojugular reflux observed when pressing over the liver
Extremities: Lower extremities edema (ankles, legs)

Comments

The patient's clinical presentation is typical of congestive heart failure.

LABORATORY DATA

Hemoglobin: 11 g/dL
Hematocrit/packed cell volume: 40%
Mean corpuscular volume: 90 fL
Platelet count: 280 × 10³/μL
Sodium: 138 mmol/L
Potassium: 4.1 mmol/L
Creatinine: 85 μmol/L
Blood urea nitrogen: 5 mmol/L

Comments

The blood analysis showed only mild anemia, probably related to the congestive heart failure.

ELECTROCARDIOGRAM

Findings

The ECG showed sinus rhythm to be 80 bpm, normal atrioventricular conduction (PR interval, 160 ms), typical LBBB with a QRS duration of 135 ms, and a QRS axis of –35 degrees (Figure 4-1).

Comments

The LBBB is typical, with a QRS of 120 ms or greater; broad, notched, or slurred R wave in the lateral leads; absence of Q waves in leads I, V_5, and V_6; an upstroke of the R wave greater than 60 ms in leads V_5 and V_6; and ST and T waves opposite to the QRS polarity.

ECHOCARDIOGRAM

Findings

M-mode analysis of the left ventricle in parasternal long-axis view revealed a left ventricular end-diastolic diameter of 55 mm and a septal flash (Figure 4-2, *A*). LVEF was measured at 33% using the biplane Simpson method (see Figure 4-2, *B*). A mild mitral regurgitation also was observed (not shown). The atria were not dilated (diameter 3.2 cm and area 15 cm²).

Comments

Although left ventricular function is impaired, the left ventricle is not dilated (<33 mm/m²).

Findings

On the echocardiogram, the pulmonary preejection time was measured from the beginning of QRS complex to the beginning of the pulmonary flow velocity curve recorded by pulse-wave Doppler in the left parasternal view at 85 ms (Figure 4-3, *A*). The aortic preejection time measured from the beginning of QRS complex to the beginning of

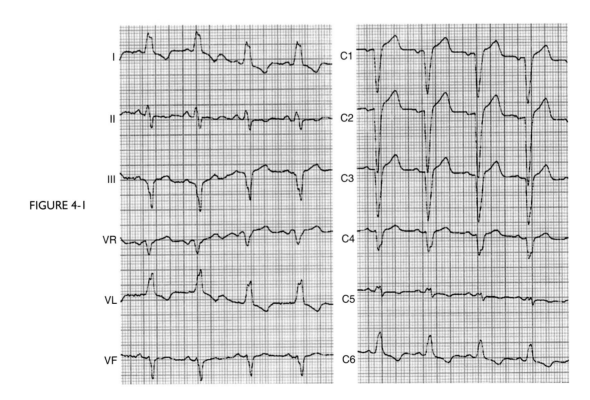

FIGURE 4-1

the aortic flow velocity curve recorded by pulse wave Doppler in the apical five-chamber view was 183 ms (Figure 4-3, *B*). The intraventricular mechanical delay was 98 ms, demonstrating interventricular dyssynchrony. Major atrioventricular dyssynchrony was demonstrated by left ventricular filling time over the RR cycle length ratio less than 40% (128/709 ms = 18%) (Figure 4-3, *C*). The apical four-chamber view showed (in *red*) the delayed motion of the anterolateral left ventricular wall (Figure 4-3, *D*). Delay between septal *(red arrow)* and anterolateral *(yellow arrow)* left ventricular walls of 301 ms demonstrated intraventricular dyssynchrony (Figure 4-3, *E*).

Comments

Echocardiography demonstrated mechanical dyssynchrony at the atrioventricular, interventricular, and intraventricular levels. Particularly, the intra–left ventricular dyssynchrony is extremely severe, with very late activation of the lateral wall.

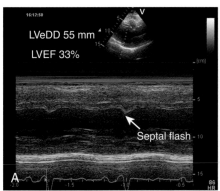

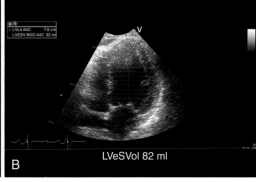

FIGURE 4-2

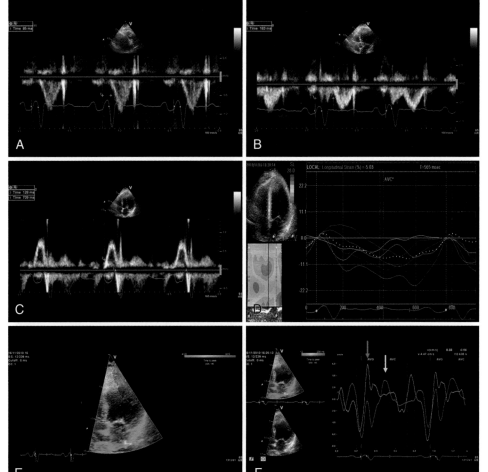

FIGURE 4-3

CATHETERIZATION

Coronary Angiography

Findings

Catheterization revealed normal coronary arteries with no stenosis.

Comments

Given the fact that the most common cause of left ventricular dilation is represented by coronary artery disease, a coronary angiography should always be performed to rule out coronary stenosis (an exercise test often is not helpful in patients with an LBBB pattern on the ECG). Usually, significant stenosis of the left anterior descending artery or of more than two other arteries is necessary to induce cardiomyopathy.

FOCUSED CLINICAL QUESTIONS AND DISCUSSION POINTS

Question

What is the incidence of LBBB in the general population?

Discussion

In the general population, the prevalence of LBBB is estimated to be 0.3% to 1.2%, higher in men than women. In most cases, LBBB is associated with structural heart diseases (e.g., ischemic, dilated or valvular cardiomyopathies, and hypertension). The incidence increases with age. However, LBBB can be observed in 0.1% of healthy individuals. Epidemiologic studies demonstrated that this pattern is associated with a worse outcome and increased all-cause mortality.

Question

In the case of persistence of the symptoms and of impaired LVEF despite optimal medical therapy, would the patient be eligible for cardiac resynchronization therapy defibrillator (CRT-D) implantation?

Discussion

A class I, level A indication of CRT implantation is optimal medical therapy, symptomatic heart failure with NYHA III or IV functional class, typical LBBB pattern with QRS of 120 ms or greater, and sinus rhythm of LVEF of 35% or less; left ventricular dilation is not a required criterion anymore.[6]

For this indication, the CRT pacemaker (CRT-P) and CRT-D have similar levels of evidence. Patients with a secondary indication for an implantable cardioverter-defibrillator (ICD) should be implanted with a CRT-D device. A reasonable expectation of survival longer than 1 year with good functional status is required for CRT-D implantation.

A CRT-D device would be preferentially implanted (rather than a CRT-P device) in patients with mildly symptomatic heart failure and larger QRS complexes 150 ms or longer.

Question

What is the impact of QRS duration on clinical events reduction with CRT?

Discussion

Traditionally, guidelines recommend CRT implantation in patients with symptomatic heart failure (NYHA class III or IV) and QRS complex duration of 120 ms or longer. This recommendation was based on the inclusion criteria of the first two major clinical trials on CRT—the Cardiac Resynchronization Heart Failure (CARE-HF)[2] study and the Comparison of Medical Therapy, Pacing and Defibrillation in Heart Failure (COMPANION)[1] study. However, most patients included in recent CRT studies specifying an inclusion criteria of QRS duration of 120 ms or longer had a QRS wider than 150 ms.

Recently, the Resynchronization Reverses Remodeling in Systolic Left Ventricular Dysfunction (REVERSE)[5] and Multicenter Automatic Defibrillator Implantation Trial with Cardiac Resynchronization Therapy (MADIT-CRT)[7] studies extended the usual inclusion criteria of symptomatic heart failure to include patients with asymptomatic or mildly symptomatic heart failure (NYHA functional class II). Although no benefit was observed in asymptomatic patients, a significant reduction of the primary end point (i.e., heart failure clinical composite response and all-cause mortality and heart failure events, respectively) was observed in both studies.

In the REVERSE study, a prespecified subgroup analysis depending on baseline QRS duration showed that patients with a prolonged QRS complex (>150 ms) and those with pronounced interventricular dyssynchrony seemed to benefit most from resynchronization.[3] Similarly, subgroup analysis of the MADIT-CRT trial suggested that patients with a QRS of 150 ms or greater were more likely to benefit from CRT-D than those with thinner QRS complexes.[11] The recently published Resynchronization–Defibrillation for Ambulatory Heart Failure Trial (RAFT) confirmed these results because it showed a greater benefit of CRT-D over ICD alone in patients with large QRS of 150 ms or longer.[9]

These three recent studies led to a modification of the European Society of Cardiology (ESC) guidelines in 2010, considering the implantation of a CRT device in patients with mildly symptomatic heart failure and a QRS of 150 ms or longer as a class I indication.

However, these subgroup analyses and the cost, potential complications, and high rate of nonresponders to CRT raise the question of whether this therapy should be reserved for patients with a QRS longer than 150 ms, whether symptomatic or not. This question is a matter of debate, particularly because of the recent publication of a meta-analysis[8] addressing this question and including the five previously cited studies (i.e., CARE-HF[2], COMPANION[1], REVERSE[5], MADIT-CRT[7], and RAFT[9]). A total of 5813 patients were included and analyzed, 62.3% and 37.7% of whom had severely and moderately prolonged QRS, respectively.[8] A 40% reduction in composite clinical events was observed in patients with severely prolonged QRS (risk ratio, 0.6; 95% confidence interval (CI), 0.53-0.67). Conversely, no benefit was demonstrated for patients with moderately prolonged QRS (risk ratio, 0.95; 95% CI 0.82-1.1), regardless of NYHA functional class at implantation. A significant relationship ($p <0.001$) between baseline QRS duration and risk ratio was evidenced, the benefit of CRT appearing for QRS duration of 150 ms or longer. A trend for benefit in the moderately prolonged QRS subgroup (120 to 159 ms) from the CARE-HF study was observed.[2] Of importance, in this study, patients with a QRS between 120 ms and 149 ms had to fulfill two of three echocardiogram criteria of dyssynchrony to be enrolled. Whether the benefit in the moderately prolonged QRS subgroup was driven by the patients with prolonged QRS between 150 and 159 ms or by patients with thinner QRS and overt dyssynchrony is unclear. Further studies are needed to address this issue.

Whether this meta-analysis, in addition to the subgroup analysis from each original trials, will lead to significant changes in guidelines and clinical practice is uncertain.

Along with QRS duration, QRS morphology was identified as another key predictor of CRT response and clinical outcome. Subgroup analyses from REVERSE[3] and MADIT-CRT[11] showed that LBBB pattern was associated with high probability of favorable outcome after CRT when patients with non-LBBB patterns, right BBB (RBBB), or nonspecific intraventricular conduction disturbances received no clinical benefit from CRT. These concordant data were used in the last version of the ESC guidelines on acute and chronic heart failure[6]: LBBB (with a QRS of ≥120 msec) is now the entry criteria for class I indication in patients with NYHA class II or III. Patients with a non-LBBB pattern can be considered for CRT (class IIa indication) if the QRS duration is 150 msec or greater.

Question

What are the predictors of super-response to CRT?

Discussion

Super-responders represent approximately 10% of CRT recipients. Criteria for super-response have not been clearly defined but could include an increase of LVEF of 15% to 20% compared with baseline or an LVEF of 50% or greater after therapy, associated with a decrease in NYHA class and no hospitalizations for heart failure during the follow-up.

Recently, Hsu and colleagues[4] investigated the predictors of LVEF super-response to CRT and identified six clinical, electrocardiographic, or echocardiographic criteria predicting such a response: female sex (odds ratio [OR], 1.96; 95% CI, 1.32-2.9), body mass index (BMI) less than 30 kg/m² (OR, 1.51; 95% CI, 1.03-2.2), no previous myocardial infarction (OR, 1.8; 95% CI, 1.2-2.71), QRS duration of 150 ms or greater (OR, 1.79; 95% CI, 1.17-2.73), LBBB pattern (OR, 2.05; 95% CI, 1.24-3.4), and small baseline left atrial volume index (OR, 1.47; 95% CI, 1.21-1.79).

This patient therefore has all of the criteria of super-response except the wide QRS duration.

FINAL DIAGNOSIS

This patient had congestive heart failure leading to the diagnosis of primary left ventricular dysfunction (LVEF, 33%), with mild left ventricular dilation, severe dyssynchrony, and an ECG demonstrating typical LBBB pattern and moderately prolonged QRS (135 ms).

The timeline of the development of LBBB is interesting to consider. The QRS, initially thin, progressively widens over time. In parallel, the LVEF, initially normal, becomes progressively impaired. This may support the diagnosis of dyssynchrony-induced cardiomyopathy.[10]

PLAN OF ACTION

Although the patient has a moderately prolonged QRS and may be part of a subgroup of patients who do not fully benefit from CRT, as previously explained, she has many of the criteria for super-response (i.e., sex, low BMI, no previous myocardial infarction, LBBB pattern, and small left atrium).

Furthermore, the timeline of QRS width and LVEF changes leading to cardiomyopathy secondary to severe dyssynchrony suggests a probable good response to CRT.

The important next step is to decide whether a CRT-P or CRT-D is to be implanted. The implantation of a CRT-P in this patient is a class IA indication of the ESC guidelines (NYHA class III/IV, QRS >120 ms, sinus rhythm, and LVEF ≤35%). The implantation of an ICD backup is a class IB indication of the ESC guidelines (i.e., NYHA II or III, LVEF ≤35%, nonischemic cause, and reasonable expectation of survival with good functional status for >1 year).

Because no arrhythmic events occurred previously (primary prevention) and a dyssynchronopathy was suspected, a CRT-P device was implanted in this patient in association with optimal medical therapy.

INTERVENTION

An atriobiventricular device was implanted as follows:

* Atrial lead in the right atrial appendage
* Right ventricular lead in the medial interventricular septum
* Left ventricular lead in a lateral branch of the coronary sinus

No complications occurred during the implantation. The sensing and pacing thresholds were correct at implantation and the following day.

The postprocedure ECG demonstrated sinus rhythm with synchronized biventricular pacing with a paced QRS width of 120 ms and a QRS axis of 90 degrees.

After optimization by echocardiography, the interventricular mechanical delay was 22 ms (vs. 93 ms before implantation). The delay between septal and anterolateral left ventricular walls decreased dramatically to 23 ms, demonstrating that the resynchronization was efficient. The left ventricular filling time increased to 65% after appropriate programming.

An optimal medical therapy was prescribed (i.e., angiotensin-converting enzyme inhibitors, beta blockers, spironolactone, and diuretics).

OUTCOME

Six months after implantation, the patient reported no shortness of breath during exercise (NYHA functional class I). Clinical examination did not show signs of heart failure (i.e., disappearance of the edema and normal lung sounds were noted).

Findings

The interrogation of the device showed a 98% rate of biventricular pacing. Pacing and sensing thresholds were correct, as were lead impedances. No ventricular arrhythmia was detected during the follow-up.

Echocardiography demonstrated a dramatic improvement of the LVEF to 62%. Ventricular size was normalized with a left ventricular end-diastolic diameter of 48 mm.

Comments

Patients with a moderately prolonged QRS (<150 ms) seem to respond to a lesser extent to CRT, regardless of NYHA class. However, some of these patients may be super-responders to CRT. Although specific studies are needed to identify these particular subgroups of patients, some criteria can help to predict whether the patient will respond to the therapy. Two of them are presented in this case report—the mechanical dyssynchrony and a clinical history suggestive of LBBB-induced cardiomyopathy.

LBBB induces abnormal left ventricular activation and contraction; the septum is activated early, as opposed to the lateral wall, which is activated and contracts after a considerable delay, sometimes after mitral valve opening. Clinical and animal studies demonstrated that dyssynchrony causes global ventricular abnormalities such as shortening of left ventricular filling time, septal hypoperfusion, and reduction of circumferential shortening and myocardial blood flow. These abnormalities lead to adverse electrical and structural remodeling that eventually cause an impairment in left ventricular function. Resynchronization therapy, by correcting electrical and mechanical dyssynchrony, can reverse such remodeling and lead to LVEF improvement.[10]

Selected References

1. Bristow MR, Saxon LA, Boehmer J, et al: Cardiac-resynchronization therapy with or without an implantable defibrillator in advanced chronic heart failure, *N Eng J Med* 350:2140-2150, 2004.
2. Cleland JG, Daubert JC, Erdmann E, et al: The effect of cardiac resynchronization on morbidity and mortality in heart failure, *N Engl J Med* 352:1539-1549, 2005.
3. Gold MR, Thébault C, Linde C, et al: The effect of QRS duration and morphology on cardiac resynchronization therapy outcomes in mild heart failure: results from the REsynchronization reVErses Remodeling in Systolic left vEntricular dysfunction (REVERSE) Study, *Circulation*, 126:822-829, 2012.
4. Hsu JC, Solomon SD, Bourgoun M, et al: Predictors of super-response to cardiac resynchronization therapy and associated improvement in clinical outcome: The MADIT-CRT (Multicenter Automatic Defibrillator Implantation Trial with the Cardiac Resynchronization Therapy) Study, *J Am Coll Cardiol* 59: 2366-2373, 2012.
5. Linde C, Abraham WT, Gold MR, et al: Randomized trial of cardiac resynchronization therapy in mildly symptomatic heart failure patients and in asymptomatic patients with left ventricular dysfunction and previous heart failure symptoms, *J Am Coll Cardiol* 52:1823-1843, 2008.
6. McMurray JJ, Adamopoulos S, Anker SD, et al: ESC guidelines for the diagnosis and treatment of acute and chronic heart failure 2012: the Task Force for the Diagnosis and Treatment of Acute and Chronic Heart Failure 2012 of the European Society of Cardiology. Developed in collaboration with the Heart Failure Association (HFA) of the ESC, *Eur Heart J* 14:803-869, 2012.
7. Moss AJ, Hall WJ, Cannom DS, et al: Cardiac resynchronization therapy for the prevention of heart failure events, *N Eng J Med* 361:1329-1338, 2009.
8. Sipahi I, Carrigan TP, Rowland DY, et al: Impact of QRS duration on clinical event reduction with cardiac resynchronization therapy, *Arch Intern Med* 171:1454-1462, 2011.
9. Tang AS, Wells GA, Talajic M, et al: Cardiac resynchronization therapy for mild to moderate heart failure, *N Engl J Med* 363: 2385-2395, 2010.
10. Vaillant C, Martins RP, Donal E, et al, *J Am Coll Cardiol* 61: 1089-1095, 2013.
11. Zareba W, Klein H, Cygankiewicz I, et al: Effectiveness of cardiac resynchronization therapy by QRS Morphology in the Multicenter Automatic Defibrillator Implantation Trial–Cardiac Resynchronization Therapy (MADIT-CRT), *Circulation* 123: 1061-1072, 2011.

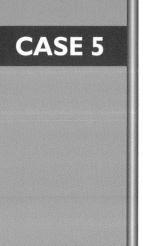

CASE 5

Cardiac Resynchronization Therapy in Patients with Right Heart Failure Resulting from Pulmonary Arterial Hypertension

Maria Rosa Costanzo

Age	Gender	Occupation	Working Diagnosis
79 Years	Female	Retired Homemaker	Worsening Right Heart Failure Resulting from Right Ventricular Apical Pacing

HISTORY

In 1985 this previously healthy patient had a syncopal episode while driving. Presumably she was found to have high-degree atrioventricular block that was treated with implantation of a permanent dual-chamber pacemaker. Except for the diagnosis of moderate chronic obstructive pulmonary disease, the patient's clinical course was uneventful until 2006, when she was hospitalized for acutely decompensated heart failure. During this hospitalization she underwent coronary angiography, which demonstrated the absence of coronary artery disease, and right heart catheterization, which demonstrated the following intracardiac pressures: right atrial, 18 mm Hg; pulmonary arterial, 88/34/53 mm Hg; and pulmonary artery wedge pressure, 25 mm Hg. Cardiac output was not measured, and hemodynamic response to vasodilators was not evaluated. Sildenafil was initiated at a twice daily dose of 50 mg.

Early in 2008 the patient required admission to the hospital for progressive exertional dyspnea, with more than 5 kg weight gain, increased jugular venous pressure, and anasarca. Admission weight was 117 kg, and renal function was severely compromised (blood urea nitrogen, 78 mg/dL; serum creatinine, 2.7 mg/dL). Transthoracic echocardiogram revealed mild left ventricular systolic dysfunction, mild-to-moderate mitral regurgitation into an enlarged left atrium, a markedly enlarged and hypokinetic right ventricle, severe tricuspid regurgitation into an enlarged right atrium, and an estimated pulmonary artery systolic pressure of greater than 65 mm Hg. To determine the appropriate therapy, hemodynamics were measured at baseline and after administration of excalating doses of inhaled nitric oxide (Table 5-1).

Based on these findings indicative of severe fluid overload, isolated venovenous ultrafiltration was initiated at a rate of 100 mL/hr and continued for 5 days. Weight and renal function changes observed with extracorporeal fluid removal were as shown in Table 5-2.

Before discharge the patient was placed on oxygen by nasal cannula at 2 L/min and on nightly bilevel positive airways pressure (BiPAP). The sildenafil dose was 20 mg three times daily, the endothelin receptor antagonist bosentan was initiated at a dose of 125 mg orally twice daily. At the follow-up office visit the patient reported improvement in exertional dyspnea and physical examination revealed a decrease in jugular venous pressure to 8 cm H_2O, absence of pulmonary crackles, and minimal lower extremity edema.

The patient continued to improve until July 2009, when she reported increasing fatigue and was found to have atrial fibrillation. With the initiation of amiodarone, sinus rhythm was spontaneously restored. In March 2010, because of malfunction and generator battery depletion of the existing pacemaker, the patient underwent implantation of a dual-chamber permanent pacemaker and placement of two new right atrial and ventricular leads. Three months after implantation of the device, atrial fibrillation recurred, but at controlled ventricular rates of approximately 75 bpm, and sinus rhythm was restored with electrical cardioversion. Atrial fibrillation recurred in October 2010, and sinus rhythm was once again restored with electrical cardioversion. Yet another recurrence of atrial fibrillation was refractory to electrical cardioversion; over the subsequent 3 months, ventricular rates increased from 110 to 120 bpm. Over the ensuing weeks the patient experienced worsening exertional dyspnea and peripheral edema, which became

TABLE 5-1   Hemodynamic Values at Baseline and after Administration of Inhaled Nitric Oxide

Hemodynamics	Baseline	NO to 80 ppm
BP (mm Hg)	93/61	71/46
RA (mm Hg)	21	18
PA (mm Hg)	71/26/45	63/21/42
PAWP (mm Hg)	12	16
TPG (mm Hg)	33	26
CO (L/min), Fick	5.2	6.1
CI (L/min/m²), Fick	2.5	2.9
PVR (Wood units)	6.4	4.3
PVRI (Wood units/m²)	13.2	9.0

BP, Arterial blood pressure; *CI,* Cardiac index; *CO,* cardiac output; *NO,* nitric oxide; *PA,* pulmonary arterial pressure; *PPM,* parts per million; *PAWP,* pulmonary artery wedge pressure; *PVR,* pulmonary vascular resistance; *PVRI,* pulmonary vascular resistance index; *RA,* right atrial pressure; *TPG,* transpulmonary gradient.

TABLE 5-2   Weight and Renal Function Changes Observed with Extracorporeal Fluid Removal

Factors Measured	Day 1	Day 2	Day 3	Day 4	Day 5
Weight (kg)	117	114.5	112	109	104
Blood urea nitrogen (mg/dL)	78	60	45	40	34
Serum creatinine (mg/dL)	2.7	2.4	2.0	1.4	1.1

increasingly more difficult to control despite frequent intensification of diuretic therapy. Early in December 2010 the patient underwent ablation of the atrioventricular node, which was associated with improvement in the signs and symptoms of congestion lasting until the end of 2011. Early in 2012 the patient began to experience worsening exertional dyspnea, weight gain, fatigue, and peripheral edema despite frequent adjustments of diuretic therapy.

Comments

The patient had true pulmonary arterial hypertension as demonstrated by the coexistence of the three hemodynamic variables that define this disease entity: a mean pulmonary arterial pressure greater than 25 mm Hg at rest, pulmonary artery wedge pressure less than 15 mm Hg, and pulmonary vascular resistance greater than 3 Wood units. The cause of pulmonary arterial hypertension in this patient is unknown, but factors such as obesity, obstructive sleep apnea, and

thyroid disease have been shown to contribute to its severity.[8]

Notably, after the first right heart catheterization, the phosphodiesterase inhibitor sildenafil was initiated without knowledge of the patient's pulmonary vascular resistance or hemodynamic response to vasodilator administration. Practice guidelines recommend that drugs specific for pulmonary arterial hypertension be initiated only after a complete hemodynamic evaluation to avoid potentially deleterious effects in patients with pulmonary arterial hypertension secondary to left heart disease.[8]

In this patient, severe pulmonary arterial hypertension is the principal cause of right ventricular dysfunction manifested by the physical findings of venous congestion and peripheral edema, the elevated right atrial pressure, and echocardiographic evidence of right ventricular enlargement and decreased systolic function.[8] Recent studies demonstrated that increased central venous pressure is a key determinant of worsening renal function because transmission of the elevated venous pressure to the renal veins further impairs the glomerular filtration rate by reducing net filtration pressure. On hospital admission the patient had severe renal impairment, which improved with extracorporeal fluid removal.[1] Loop diuretics, the most commonly used medications to reduce congestion, block sodium chloride uptake in the macula densa, independent of any effect on sodium and water balance, thereby stimulating the renin-angiotensin-aldosterone system. This pathophysiology and the growing literature documenting the adverse consequences of diuretic use on acute heart failure outcomes has led to exploration of other approaches.[1] Fluid removal by ultrafiltration at a rate that does not exceed the interstitial fluid mobilization rate of 14 to 15 mL/min avoids further activation of the renin-angiotensin-aldosterone system. Moreover, for the same fluid volume, more sodium is removed by isotonic ultrafiltration than by diuretic-induced hypotonic diuresis. In this patient, venovenous ultrafiltration was associated with a progressive reduction in weight and improvement in renal function.[2]

After approximately 12 months of clinical stability, the patient's disease progression accelerated, as suggested by the increasing burden of atrial fibrillation. In addition, because the patient has right ventricular dysfunction, she tolerates rapid ventricular rates especially poorly. As in this patient, atrial fibrillation occurs in the majority of individuals in the setting of structural heart disease. Changes in metabolic, mechanical, neurohormonal, and inflammatory factors associated with heart failure contribute to the development of atrial fibrillation. However the mechanisms linking these factors to the development of the substrate for atrial fibrillation and its progression from paroxysmal to permanent are not completely understood. A recent Euro Heart Survey analysis documented that paroxysmal atrial fibrillation progressed to persistent forms in 178 of 1219 (15%)

patients. On multivariable analysis, hypertension, age older than 75 years, previous transient ischemic attack, chronic obstructive pulmonary disease, and heart failure independently predicted progression of atrial fibrillation from paroxismal to persistent. Using the regression coefficient as a benchmark, the investigators developed a score to predict the risk for atrial fibrillation progression. Based on the presence of heart failure (2 points), history of chronic obstructive pulmonary disease (1 point), and age older than 75 years, the patient had a score of 4, indicative of moderate-to-high risk for progression from paroxysmal to persistent atrial fibrillation.[3]

The patient tolerates rapid ventricular rates poorly. This is typical of patients with right ventricular failure. In normal individuals, 85% of the blood volume is stored in the venous circulation and 15% in the arterial circulation. Patients with right ventricular failure have a larger proportion of the blood volume stored in the venovenous circulation, which renders them especially susceptible to intraarterial volume depletion. This risk is further accentuated if conditions such as atrial fibrillation with rapid ventricular response further compromise filling of the left ventricle.[3]

CURRENT MEDICATIONS

The patient's current medications are torsemide 60 mg twice daily, hydrochlorothiazide 25 mg once daily 30 to 60 minutes before taking the torsemide, spironolactone 50 mg in the morning and 25 mg in the evening 30 to 60 minutes before taking the torsemide, potassium chloride 30 mEq daily, sildenafil 20 mg three times daily, bosentan 125 mg twice daily, warfarin 7.5 mg daily, aspirin 81 mg daily, levothyroxine 75 mcg daily, omeprazole 20 mg daily, and fluticasone-salmeterol 250/50 mcg, one inhalation twice daily.

Comments

The loop diuretic used in this patient is torsemide. It is preferred over furosemide because it has better oral bioavailability (unpredictable for furosemide, 100% for torsemide) and longer half-life (2.5 vs. 6.5 hours), which reduces the length of time of postdiuretic renal sodium retention. With chronic loop diuretic therapy the distal tubular cells adapt to reabsorb sodium more efficiently, thus reducing the natriuresis produced by loop diuretics. Because thiazide diuretics and aldosterone antagonists have a longer half-life than loop diuretics, the patient was instructed to take these medications before the loop diuretic to mitigate the effects of distal tubular adaptation to loop diuretics and thus maintain the effectiveness of torsemide.[4]

The patient's therapy for pulmonary arterial hypertension included the phosphodiesterase inhibitor sildenafil and the nonselective endothelin antagonist bosentan.

The presence of severe right ventricular failure warrants consideration of the addition of a prostacyclin preparation. This was not used in this patient because of concerns that this type of medication may increase intrapulmonary shunting when left ventricular systolic function is below normal and left cardiac filling pressures rise in response to inhaled nitric oxide.[8]

Therapy also did not include antiarrhythmic agents. The authors of the Euro Heart Survey analysis found that use of antiarrhythmic agents did not prevent progression of atrial fibrillation in high-risk patients and suggested that in these patients therapy should be aimed at controlling heart rate rather than rhythm.[2] In this patient a rate control agent, such as diltiazem, was not used because its negative inotropic action could worsen the systolic function of the already compromised right ventricle and increase fluid retention.[8]

CURRENT SYMPTOMS

The patient's current symptoms are dyspnea with minimal exertion, 5.4 kg weight gain, fatigue, increased oxygen requirements.

Comments

After ablation of the atrioventricular node the patient had a period of symptomatic improvement before experiencing the current clinical deterioration. This observation raises the question of which factor(s) produced the initial improvement and why such improvement was not sustained beyond 12 months. With right ventricular pressure overload, which in this patient's case is due to pulmonary arterial hypertension, leftward bowing of the interventricular septum during diastole causes decreased left ventricular filling, chamber size, compliance, and contractility. Atrial fibrillation with rapid ventricular response further compromises left ventricular filling, thus increasing left cardiac filling pressure and decreasing forward cardiac output.[9] This hemodynamic deterioration is the likely culprit of the worsening heart failure symptoms experienced by the patient. It is plausible that the clinical improvement occurring immediately after atrioventricular node ablation resulted from improvement in left ventricular filling permitted by slower heart rates.[9]

It is more difficult to explain why the clinical improvement occurring after atrioventricular node ablation persisted for almost 12 months. A recent study demonstrated that right ventricular pressure overload results in both myocardial and electrical remodeling.[6] The effects of the latter—conduction slowing and action potential prolongation—contribute to the lengthening of right ventricular contraction duration and marked delay in right ventricular peak myocardial shortening and, consequently, in the onset of diastolic relaxation in contrast to the septum and the left ventricle.[6] This interventricular mechanical dyssynchrony decreases left ventricular filling and stroke volume. Therefore left ventricular dysfunction, initially caused by left ventricular compression by the diastolic bowing of the septum, is maintained and amplified by low left ventricular preload and underfilling. It has been suggested that in patients with right ventricular pressure overload the interventricular delay in systolic contraction and diastolic relaxation may be improved with preexcitation of the right ventricle with right ventricular pacing.[6] Therefore it is possible that the clinical improvement occurring in the patient after atrioventricular node ablation can be explained by the fact that, for a time, right ventricular pacing may have decreased diastolic interventricular delay and improved left ventricular filling and stroke volume.

After an extended period of relative clinical stability, the patient experienced a decline in functional capacity and worsening signs and symptoms of congestion. This clinical deterioration may be due to the detrimental effects of prolonged right ventricular apical pacing on cardiac structure and left ventricular function.[10] This may be related to the abnormal electrical and mechanical activation pattern of the ventricles caused by right ventricular apical pacing. Several large, randomized clinical trials of pacing mode selection have suggested an association between a high percentage of right ventricular apical pacing and worse clinical outcomes. Pertinent to this case is the fact that the negative effects of apical right ventricular pacing may be more pronounced in patients with underlying conduction disease and those who underwent atrioventricular node ablation.[10]

PHYSICAL EXAMINATION

BP/HR: 92/60 mm Hg/115 bpm
Height/weight: 172 cm/100 kg
Neck veins: Jugular venous pressure 11 to 12 cm H_2O at 45 degrees
Lungs/chest: Decreased breath sounds and fine crackles at the lung bases
Heart: Diffuse point of maximum impulse, right ventricular lift, regular rhythm, increased P_2 heart sound, right-sided third heart sound (S_3)
Abdomen: Moderately distended, liver span 15 cm, active bowel sounds
Extremities: Bilateral venous stasis changes, 3+ pitting edema

Comments

The patient's physical examination findings are consistent with a "wet and cold" hemodynamic profile, in which a low cardiac output, suggested by a low systolic blood pressure, is associated with signs of fluid overload, manifested by an elevated jugular venous pressure, enlarged liver, and marked peripheral edema.

The right ventricular lift and the increased pulmonary component of the second heart sounds (S_2) are consistent with marked right ventricular enlargement and dysfunction and with severe pulmonary arterial hypertension.[8]

LABORATORY DATA

Hemoglobin: 12.2 g/dL
Hematocrit/packed cell volume: 38.1%
Mean corpuscular volume: 90.9 fL
Platelet count: $256 \times 10^3/\mu L$
Sodium: 137 mEq/L
Potassium: 5.5 mEq/L
Creatinine: 1.3 mg/dL
Blood urea nitrogen: 43 mg/dL

Comments

The elevated blood urea nitrogen/creatinine ratio is a manifestation of the effects of an elevated central venous pressure on renal function. As explained earlier, an increase in central venous pressure produces a reduction in renal blood flow. The renal reabsorption of urea increases with decreasing renal blood flow. Therefore in this patient the elevation of blood urea nitrogen is due to increased renal reabsorption of urea resulting from the decrease in renal blood flow produced by the elevated central venous pressure.[1]

The patient's serum potassium level is in the upper limits of normal as a result of the use of the potassium-sparing diuretic spironolactone in a patient with significant renal dysfunction.

According to the Modified Diet in Renal Disease (MDRD) equation, the patient's estimated glomerular filtration rate is 40 mL/min/1.73 m², consistent with moderate reduction in renal function. North American and European practice guidelines for the treatment of heart failure in adults include specific recommendations for the monitoring, prevention, and treatment of hyperkalemia in patients receiving aldosterone antagonists.[7]

ELECTROCARDIOGRAM

Findings

A 12-lead electrocardiogaram was obtained in November 2010, shortly before the patient underwent atrioventricular node ablation (Figure 5-1). The tracing showed atrial fibrillation with a ventricular rate of approximately 115 bpm. In addition, a leftward axis, right bundle branch block, and nonspecific T waves changes in the inferior leads were noted.

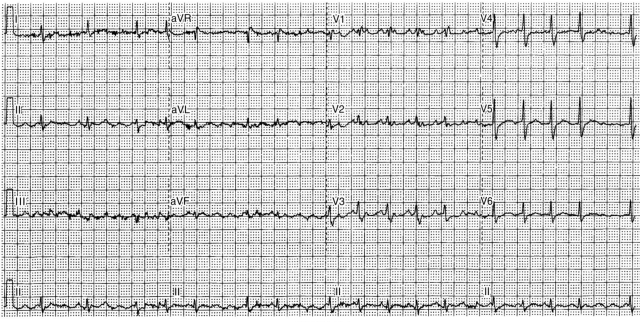

FIGURE 5-1

Comments

Atrial fibrillation with rapid ventricular response was associated with hemodynamic instability and worsening signs and symptoms of right ventricular failure because this arrhythmia further compromises left ventricular diastolic filling and aggravates venous congestion.

Some typical electrocardiographic features of pulmonary arterial hypertension are not seen in the patient's tracing. Right atrial enlargement cannot be appreciated because of the presence of atrial fibrillation. Right axis deviation and right ventricular hypertrophy with a strain pattern also are absent.

ECHOCARDIOGRAM

Findings

The echocardiogram showed tricuspid annular systolic velocity before and after upgrade to cardiac resynchronization therapy (Figure 5-2, *A*), right ventricular area change before upgrade to cardiac resynchronization therapy (Figure 5-2, *B*), and right ventricular area change after upgrade to cardiac resynchronization therapy (Figure 5-2, *C*).

Comments

Right ventricular pressure overload is associated with negative left ventricular remodeling. On the other hand, left ventricular function greatly influences right ventricular systolic function. Left ventricular contraction is responsible for as much as 40% of right ventricular systolic pressure and cardiac output. In this patient the improved left ventricular performance resulting from cardiac resynchronization therapy appears to have increased right ventricular contractility, which, in turn, is associated with reduction in central venous pressure and in the signs and symptoms of right ventricular failure.

COMPUTED TOMOGRAPHY

Findings

Noncontrast computed tomography of the chest at the level of the main pulmonary artery demonstrated markedly enlarged main, right, and left pulmonary arteries (Figure 5-3).

Comments

The computed tomography findings are consistent with the diagnosis of pulmonary arterial hypertension. Pulmonary arterial hypertension is characterized by intimal hypertrophy and fibrosis, smooth muscle hypertrophy, vasoconstriction, and adventitial proliferation with thrombosis in situ. These changes occur primarily in the small pulmonary arterioles and cause progressive dilation of the larger pulmonary vessels.

Tricuspid annular systolic velocity

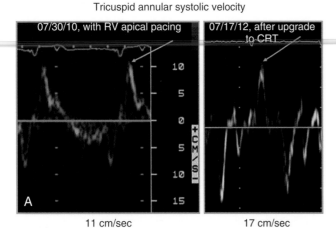

11 cm/sec   17 cm/sec

RV area change 20%
7/30/10, with RV apical pacing

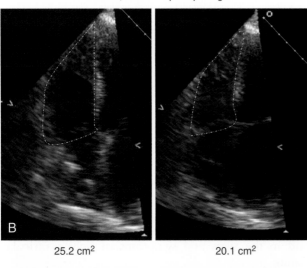

25.2 cm²   20.1 cm²

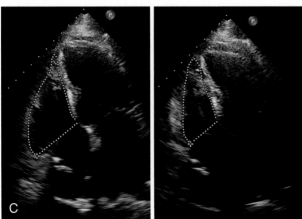

FIGURE 5-2   **A** to **C**.

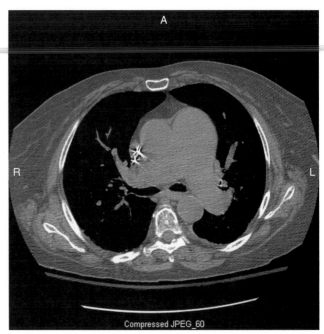

FIGURE 5-3

HEMODYNAMICS

Findings

Hemodynamic studies revealed systemic arterial hypotension, elevated right and left cardiac filling pressures, and severe pulmonary arterial hypertension (Table 5-3).

Comments

In contrast to the improvement obtained with optimization of pharmacologic treatment, the patient's hemodynamic picture is now definitely worse. Noteworthy is the marked increase in pulmonary artery wedge pressure, which suggests progression of left ventricular dysfunction. The most plausible reason for this decrease in left ventricular performance is the detrimental effect of persistent apical right ventricular pacing on the electrical and mechanical activation pattern of the left ventricle.[10]

FOCUSED CLINICAL QUESTIONS AND DISCUSSION POINTS

Question

Why did the patient's atrial fibrillation progress from paroxysmal to persistent?

Discussion

The patient is at an increased risk for atrial fibrillation progression from paroxysmal to persistent because of

TABLE 5-3 **Comparison of Hemodynamic Monitoring Results before Atrial Fibrillation and before Upgrade to Cardiac Resynchronization Therapy**

Factors Measured	Before Onset of AF	Before Upgrade to CRT
BP (mm Hg)	110/70	92/60
RA (mm Hg)	2	13
PA (mm Hg)	32/13/22	59/36/43
PAWP (mm Hg)	5	27
TPG (mm Hg)	17	16
CO (L/min)	3.8	4.1
CI (L/min/m²)	2.0	2.0
PVR (Wood units)	4.5	3.9
PVRI (Wood units/m²)	8.4	7.9

AF, Atrial fibrillation; *BP,* arterial blood pressure; *CI,* cardiac index; *CO,* cardiac output; *CRT,* cardiac resynchronization therapy, *PA,* pulmonary arterial pressure; *PAWP,* pulmonary artery wedge pressure; *PVR,* pulmonary vascular resistance; *PVRI,* pulmonary vascular resistance index; *RA,* right atrial pressure; *TPG,* transpulmonary gradient.

her older age, underlying chronic obstructive pulmonary disease, and right heart failure. Although knowledge is increasing about the risk factors for atrial fibrillation progression, the specific electrophysiologic substrates favoring such evolution are incompletely understood. The scheme proposed by the Euro Heart Survey Investigators to predict atrial fibrillation progression bears a striking resemblance to the CHADS2 score used to predict thromboembolic events.[3] Both reflect the advanced age of patients with atrial fibrillation and their high comorbidity burden, highlighting the fact that congestive heart failure, hypertension, previous stroke or transient ischemic attack, pulmonary disease, and diabetes are associated with a substrate favoring both the progression of atrial fibrillation and the development of complications associated with this arrhythmia.[3] Another unresolved issue is the optimal treatment of paroxysmal atrial fibrillation at high risk for progression. Even less is known about selection of treatment for patients who develop atrial fibrillation in the setting of right heart failure caused by pulmonary arterial hypertension. The patient presented here was a poor candidate for both calcium channel blockers because of her severe right heart failure and congestion, and amiodarone, because of the fear that possible pulmonary complications may prove fatal in the setting of underlying pulmonary disease and severe pulmonary arterial hypertension. Although atrioventricular node ablation was the best option in this patient's situation, it ultimately exposed her to the detrimental effects of continuous apical right ventricular pacing.[10]

Question

Does pressure-induced right ventricular failure affect left ventricular function?

Discussion

It is known that right ventricular pressure overload leads to leftward bowing of the interventricular septum during diastole, thereby causing decreased left ventricular chamber size, compliance, and contractility. However, the impaired left ventricular function in this setting may not simply be the result of geometric effects of right vetricular enlargement and left ventricular chamber distortion. Electrophysiologic effects of right ventricular remodeling, such as conduction slowing and action potential prolongation, lengthen right ventricular contraction and delay the onset of diastolic relaxation with respect to the septum and the left ventricle.[6] This interventricular dyssynchrony reduces left ventricular filling and stroke volume. In clinical observations and animal studies of pulmonary hypertension, ventricular interdependence was further manifested by left ventricular "atrophic" electrical and mechanical remodeling. Because interventricular delay in systolic contraction and diastolic relaxation occur in patients with right ventricular pressure overload, pre-excitation of the right ventricle with right ventricular pacing may minimize diastolic interventricular delay and improve left ventricular filling and stroke volume.[6] Attenuation of "atrophic" left ventricular remodeling by right ventricular pacing may explain the clinical and hemodynamic improvement experienced by the patient in the 12-month period between atrioventricular node ablation and recurrent clinical deterioration. Right ventricular outflow tract pacing, septal pacing, and bundle of His pacing have been proposed as alternatives to right ventricular apical pacing based on the hypothesis that closer proximity of the pacing site to the normal conduction system may result in less electrical activation delay and mechanical dyssyncrony.[10] In this respect, however, not all studies have been uniformly positive. In a randomized study of 98 patients with atrioventricular block, no difference in left ventricular ejection fraction and exercise capacity occurred after 18 months of follow-up between patients treated with septal versus apical right ventricular pacing.[10] In addition, in the patient described here, an alternative right ventricular pacing site would have probably been unattainable because of the difficulties in lead positioning and concerns about lead stability and threshold caused by the very large, pressure-overloaded right ventricle.

Question

What is the likelihood that upgrade from right ventricular pacing to cardiac resynchronizaation therapy (CRT) will improve the patient's clinical and hemodynamic condition?

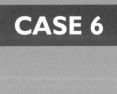

CASE 6

Role of Optimal Medical Therapy

Chin Pang, Chan and Cheuk-Man Yu

Age	Gender	Occupation	Working Diagnosis
51 Years	Male	Professional Driver	Ischemic Dilated Cardiomyopathy

HISTORY

The patient was a nonsmoker. He had experienced a myocardial infarction in 2003. A coronary angiogram performed in 2003 showed severe left main artery disease and triple vessel disease. He underwent coronary artery bypass grafting (CABG) the same year. Echocardiography was done 6 months after CABG showed left ventricular ejection fraction (LVEF) of 25%. He was diagnosed with New York Heart Association (NYHA) class III disease, and electrocardiography showed sinus rhythm with a left bundle branch block pattern. QRS duration was 150 msec, and no history of ventricular arrhythmia was reported. In view of persistent left ventricular systolic dysfunction and underlying wide QRS duration, cardiac resynchronization therapy with defibrillator (CRT-D) backup was performed. The procedure was uneventful, and the left ventricular lead was inserted in the posterolateral branch of the coronary sinus. He was subsequently followed regularly by the combined heart failure and device clinic.

The patient returned 6 months after CRT-D implantation and was found to be clinically still in NYHA class III. Device interrogation showed that he received 85% biventricular pacing. Other parameters were unremarkable. Follow-up echocardiographic examination showed an LVEF of 25%.

Comments

The patient was both clinically and echocardiographically a CRT nonresponder. It was necessary to explore the potential cause of lack of CRT response.

CURRENT MEDICATIONS

The patient's medications are aspirin 80 mg daily, metoprolol controlled-release 12.5 mg daily, ramipril 1.25 mg daily, furosemide 20 mg daily, and simvastatin 20 mg daily.

Comments

The patient received most of the guideline-recommended medications. However, the dosage was not optimal.

CURRENT SYMPTOMS

The patient experienced persistent heart failure symptoms after CRT-D implantation.

Comments

The cause of the patient's nonresponse to CRT needs to be identified. It is likely due to suboptimal biventricular pacing and suboptimal medical therapy.

PHYSICAL EXAMINATION

BP/HR: 113/45 mm Hg/84 bpm
Height/weight: 164 cm/62 kg
Neck veins: Distended jugular vein
Lungs/chest: Bilateral lung base crepitations
Heart: Heart sounds are normal and no murmur
Abdomen: Soft and nontender
Extremities: Normal perfusion

Comments

The patient was clinically in NYHA class III heart failure.

LABORATORY DATA

Hemoglobin: Within normal range
Hematocrit/PCV: Within normal range
MCV: Within normal range
Platelet count: Within normal range
Sodium: Within normal range
Potassium: Within normal range

Creatinine: Within normal range
Blood urea nitrogen: Within normal range

ELECTROCARDIOGRAM

Findings

The electrocardiogram revealed sinus rhythm with inadequate biventricular pacing (Figure 6-1) and adequate biventricular pacing after medical therapy (Figure 6-2).

Comments

It is necessary to confirm this is biventricular capturing.

CHEST RADIOGRAPH

Findings

The chest radiograph revealed cardiomegaly with no evidence of congestion. All leads were in situ.

ECHOCARDIOGRAM

Findings

The echocardiogram in apical four chamber view revealed dyschronous contraction resulting from lack of biventricular pacing (Figure 6-3).

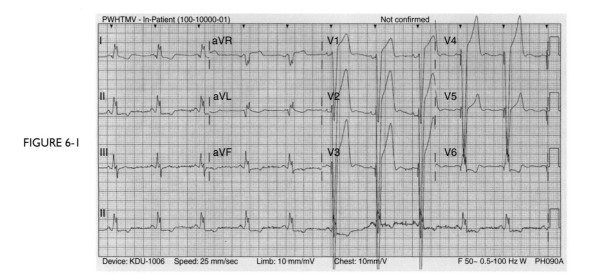

FIGURE 6-1

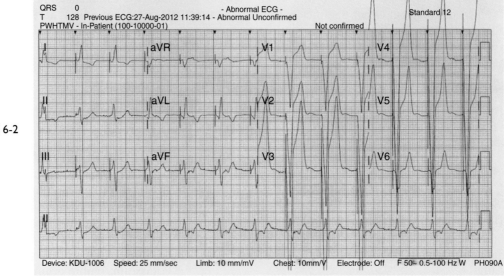

FIGURE 6-2

Findings

The apical four chamber view showed improved LVEF and significantly less left ventricular cavity dilation after optimal medical therapy (Figure 6-4).

FOCUSED CLINICAL QUESTIONS AND DISCUSSION POINTS

Question

What are the potential causes of CRT nonresponder in this patient?

Discussion

Two obvious factors contributed to the patient's illness—inadequate biventricular pacing and suboptimal medical therapy with an inadequate dosage of medication.

Question

What should be done to maximize CRT response?

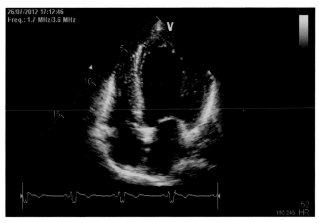

FIGURE 6-3   See *expertconsult.com* for video.

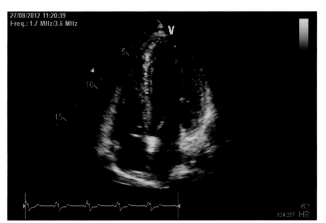

FIGURE 6-4   See *expertconsult.com* for video.

Discussion

The dosage of metoprolol (Betaloc), a beta blocker, should be increased for two reasons. First we should try to titrate up the dosage of medication to guideline-recommended dosage and the current prescribed dose was too low. Second, the increase of beta blocker can slow intrinsic heart rate while increasing the percentage of biventricular pacing. Higher percentage of biventricular pacing has been shown to correspond to increased CRT treatment efficacy.

Question

Is any other medical therapy appropriate to be added for this patient?

Discussion

An aldosterone receptor blocker[4] and digoxin[2] can be added according to current recommendations.

FINAL DIAGNOSIS

The patient's final diagnosis is suboptimal medical therapy leading to CRT nonresponse.

PLAN OF ACTION

The plan of action in this patient was escalation of medical therapy.

INTERVENTION

The dosages of the beta blocker and ramipril were increased, and digoxin and aldactone were added.

OUTCOME

Further device interrogation showed that biventricular pacing percentage approached 100%, and the latest echocardiography showed the LVEF to be approximately 40%. Clinically the patient was in NYHA class II.

Findings

This case illustrates the importance of optimal medical therapy in patients with CRT. Current device guidelines suggest it is mandatory to give optimal medical therapy before CRT implantation.[1] Also, study has led to the suggestion that patients receiving CRT without optimal medical therapy were associated with less echocardiographic and clinical improvement.[3]

Selected References

1. Digitalis Investigation Group: The effect of digoxin on mortality and morbidity in patients with heart failure, *N Engl J Med* 336:525-533, 1997.
2. Epstein AE, DiMarco JP, et al: American College of Cardiology/American Heart Association task force on practice guidelines (Writing committee to revise the ACC/AHA/NASPE 2002 guideline update for implantation of cardiac pacemakers and antiarrhythmia devices); American association for thoracic surgery; Society of thoracic surgeons. ACC/AHA/HRS 2008 guidelines for device-based therapy of cardiac rhythm abnormalities, *J Am Coll Cardiol* 51:e1-e62, 2008.
3. Fung JW, Chan JY, Kum LC, et al: Suboptimal medical therapy in patients with systolic heart failure is associated with less improvement by cardiac resynchronization therapy, *Int J Cardiol* 115: 214-219, 2007.
4. Pitt B, Remme W, Zannad F, et al: Eplerenone, a selective aldosterone blocker, in patients with left ventricular dysfunction after myocardial infarction. Eplerenone Post-Acute Myocardial Infarction Heart Failure Efficacy and Survival Study Investigators, *N Engl J Med* 348:1309-1321, 2003.

SECTION 2

Expanding Indications of Cardiac Resynchronization Therapy

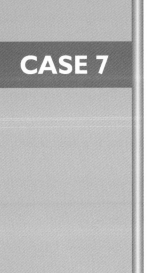

CASE 7

Efficacy of Cardiac Resynchronization Therapy in New York Heart Association II

Matthew T. Bennett and Anthony S. L. Tang

Age	Gender	Occupation	Working Diagnosis
66 Years	Female	Housewife	Nonischemic Cardiomyopathy

HISTORY

The patient is a 66-year-old woman who first came to medical attention for her heart disease 3 years ago. She had been on a cruise when she initially noticed some functional limitation. She began to have difficulty climbing the stairs and found it necessary to use the elevator. By the end of the cruise she had pedal edema to the midcalf and had to sleep semirecumbant because of shortness of breath while lying flat.

On her return home, she went to see her family doctor, who ordered an echocardiogram. This showed an ejection fraction of 20%. There was trivial mitral regurgitation. The left ventricular mass index was 153 g/m². The left ventricular end-systolic and end-diastolic dimensions were 44 and 66 mm, respectively. An electrocardiogram (ECG) demonstrated normal sinus rhythm at 77 bpm with left bundle branch block (LBBB) and left axis deviation.

She was initially treated with a diuretic (furosemide [Lasix]) and an angiotensin-converting enzyme inhibitor (ramipril). When she became euvolemic a beta blocker was added (carvedilol) and titrated up to target doses.

She underwent a coronary angiogram, which showed no evidence of flow-limiting coronary artery disease.

Her past medical history included smoking (she stopped smoking 3 years ago, after smoking one pack per day for 20 years). She had a history of breast cancer for which she was treated with chemotherapy (including doxorubicin) and radiation. She drinks 1 to 2 glasses of wine on weekend evenings. She has no family history of cardiomyopathy.

The workup for her heart failure revealed no evidence of human immunodeficiency virus, thyroid disease, hemochromatosis, or amyloidosis. She had no recent history of viral infection.

After 9 months of therapy a repeat echocardiogram was performed and showed an ejection fraction of 30%.

Her symptoms had improved such that she denied any functional limitation. An exercise stress test was performed to assess her functional ability objectively. She performed a bicycle stress test and was able to perform 3.8 metabolic equivalents. This was deemed to be below expected for her age and gender.

She was referred for a biventricular implantable cardioverter-defibrillator (ICD), but she initially refused because she felt well. During the subsequent 2 years she had one hospitalization for heart failure. At that time her weight was 5 kg over her usual dry weight. She was admitted for a total of 3 days and after intravenous diuretics was back to her baseline weight and functional status.

At a recent visit to the cardiac function clinic it was recommended again that she consider a cardiac resynchronization therapy defibrillator (CRT-D). She wished to discuss it further and was referred to a cardiac electrophysiologist.

Comments

This woman is a 66-year-old woman with nonischemic (presumably chemotherapy induced) cardiomyopathy. Although she denies functional limitation, her exercise stress test demonstrates mild functional limitation (New York Heart Association class II [NYHA]).

CURRENT MEDICATIONS

The patient takes ramipril 10 mg, carvedilol 25 mg, and spironolactone 12.5 mg in the morning and carvedilol 25 mg in the evening.

Comments

The patient appears to be on optimal medical therapy.

Current Symptoms

The patient currently denies orthopnea and paroxysmal nocturnal dyspnea. She is now able to walk eight blocks on the flat surfaces. However, she no longer rides her bike or does aerobics and she takes the elevator instead of the stairs when at the mall.

Comments

This patient has NYHA II heart failure symptoms despite medical therapy. Often, patients will habituate to their functional limitation and feel well. They may not realize that they have changed their lifestyle to accommodate the change in their functional decline.

PHYSICAL EXAMINATION

BP/HR: 88/54 mm Hg (left arm, seated position)/53 bpm at rest
Height/weight: 172.5 cm/80.5 kg
Neck veins: 2 cm above the sternal angle, positive abdominojugular reflux
Lungs/chest: Good breath sounds, no crepitations nor wheezes
Heart: Normal first heart sound (S_1), paradoxically split second heart sound (S_2), no third (S_3) or fourth (S_4) heart sounds, no audible murmurs
Abdomen: No hepatosplenomegaly, no aortic enlargement
Extremities: Warm, well perfused; grade 2 pedal edema

Comments

The patient appears mildly volume overloaded.

LABORATORY DATA

Hemoglobin: 139 g/L
Hematocrit/packed cell volume: 0.43%
Mean corpuscular volume: 88 fL
Platelet count: 219 × 10³/μL
Sodium: 140 mmol/L
Potassium: 5.6 mmol/L
Creatinine: 115 μmol/L
Blood urea nitrogen: 7 mmol/L

Comments

The blood work shows renal insufficiency (a chronic problem) and mild hyperkalemia (likely from the spironolactone).

ELECTROCARDIOGRAM

Findings

The 12-lead ECG shows sinus rhythm at a rate of 84 bpm and LBBB (Figure 7-1).

Comments

The patient's LBBB QRS duration is 168 msec.

ECHOCARDIOGRAM

Findings

The parasternal long axis shows left ventricular dilation with left ventricular end-diastolic and end-systolic dimensions of 60 and 49 mm, respectively (Figure 7-2).

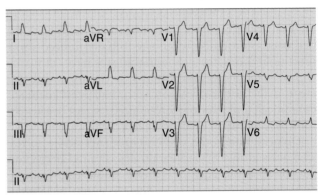

FIGURE 7-1

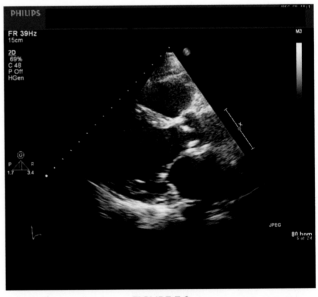

FIGURE 7-2

Comments

The left ventricle is mildly enlarged.

Findings

The left ventricular ejection fraction was calculated to be 22% by Simpson's biplane method. Mild mitral regurgitation was present (Figure 7-3).

Comments

The ejection fraction is significantly reduced.

FOCUSED CLINICAL QUESTIONS AND DISCUSSION POINTS

Question

Is there any benefit in the implantation of a biventricular pacing device in this woman?

Discussion

Both the Comparison of Medical Therapy, Pacing, and Defibrillation in Heart Failure (COMPANION) and Cardiac Resynchronization in Heart Failure (CARE-HF) trials have shown efficacy of biventricular pacing in patients with NYHA III and IV heart failure. In the COMPANION trial, Bristow and colleagues[1] randomized 1520 patients with a QRS duration greater than 120 msec and an ejection fraction of less than 35% to standard medical therapy alone or in combination with

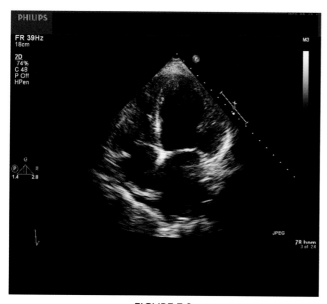

FIGURE 7-3

a biventricular pacemaker or biventricular defibrillator. Overall, reduction in death from, or hospitalization for, heart failure by 34% in the biventricular pacemaker group and 40% in the biventricular ICD group were reported.

In CARE-HF, Cleland and colleagues[2] randomized 813 patients with NYHA III and IV heart failure, an ejection fraction of 35% or less, a QRS duration of 120 msec or greater (other measures of dyssynchrony were required if the QRS duration was <150 msec), and left ventricular dilation to optimal medical therapy with or without biventricular pacing. The occurrence of death or hospitalization for a major cardiovascular event was reduced by 37% in the patients with biventricular pacing. In addition, a reduction in mortality by 36% was seen.

Both the Multicenter Automatic Defibrillator Implantation With Cardiac Resynchronization Therapy (MADIT-CRT) study and the Resynchronization–Defibrillation for Ambulatory Heart Failure Trial (RAFT) examined the efficacy of biventricular defibrillators in patients with less symptomatic heart failure.[3,4] In MADIT-CRT, 1820 patients with an ejection fraction of 30% or less, a QRS of 130 msec or greater, and NYHA I or II heart failure symptoms were randomized to a biventricular ICD or ICD alone. The primary end point of death from any cause or heart-failure event occurred more frequently in the ICD alone group than the biventricular ICD group (25.3% vs. 17.2%).[3]

In the RAFT trial, 1798 patients with NYHA II and III heart failure, an ejection fraction of 30% or less, and a QRS of 120 msec or greater were randomized to an ICD alone or ICD plus biventricular pacing. After the mean follow-up of 40 months, the primary outcome of all-cause death or hospitalization for heart failure had occurred in 40.3% of the ICD group and 33.2% of the biventricular ICD group.

Question

Is the reduction in events with biventricular pacing seen with symptom reduction and mortality reduction or both?

Discussion

In both the MADIT-CRT trial and RAFT a reduction in heart failure in the biventricular ICD group (MADIT-CRT: relative risk reduction [RRR] = 41% in heart failure events; RAFT: RRR = 32% in heart failure hospitalizations) was seen.[3,4] In RAFT, a 25% reduction in the risk for death was seen in the biventricular ICD group in contrast to the ICD alone group. However, no reduction in mortality in the biventricular ICD group in contrast to the ICD alone group was seen in the MADIT-CRT trial.

Question

Which patients with NYHA II heart failure appear to derive the most benefit from biventricular pacing? Is it expected that the patient in this case will derive benefit?

Discussion

In the MADIT-CRT trial, several prespecified subgroups were analyzed in regard to the efficacy of biventricular ICD therapy on the primary outcomes. It appeared that biventricular ICD therapy conferred a greater benefit in women than men and in patients with a QRS greater than 150 msec than in patients with a QRS less than 150 msec.[3]

In the RAFT trial, biventricular ICD therapy appeared to have a greater efficacy in the patients with QRS duration greater than 150 msec than in patients with a QRS duration less than 150 msec and in patients with an LBBB QRS morphology than with other morphologies.[4]

This patient fits the enrollment criteria for these two trials. In addition, she has an LBBB QRS morphology with a QRS of greater than 150 msec. This portends a good response to biventricular pacing. In addition, her gender would support a greater improvement with biventricular pacing.

FINAL DIAGNOSIS

This patient is 66 years old and has nonischemic (presumably anthracycline induced) cardiomyopathy. She feels well but has had a heart failure admission and had functional limitation on her exercise stress test. Her ECG shows LBBB with a QRS duration of 168 msec.

PLAN OF ACTION

After a discussion with the patient regarding the risks and benefits of implantation of CRT-D or ICD, the patient wished to proceed with a CRT-D.

INTERVENTION

CRT-D was undertaken; the coronary sinus venogram identified a suitable posterolateral coronary sinus branch within which a left ventricular lead was inserted (Figure 7-4). Initially, the lead was inserted without the use of an angioplasty wire but could not be fully inserted (Figure 7-5). Therefore an angioplasty wire (Figure 7-6) was used to facilitate more fully advanced

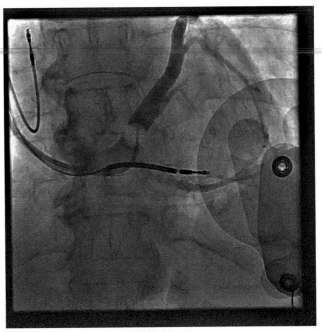

FIGURE 7-4

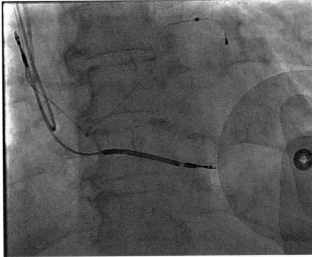

FIGURE 7-5

lead placement (Figure 7-7). The final position is identified on the posteroanterior and lateral radiographs (Figures 7-8 and 7-9).

OUTCOME

The patient returned to the clinic 1 month after the procedure. She was feeling much better despite having denied any functional limitation previously.

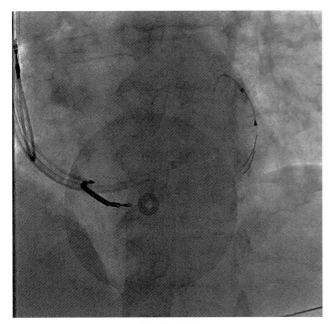

FIGURE 7-6

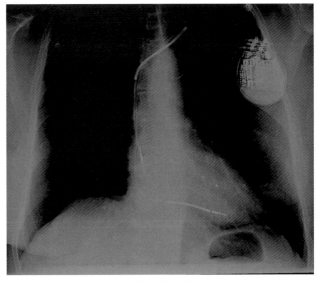

FIGURE 7-8

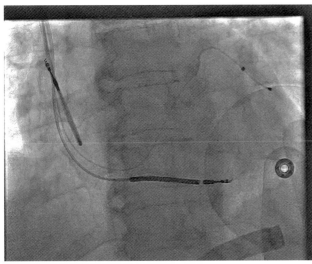

FIGURE 7-7

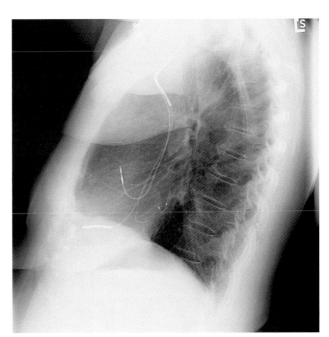

FIGURE 7-9

Selected References

1. Bristow MR, Saxon LA, Boehmer J, et al: Cardiac-resynchronization therapy with or without an implantable defibrillator in advanced chronic heart failure, *N Engl J Med* 350:2140-2150, 2004.
2. Cleland JG, Daubert JC, Erdmann E, et al: The effect of cardiac resynchronization on morbidity and mortality in heart failure, *N Engl J Med* 352:1539-1549, 2005.
3. Moss AJ, Hall WJ, Cannom DS, et al: Cardiac-resynchronization therapy for the prevention of heart-failure events, *N Engl J Med* 361:1329-1338, 2009.
4. Tang AS, Wells GA, Talajic M, et al: Cardiac-resynchronization therapy for mild-to-moderate heart failure, *N Engl J Med* 363:2385-2395, 2010.

Pacemaker Indication

Chin Pang, Chan and Cheuk-Man Yu

Age	Gender	Occupation	Working Diagnosis
73 Years	Male	Retired Chef	Complete Heart Block

HISTORY

The patient was a nonsmoker and enjoyed good health in the past. He had a history of new-onset dizziness and one episode of syncope. He was admitted to the hospital, and electrocardiogram (ECG) showed complete heart block with ventricular escape rate about 40 bpm. Clinically, he was not in heart failure, and echocardiography demonstrated normal left ventricular systolic function. Because there was no reversible cause, a dual-chamber pacemaker was implanted. The right ventricular lead was fixed at the right ventricular apex, and the right atrial lead was fixed at the right atrial appendage. The procedure was uneventful, and he was discharged.

One month after discharge, the patient reported a decrease in exercise tolerance and dyspnea.

CURRENT MEDICATIONS

The patient is on no medications.

CURRENT SYMPTOMS

The patient experienced a decrease in exercise tolerance and dyspnea.

Comments

It is likely new-onset heart failure symptoms occurred after device implantation.

PHYSICAL EXAMINATION

BP/HR: 120/64 mm Hg/74 bpm, atrial sensing with ventricular pacing rhythm
Height/weight: 170 cm/50 kg
Neck veins: Mildly distended

Lungs/chest: Fine crepitation over bilateral lung bases
Heart: Normal heart sounds, no murmur
Abdomen: Soft and nontender, no evidence of organomegaly
Extremities: Warm and normal perfusion

Comments

Physical examination revealed evidence of heart failure.

LABORATORY DATA

Hemoglobin: Within normal range
Hematocrit/packed cell volume: Within normal range
Mean corpuscular volume: Within normal range
Platelet count: Within normal range
Sodium: Within normal range
Potassium: Within normal range
Creatinine: Within normal range
Blood urea nitrogen: Within normal range

ELECTROCARDIOGRAM

Findings

Atrial sensing and ventricular pacing rhythm, dependent pacing rhythm.

Comments

The ECG showed dependent pacing rhythm.

CHEST RADIOGRAPH

Findings

The chest radiograph did not show any abnormalities.

Comments

It is necessary to rule out pulmonary disease and see any evidence of congestive heart failure.

ECHOCARDIOGRAM

Findings

Echocardiography revealed decreased systolic function and dyssynchronous contraction (Figures 8-1 and 8-2).

Findings

The echocardiogram also shows improved systolic function and synchronous contraction after upgrade (Figure 8-3).

MAGNETIC RESONANCE IMAGING

It is contraindicated to proceed to magnetic resonance imaging (MRI) with a history of non–MRI-compatible pacemaker implantation.

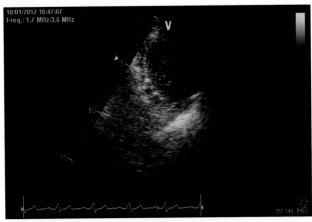

FIGURE 8-1 Short axis view. See *expertconsult.com* for video.

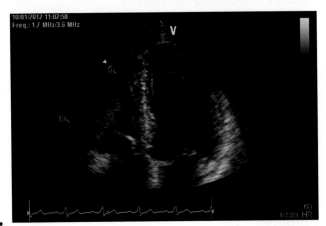

FIGURE 8-2 Apical four chamber view. See *expertconsult.com* for video.

CATHETERIZATION

Catheterization is an appropriate option in this patient.

HEMODYNAMICS

Hemodynamic studies revealed left ventricular end-diastolic pressure of approximately 14 mm H_2O.

Findings

The findings on coronary angiogram were normal.

Comments

It is necessary to rule out underlying ischemic heart disease.

FOCUSED CLINICAL QUESTIONS AND DISCUSSION POINTS

Question

What is the clinical diagnosis?

Discussion

Clinically, the patient's symptoms are compatible with a diagnosis of heart failure. It is necessary to exclude other causes, such as pulmonary disease and undiagnosed ischemic heart disease.

Question

For device interrogation, which pacing parameter is particularly useful to establish the potential diagnosis?

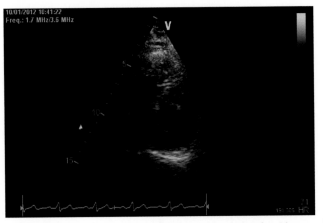

FIGURE 8-3 Short axis view. See *expertconsult.com* for video.

Discussion

Pacing burden is the most important parameter in this case. Pacing burden is directly related to the risk for development of pacing-induced left ventricular systolic dysfunction.

Question

What kinds of investigation are indicated?

Discussion

Echocardiography is essential to establish the diagnosis; in this case it showed evidence of deterioration of systolic function and enabled assessment of the degree of systolic dyssynchrony in this patient. Also, coronary angiogram is indicated in this case and it is important to rule out ischemia-related cardiac dysfunction.

Question

What is the potential treatment for this condition?

Discussion

The cause of systolic dysfunction in this patient is abnormal pacing; therefore upgrading to biventricular pacing was recommended.

FINAL DIAGNOSIS

The final diagnosis in this case is pacing-induced left ventricular systolic dysfunction with clinical features of heart failure.

PLAN OF ACTION

The plan of action for this patient was to correct the underlying dyssynchrony and upgrade to cardiac resynchronization therapy with a pacemaker (CRT-P).

INTERVENTION

The intervention for this patient was to upgrade to biventricular pacing.

OUTCOME

Postimplantation echocardiography showed improved systolic function, and the degree of dyssynchrony was minimal. Clinically, significant improvement was seen and exercise tolerance was improved.

Comments

This case illustrates the potential risk for pacing-induced left ventricular dysfunction. The risk is particularly high if the patient has an underlying history of systolic dysfunction.[4] The cause is mainly pacing-induced mechanical dyssynchrony. Recent studies demontrated that right ventricular pacing causes deterioration of systolic function after 2 years but systolic function was preserved if the patient received biventricular pacing at baseline.[1,5] Although baseline systolic function was normal in both groups, the risk for deterioration was related to the degree of pacing burden. As a result, current guidelines recommend implantation of a biventricular pacemaker for those with underlying systolic dysfunction and dependent pacing. Also, guidelines suggest upgrading the device to biventricular pacing on evidence of pacing-induced systolic dysfunction by conventional right ventricular pacing.[2,3]

Selected References

1. Chan JY, Fang F, Zhang Q, et al: Biventricular pacing is superior to right ventricular pacing in bradycardia patients with preserved systolic function: 2-year results of the PACE trial, *Eur Heart J* 32:2533-2540, 2011.
2. Epstein AE, DiMarco JP, Ellenbogen KA, et al: American College of Cardiology/American Heart Association Task Force on Practice Guidelines (Writing Committee to Revise the ACC/AHA/NASPE 2002 Guideline Update for Implantation of Cardiac Pacemakers and Antiarrhythmia Devices); American Association for Thoracic Surgery; Society of Thoracic Surgeons. ACC/AHA/HRS 2008 guidelines for device-based therapy of cardiac rhythm abnormalities, *J Am Coll Cardiol* 51:e1-e62, 2008.
3. Vardas PE, Auricchio A, Blanc JJ, et al: European Society of Cardiology; European Heart Rhythm Association. Guidelines for cardiac pacing and cardiac resynchronization therapy: The Task Force for Cardiac Pacing and Cardiac Resynchronization Therapy of the European Society of Cardiology. Developed in collaboration with the European Heart Rhythm Association, *Eur Heart J* 28:2256-2295, 2007.
4. Wilkoff BL, Cook JR, Epstein AE, et al: Dual-chamber pacing or ventricular backup pacing in patients with an implantable defibrillator: the Dual Chamber and VVI Implantable Defibrillator (DAVID) Trial, *JAMA* 288:3115-3123, 2002.
5. Yu CM, Chan JY, Zhang Q, et al: Biventricular pacing in patients with bradycardia and normal ejection fraction, *N Engl J Med* 361:2123-2134, 2009.

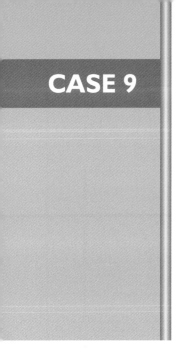

CASE 9

Intercommissural Lead Placement into a Right Ventricular Coronary Sinus

Christopher J. McLeod

Age	Gender	Occupation	Working Diagnosis
61 Years	Male		Ebstein's Anomaly with High-Grade Atrioventricular Block

HISTORY

A 61-year-old man with a history of Ebstein's anomaly, which initially went to had repaired in 1997; he then underwent tricuspid valve replacement with a 35-mm bioprosthesis in 2001. The initial surgery also involved an intraoperative ablation of an accessory pathway and right atrial maze procedure. For recurrent paroxysmal atrial fibrillation, he underwent a successful pulmonary vein isolation procedure in 2004. The electrophysiologic study performed at that time revealed severe sinus node dysfunction, but he remained asymptomatic. It was also noted that the tricuspid valve prosthesis was implanted proximal (atrial) to the coronary sinus.

Comments

It is not uncommon for the bioprosthetic valve to be sewn on the atrial aspect of the coronary sinus in repair of Ebstein's anomaly. This is performed to avoid injury to the compact atrioventricular node.

CURRENT MEDICATIONS

The patient takes aldactone, furosemide (Lasix), warfarin, losartan (Cozaar), atorvastin (Lipitor), and aspirin.

CURRENT SYMPTOMS

More frequent spells of presyncope continued, but no frank syncope occurred. The patient also described infrequent tingling of the face and arm.

PHYSICAL EXAMINATION

BP/HR: 116/66 mm Hg/52 bpm and regular
Height/weight: 169 cm/93 kg
Neck veins: No jugular venous pressure elevation
Lungs/chest: Clear
Heart: Moderate right ventricular heave, with a regular heart rate; second heart sound (S_2) normal/split. 1/6 systolic murmur at the left sternal border; no diastolic murmur or gallop
Abdomen: Soft, nontender, with no organomegaly
Extremities: No cyanosis, no edema

Comments

No clinical evidence of overt right heart failure or systemic desaturation was found.

LABORATORY DATA

Hemoglobin: 14.4 g/dL
Mean corpuscular volume: 92.2 fL
Platelet count: 202×10^9/L
Sodium: 142 mmol/L
Potassium: 4.2 mmol/L
Creatinine: 0.9 mg/dL
Blood urea nitrogen: 16 mg/dL

ELECTROCARDIOGRAM

Findings

Electrocardiography revealed marked sinus bradycardia with right bundle branch block and a ventricular rate of

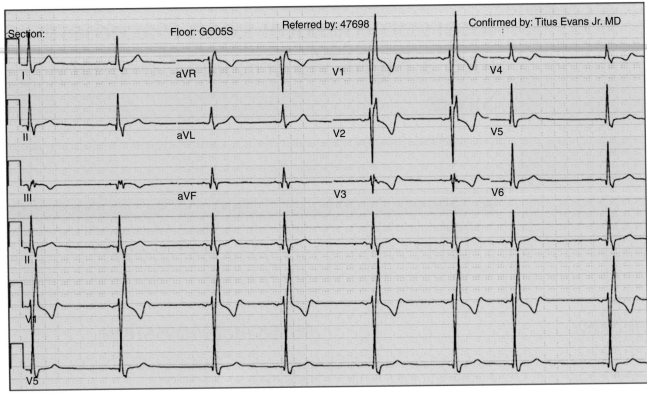

FIGURE 9-1

45 bpm (Figure 9-1). A sinus arrhythmia is present, in addition to a premature atrial complex.

CHEST RADIOGRAPH

Findings

A chest radiograph revealed a normal-sized heart with a prominent right ventricular contour (Figure 9-2) and clear lung fields. A bioprosthetic valve ring was evident.

EXERCISE TESTING

The exercise test was a maximal test and was negative for ischemia. His exercise capacity was poor (5.5 metabolic equivalents), with a hypotensive response to exercise. In addition, a limited heart rate response of 81 bpm (peak), with frequent premature atrial and ventricular contractions (PACs and PVCs), was noted.

ECHOCARDIOGRAM

Findings

The echocardiogram showed normal left ventricular chamber size and systolic function, moderate right ventricular enlargement, and a moderate decrease in right ventricular systolic function. The patient had undergone 35-mm Carpentier-Edwards tricuspid prosthetic valve replacement. The mean gradient was 4 mm Hg at a heart rate of 42 bpm. Trace tricuspid regurgitation was noted. Mobile echodensity was seen in the right ventricle attached at the midventricular septum. The location and characteristics were suggestive of a residual chord.

PHYSIOLOGIC TRACINGS

Findings

Event monitor tracings showed atrial premature contractions in a bigeminal pattern; varying P wave morphologies, a 2-second pause after a supraventricular premature contraction, and a single premature ventricular contraction (Figure 9-3). High-grade atrioventricular block is noted with a 4.1-second pause.

FOCUSED CLINICAL QUESTIONS AND DISCUSSION POINTS

Question

Should epicardial lead placement be recommended?

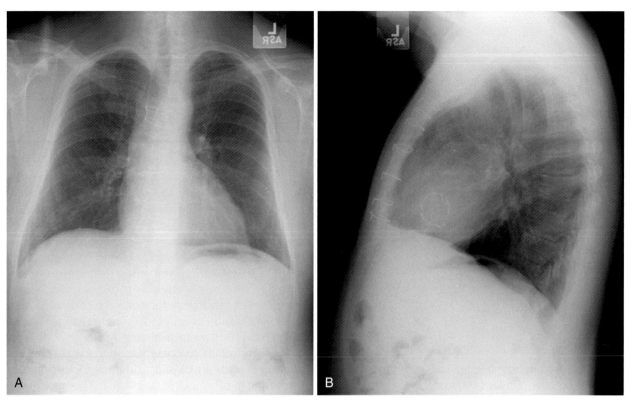

FIGURE 9-2

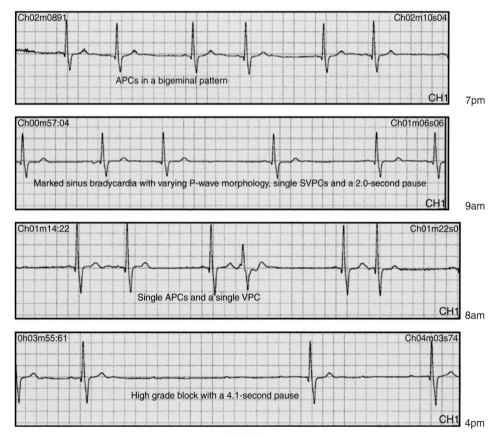

FIGURE 9-3

Discussion

Epicardial lead placement is mandatory in certain scenarios—that is, intracardiac shunting, Glenn anastamosis (i.e., bidirectional cavopulmonary), or mechanical tricuspid valve. In this situation, we did not consider epicardial lead placement because a bioprosthetic valve can be ultimately crossed by conventional pacing leads. It is also important to note that in this population of patients who have undergone one or more cardiac operations, the epicardium has significant amounts of scar tissue that preclude effective long-term epicardial pacing. Epicardial pacing in children with virgin epicardial ventricular or atrial surfaces has better long-term lead performance.[3]

Question

Could single-chamber atrial lead placement provide sufficient pacing support?

Discussion

Despite event monitor tracing showing evidence of high-grade atrioventricular block, intraatrial block must be considered in these patients. Repair of Epstein's anomaly often involve resection and plication of large areas of redundant atrial myocardium. This leaves significant scarring within the atrium, and functional or anatomic block from the sinus node to the atrioventricular node may be present. Atrioventricular nodal function can remain normal in patients seen to have high-grade atrioventricular block. To assess this properly, multiple atrial lead positions should be attempted, with pacing close to the atrioventricular node, ideally on the septum. If pacing close to the node shows no evidence of atrioventricular block, the diagnosis is intraatrial block and a ventricular lead potentially can be avoided. This feature of intraatrial conduction delay also can be seen after other congenital heart disease operations.

Question

Should a right ventricular lead be placed through the tricuspid prosthesis?

Discussion

Conceptually, it remains logical to avoid placing a lead through a bioprosthetic valve. Not infrequently, it is seen to negatively affect tricuspid valve integrity and function. Recently, however, a study looking at this particular question has shown that transvalvular device lead placement across bioprosthetic valves is not associated with an increased incidence of significant prosthetic tricuspid regurgitation. This, however, has to be balanced against the need for a repeat operation in patients with congenital disease who have undergone one or more operations in which mediastinal and pericardial fibrosis and adhesions make further operations much higher risk.[2]

Question

Is it appropriate to consider coronary sinus lead placement, despite the prosthetic valve being sewn on the atrial aspect of the coronary sinus?

Discussion

In this patient, to pace the ventricle, it was necessary to cross the tricuspid valve for right ventricular apical pacing or coronary sinus pacing. However, it was postulated that several inherent differences exist in coronary sinus lead placement versus right ventricular apical placement. Right ventricular dyssynchrony caused by right ventricular apical pacing can potentially aggravate tricuspid regurgitation. In addition, left ventricular pacing in the context of cardiac resynchronization therapy (CRT) has been noted to confer a beneficial effect on tricuspid regurgitation.[1]

It is important to recognize that the current coronary sinus leads are thinner and more pliable than conventional right apical pacing leads. This makes them more amenable to intercommissural placement and avoidance of the leaflet edges. Intracardiac echocardiography at the time of lead placement can aid in both apical and coronary sinus placement to avoid the leaf edges and place the lead between the commissures. It is also important to note that the coronary sinus leads are not subject to as much diastolic and systolic cardiac motion as right ventricular apical leads. Their position within the atrioventricular groove thus can reduce the potential for leaflet trauma. If this approach is adopted, acute monitoring of the results and tricuspid regurgitation with intracardiac echocardiography allows for confirmation of optimal lead placement.

FINAL DIAGNOSIS

The final diagnosis was symptomatic sinus node and atrioventricular node dysfunction.

PLAN OF ACTION

Pacemaker insertion was recommended, with assessment of intraatrial delay through pacing at various sites within the right atrium.

INTERVENTION

To avoid prosthetic valve dysfunction, we planned to sequentially attempt atrial lead–only pacing, intracardiac echocardiography-guided right ventricular pacing,

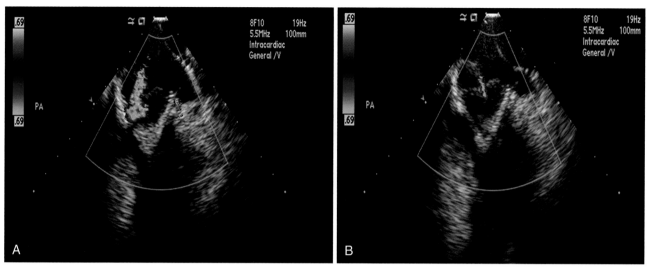

FIGURE 9-4

or coronary sinus pacing. First, the possibility of intraatrial conduction block was considered, and therefore various atrial lead positions were tried to assess conduction across any possible intraatrial delay sites. No evidence of intraatrial conduction delay was found, and the atrial lead was placed with acceptable thresholds slightly inferior to the superior vena cava junction. Atrioventricular nodal function was tested and found to be poor, with Wenckebach occurring at pacing rates above 600 ms (90 bpm), confirming the absolute need for a ventricular lead. To examine the effect of passing a pacing lead through the tricuspid valve, intracardiac ultrasound images were obtained after inserting a pacemaker lead across the valve toward the right ventricular apex. This resulted in significant tricuspid regurgitation, as noted in Figure 9-4, *A*. Thus an alternative approach was taken in which a thin (5.7-French, EASYTRAK 2, Boston Scientific, Natick, Mass) pacing wire was specifically guided between the commissure of the anterior and posterior prosthetic tricuspid valve leaflets into the coronary sinus, located just distal to the prosthesis in the basilar segment of the right ventricle (Figures 9-5 and 9-6). Subsequent intracardiac imaging performed after all wires were pulled revealed a very satisfactory placement with no tricuspid regurgitation noted, as seen in Figure 9-4, *B*.

OUTCOME

Acutely, a dual-chamber permanent pacemaker was implanted, with no tricuspid regurgitation. At his 1-year follow-up, the patient reported complete resolution of all presyncopal symptoms and an excellent exercise tolerance—biking about 5 miles without notable limitation. There was no evidence of lead dislodgement in the chest radiograph, and transthoracic echocardiography

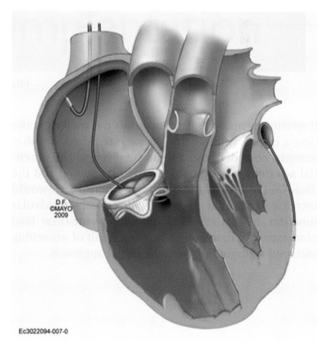

Ec3022094-007-0

FIGURE 9-5

demonstrated no prosthetic tricuspid valve dysfunction and specifically no tricuspid regurgitation. The mean gradient was unchanged at 3 mm Hg. The lead was easily seen going across the prosthesis and into the coronary sinus. Device thresholds were all stable.

This case is pertinent to a discussion of CRT, even though this patient did not require CRT. The issues faced in patients with a congenital cardiac anomaly are much different from those without and require a careful and thoughtful approach to best lead placement. In addition, many congenital anomalies may result in severe systemic ventricular dysfunction. Even

CASE 10

Right Ventricular Pacing–Related Cardiomyopathy

Joseph J. Gard and Samuel J. Asirvatham

Age	Gender	Occupation	Working Diagnosis
62 Years	Male	Physician	Progressive Left Ventricular Dysfunction Resulting from Chronic Right Ventricular Pacing

HISTORY

A 62-year-old nonsmoking man was referred for upgrade of his dual-chamber pacing system to a cardiac resynchronization therapy (CRT) pacing system. The dual-chamber pacing system had been implanted 4 years earlier. The initial indication for cardiac pacing was complete heart block that developed roughly 8 hours after radiofrequency ablation of the cavotricuspid isthmus for the treatment of symptomatic atrial flutter. The components of this initial pacing system were a St. Jude Medical Victory XL DR 5816, a Medtronic bipolar screw-in atrial lead 5568-53, and a Medtronic bipolar screw-in ventricular lead 4076-58. At the time the initial pacing system was implanted, his left ventricular size and ejection fraction (60%-65%) were normal. On device interrogation he routinely paced more than 99% of the time.

The patient developed fatigue, exercise intolerance, and dyspnea on exertion. After atrial flutter ablation, he was started on flecainide for symptomatic paroxysmal atrial fibrillation. His other pertinent medical history included dyslipidemia and hypertension. His ejection fraction was reassessed. His left ventricular ejection fraction by radionuclide angiogram was 38%. An ischemic cause for his cardiomyopathy was ruled out by elective coronary angiography.

CURRENT MEDICATIONS

The patient's daily medications were aspirin 81 mg, cetirizine 10 mg, dutasteride 0.5 mg, enalapril 5 mg, escitalopram 10 mg, flecainide 50 mg, hydrochlorothiazide 25 mg, and simvastatin 80 mg.

Comments

Flecainide is generally avoided in patients with conduction system disease. Flecainide slows conduction that can further widen the QRS complex from baseline, leading for further ventricular dyssynchrony. Flecainide also should be avoided in patients with coronary or structural heart disease because of the increased risk for malignant tachyarrhythmias. Flecainide was discontinued in this patient for these reasons.

CURRENT SYMPTOMS

The patient's symptoms included fatigue, exercise intolerance, and dyspnea on exertion.

PHYSICAL EXAMINATION

BP/HR: 140/94 mm Hg/60 bpm
Height/weight: 180.0 cm/100.60 kg
Neck veins: No jugulovenous pressure distention
Lungs/chest: Normal breath sounds bilaterally
Heart: Regular rate and rhythm with wide paradoxical splitting of the second heart sound (S$_2$); faint murmur of tricuspid regurgitation
Abdomen: Soft, nontender, nondistended
Extremities: Normal

LABORATORY DATA

Hemoglobin: 14.7 g/dL
Hematocrit/packed cell volume: 43.2

Mean corpuscular volume: 91.1 fL
Platelet count: 212 × 10³/μL
Sodium: 143 mmol/L
Potassium: 4.1 mmol/L
Creatinine: 1.1 mg/dL

ELECTROCARDIOGRAM

Findings

An electrocardiogram demonstrating atrioventricular sequential dual-chamber pacing at a rate of 60 bpm (Figure 10-1) and QRS duration of 182 ms.

Comments

The morphology of the paced QRS is consistent with a right ventricular apical location. The paced left bundle branch (LBB) morphology suggests right ventricular origin. The predominant positive voltage in lead I is due to right-to-left activation. The apical position is supported by the completely negative morphology in V4 (apical lead) resulting from ventricular activation away from the apex.

CHEST RADIOGRAPH

Findings

Chest radiography was performed in posteroanterior (Figure 10-2, *A*) and lateral (Figure 10-2, *B*) views. The left infraclavicular pacemaker has leads positioned in the right atrial appendage and the right ventricular septum.

FOCUSED CLINICAL QUESTIONS AND DISCUSSION POINTS

Question

What anatomic landmarks are relevant for successful and efficient deployment of a left ventricular lead?

Discussion

A thorough understanding of the coronary venous system anatomy is critical for success with placement of left ventricular leads.[4,5] The coronary sinus ostium enters the inferior septal aspect of the right atrium between the tricuspid valve and the inferior vena cava. The fat of the avioventricular groove is typically apparent by fluoroscopy in the right anterior oblique (RAO) view as a landmark to aid in anticipating the location of the coronary sinus ostium. A steerable catheter can be used to engage the coronary sinus ostium, by pulling back the catheter from the right ventricle while torquing it septally (i.e., counterclockwise torque from superior access site). This withdrawal from the right ventricle is observed in the RAO view until the catheter is observed to sway back and forth when the ostium is engaged. At this point the left anterior oblique view can be used to confirm advancement into the coronary venous system within the left heart.[1]

The relevant components of the coronary venous system include the coronary sinus, great cardiac vein, anterior interventricular vein, middle cardiac vein, and lateral vein(s). A thebesian valve can be present at the coronary sinus ostium. This thebesian valve can present a technical challenge to coronary sinus cannulation that often can be negotiated by entering the inferior margin of the coronary sinus. Blood draining from the inferior interventricular septum returns to the coronary sinus via

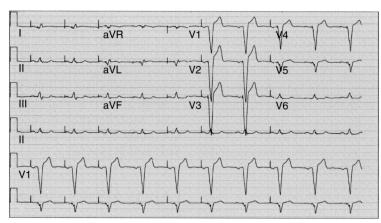

FIGURE 10-1

the middle cardiac vein. The coronary sinus becomes the great cardiac vein. A left ventricular lead in a lateral or posterolateral vein is generally the preferred location for biventricular pacing. The Vieussens valve can be located at the ostium of the posterolateral vein. The Vieussens valve can be obstructive to deployment of a left ventricular lead.[3]

An understanding of the coronary venous anatomy and experience with its typical fluoroscopic layout helps avoid complications. The primary complication with implanting a left ventricular lead is dissection of the thin-walled coronary venous system. This can occur with manipulation of the lead and delivery system in the coronary sinus but also with a venogram. Comfort with the anatomy and its typical fluoroscopic layout allows the operator to anticipate how to navigate the coronary venous system and minimize mechanical trauma resulting from misdirection. Other issues that can complicate left ventricular lead implantation include phrenic nerve stimulation and positioning the lead in a nonoptimal location.

Question

How can diaphragmatic and intercostal stimulation be avoided and, if occurring after implant, be nonoperatively assessed and managed?

Discussion

Diaphragmatic and intercostal stimulation should be assessed in nonparalyzed patients before committing to a left ventricular pacing site. This is done by pacing the lead at high output, by visualizing the patient both directly and fluoroscopically, and by feeling the chest wall for diaphragmatic stimulation. This should be done throughout a full respiratory cycle because the stimulation might only transiently depend on relative anatomic positional changes during respiration. Similarly, the intercostal muscles should be palpated for stimulation during high-output pacing. If awake, the patient can be asked if he or she has a hiccups sensation. Despite careful assessment at implant, diaphragmatic and intercostal stimulation can occur after implant. The assessment after implant is similar to that during implant but because the patient is no longer in procedure, different positions of the patient can be checked.

If extracardiac stimulation occurs after implant, attempts to avoid and minimize extracardiac stimulation can be done by programming. Sometimes the left ventricular lead pacing output can be adjusted to a lower setting that no longer produces extracardiac stimulation yet is balanced against sufficient output to effectively and reliably capture. Similarly, unipolar pacing produces

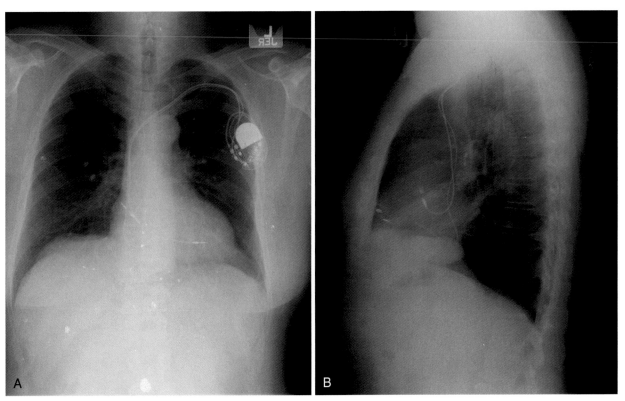

FIGURE 10-2

a larger area of stimulation than bipolar pacing; thus unipolar pacing is more likely to create extracardiac stimulation. Modern biventricular pacing systems offer multiple programmable pacing vectors that can be used for additional pacing options in the management of issues with capture threshold and extracardiac stimulation.

Question

What QRS morphology is anticipated with biventricular pacing from the posterolateral vein and right ventricular apex?

Discussion

The QRS morphology of biventricular pacing is anticipated to be a hybrid of the QRS of left ventricular and right ventricular pacing. The locations of the left ventricular and right ventricular pacing leads dictate the QRS morphology based on the myocardial activation patterns emanating from the pacing sites.

A lead in the traditional right ventricular apical septal location produces a QRS that is positive in lead I and has an LBB morphology in lead V1. The apical position leads to a superiorly directed vector and manifests with a QS pattern in the inferior leads (II, III, and aVF). Pacing from a left ventricular lead should produce a QRS with right bundle branch block morphology and a negative QS pattern in lead I (activation from left to right). Pacing from the anterior interventricular vein characteristically has a right bundle branch block (RBBB) morphology with positive deflection in the inferior leads. A negative complex in lead I becomes manifest when pacing from a lateral branch of the anterior interventricular vein.

The QRS morphology of biventricular pacing represents the hybrid of the activation patterns from the right and left ventricular leads. Biventricular pacing via the right ventricular apical and the posterolateral vein produce an atypical RBBB, and the inferior leads manifest biphasic or isoelectric QRS morphology. Activation from the left leads to a negative complex in lead I that also may be isoelectric depending on the balance of activation from the right and left ventricular leads. The QRS duration is generally shorter with biventricular pacing than with single-site pacing. The electrocardiographic manifestation of biventricular pacing has been nicely further detailed in the literature.[2]

FINAL DIAGNOSIS

At this point, the working diagnosis was cardiomyopathy suspected to be due to right ventricular pacing for complete atrioventricular block.

PLAN OF ACTION

The patient was referred for upgrade of his atrioventricular sequential dual-chamber pacing system to a CRT pacing system with the addition of a left ventricular lead.

INTERVENTION

The patient's atrioventricular sequential dual-chamber pacing system was upgraded to a CRT-pacemaker system. A Guidant bipolar tined left ventricular lead EASY-TRAK 2 IS-1 4543 was deployed, and his generator was exchanged for a Medtronic InSync III 8042.

Extensive fibrosis was noted at the previous generator site. Careful dissection allowed the generator and redundant leads to be freed from the pocket. Intravenous contrast injection demonstrated near total obstruction of the proximal subclavian vein. Despite attempting access from a medial stick, the obstruction was still troubling, so a glide wire was navigated to the inferior vena cava. Serial dilations of the obstruction were made to allow passage of the coronary sinus delivery system. The coronary sinus was cannulated, and multiple potential ventricular venous pacing sites were tested. The pacing thresholds were very high, and a wide QRS morphology occurred with pacing in the posterolateral vein. The QRS morphology was improved when pacing closer to the apex and also at the inferior wall; however, these positions did not appear to be stable. The lead was ultimately placed into an anterolateral branch (as shown in Figure 10-3) with a stable appearance, satisfactory pacing and sensing thresholds, and no extracardiac stimulation at high-output pacing.

OUTCOME

In clinical follow-up the patient noted symptomatic improvement and his paced QRS duration improved (Figure 10-4) from baseline 182 to 166 ms. The paced QRS morphology is consistent with biventricular pacing via right ventricular apical lead and also a lead within the anterior interventricular vein, as evident on the chest radiograph.

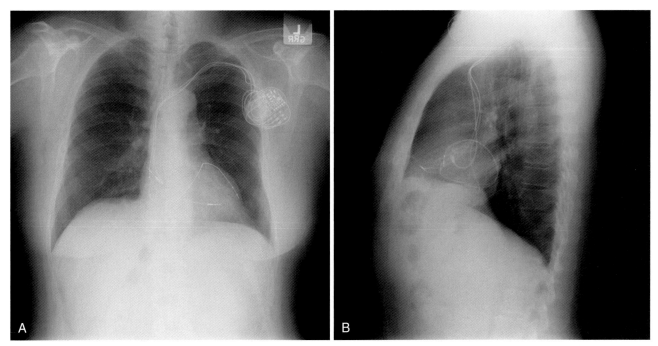

FIGURE 10-3   The new left ventricular lead and generator have been placed. The left ventricular lead appears to be in a satisfactory position, is lateral on the posteroanterior image **(A)** and appropriately anterior on the lateral image **(B),** consistent with positioning in the anterior interventricular vein.

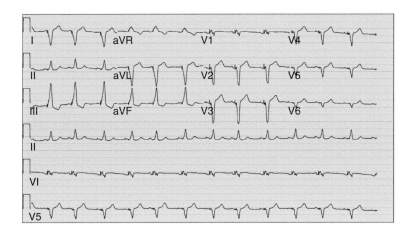

FIGURE 10-4   The QRS morphology is consistent with biventricular pacing. V1 demonstrates atypical right bundle branch morphology suggestive of some activation from the left ventricle. Lead I is strongly negative, as would be expected with left to right activation. The inferior leads, however, have a positive vector, as likely from the more superior left ventricular lead position.

Selected References

1. Asirvatham SJ: Cardiac anatomic considerations in pediatric electrophysiology, *Indian Pacing Electrophysiol J* 8(suppl. 1): S75-S91, 2008.
2. Asirvatham SJ: Electrocardiogram interpretation with biventricular pacing devices. In Hayes DL, Wang PJ, Sackner-Bernstein J, et al: *Resynchronization and defibrillation for heart failure: a practical approach*, Oxford, UK, 2008, Blackwell Publishing.
3. Corcoran SJ, Lawrence C, McGuire MA: The valve of Vieussens: an important cause of difficulty in advancing catheters into the cardiac veins, *J Cardiovasc Electrophysiol* 10:804-808, 1999.
4. Habib A, Lachman N, et al: The anatomy of the coronary sinus venous system for the cardiac electrophysiologist, *Europace* 11(suppl 5):v15-v21, 2009.
5. Stellbrink C, Breithardt OA, Franke A, et al: Technical considerations in implanting left ventricular pacing leads for cardiac resynchronisation therapy, *Eur Heart J Suppl* 6(D):D43-D46, 2004.

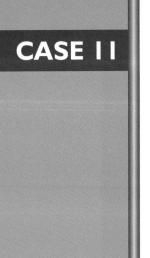

CASE 11

Successful Cardiac Resynchronization Therapy Implantation: When to Consider the Middle Cardiac Vein

Vishnu M. Chandra, Joseph J. Gard, and Samuel J. Asirvatham

Age	Gender	Occupation	Working Diagnosis
58 Years	Male	Office Worker	Heart Failure Exacerbation

HISTORY

A 58-year-old male office worker with a long-standing history of cardiomyopathy, likely after an episode of viral myocarditis 20 years previously, sought treatment for worsening shortness of breath and functional deterioration. The patient was mildly obese and not in acute respiratory distress. He had a dual-chamber pacing system because of intermittent heart block and symptomatic sinus bradycardia while on medical therapy.

Because of ventricular dysfunction with a left ventricular ejection fraction (LVEF) of 28%, an implantable cardioverter-defibrillator (ICD) was recommended. The patient also had symptomatic heart failure (New York Heart Association [class III]) despite optimal medical therapy and a left bundle branch block with QRS duration of 148 ms. Cardiac resynchronization therapy (CRT) also was recommended.

He was taken to the procedure room at his local facility for upgrade to a CRT defibrillator (CRT-D) system. However, because of inability to place the left ventricular lead, the procedure was abandoned and the patient was referred for consideration of an epicardial system or to reattempt endocardial left ventricular lead and CRT-D placement. The operative note from the outside facility mentioned difficult subclavian venous access and inability to pass a wire beyond approximately 2 cm into the coronary sinus.

Past medical history is significant for intermittent atrial fibrillation, associated with mild symptoms and managed with rate control and anticoagulation.

CURRENT MEDICATIONS

The patient was taking lisinopril 10 mg twice daily, carvedilol 25 mg three times daily, and digoxin 0.125 mg once daily.

PHYSICAL EXAMINATION

BP/HR: 142/78 mm Hg/60 bpm, regular
Jugular venous pressure: 10 cm H_2O
Heart: Cardiac auscultatory findings significant for murmurs consistent with mild tricuspid and mitral regurgitation and wide splitting of the second heart sound (S_2) with accentuated pulmonary component; no third heart sound (S_3); pacemaker site appeared to be healing normally from the recent procedure; trace pedal edema was noted

HOSPITAL AND PROCEDURAL COURSE

After discussing the options of reattempting left ventricular lead placement, surgical epicardial lead placement, and assessment for appropriateness of left ventricular assist device or cardiac transplantation, it was decided to make another attempt at placing the coronary sinus lead before considering the other options. Another attempt at a transvenous approach was favored because of the benefits it offered over epicardial pacing, including lower surgical trauma, potentially more stable pacing electrical thresholds, and greater lead stability.[6]

The patient was brought in the fasting state to the procedure room. An axillary vein puncture was done with contrast venography, and a temporary pacing lead was placed because the patient was pacemaker dependent. The coronary sinus was cannulated without difficulty and balloon venography performed.

Venography findings are shown in Figure 11-1. As noted in the operative report from the referring institution, a wire would not pass beyond approximately 2 cm into the coronary sinus.

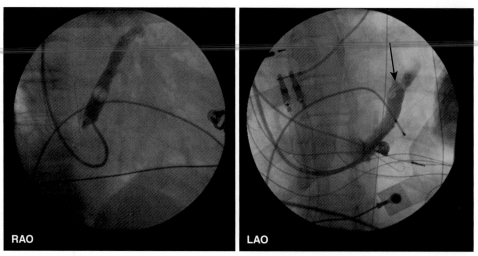

FIGURE 11-1   See *expertconsult.com* for video.

FOCUSED CLINICAL QUESTIONS AND DISCUSSION POINTS

Question

What is the likely cause of difficulty in advancing into the coronary venous system in this patient?

Discussion

Venography demonstrated a prominent Vieussens valve.[2] The Vieussens valve is a normal anatomic variant and is an intravenous valve located at the junction of the coronary sinus and the great cardiac vein. This is typically the site of takeoff for the posterolateral ventricular vein and the oblique vein of the atrium (vein of Marshall). Studies have shown that a nearly occlusive Vieussens value, as found in this patient, can prevent progression of catheters and guide wires and complicate a cardiovascular interventional procedure.[4] Therefore when various wires were passed into the coronary sinus, they would typically not advance beyond the valve and curve back into the main body of the coronary sinus.

Question

What are other potential reasons a wire will not pass freely into the branches of the coronary venous system?

Discussion

Once the coronary sinus has been cannulated, it may be extraordinarily difficult in certain patients to advance into the coronary venous system, particularly to the lateral free wall of the left ventricle. Potential reasons for this include coronary vein stenosis, intraprocedural coronary artery dissection, coronary vein dissection, and postsurgical or ablative therapy–related vein occlusion.

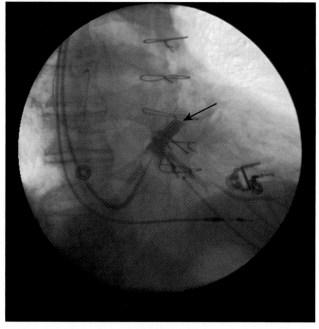

FIGURE 11-2

In cases in which the target vein is obstructed and no alternative vessels exist, balloon dilation or stenting may be necessary for successful lead implantation. Although the frequency of coronary vein stenosis is reported to be about 2.4% in one study, balloon angioplasty proved to be an effective method when used in combination with careful maneuvering of guide wires and leads for nearly all the patients.[5]

Sharp angles at which veins enter the coronary sinus can further interfere with the successful advancement of guide wires and lead into distal regions of the coronary venous system.[8]

Figure 11-2 shows venography from another patient in whom abrupt termination of the coronary sinus just distal to a posterolateral vein is noted. This patient did

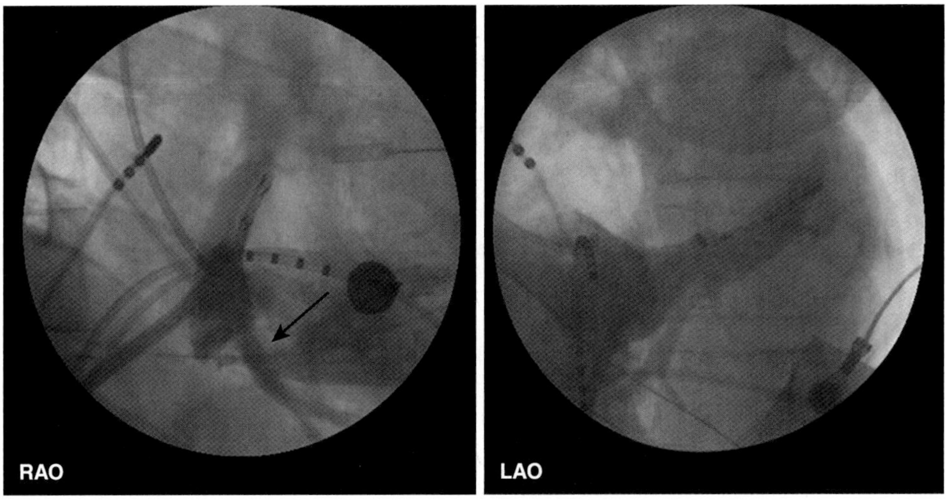

FIGURE 11-3

have prior mitral valve repair along with coronary artery bypass surgery.

Paradoxically, a very large coronary venous system also can make passing a wire into the ventricular veins difficult.

Figure 11-3 shows a large aneurysm in the coronary sinus with prominent posterior venous branches *(arrow)*. Although the coronary sinus may be easy to cannulate in such patients, presumably because of prominent flow back into the right atrium, advancing a wire without coiling it back in the large aneurysm or venous system may be difficult.

Question

What options are available for the operator caring for a patient where there is inability to pass a wire to the distal ventricular venous system and lateral wall, such as in our patient with a prominent Vieussens valve?

Discussion

The previously mentioned causes of difficulty in advancing into the lateral venous system and great cardiac vein (i.e., dissection, stenosis, and Vieussens valve) typically spare the coronary sinus ostium and proximal segment of this vein. Because the middle cardiac vein (MCV) or posterior interventricular vein arises very proximally—often immediately distal to the ostium—cannulating the MCV and advancing the lead through the collateral branch of the MCV to the lateral left ventricular wall can be an effective option to consider in such patients.[7] The primary branch of this vein courses along the posterior intraventricular groove and drains into the coronary sinus close to the right atrial orifice.[6]

How does one cannulate the MCV? Because of the proximity of the ostium of the MCV to the coronary sinus, technical difficulties arise in cannulating the MCV.

Figure 11-4 shows a useful maneuver that implanters should be familiar with for cannulating the MCV. Typically, counterclockwise torque on a preformed sheath placed from the subclavian venous system is required to enter the coronary sinus. However, continued counterclockwise torque will take the tip of the sheath toward the atrial rather than the ventricular vein. Thus the operator will need to gently withdraw the sheath back toward the ostium while placing *clockwise* torque on the sheath. In a stepwise manner, a wire is advanced to gently probe for the ostium of the MCV as this maneuver is employed. As the sheath is pulled back with clockwise torque just before falling out of the coronary sinus itself, the wire will advance into the MCV. Here it is sometimes useful to pass either a second wire or deflectable catheter to firmly gain access to the MCV. The sheath then can be pulled back to the right atrium to create a straight line between the sheath and the access of the MCV, and then the sheath is advanced, subselecting the MCV.

INTERVENTION

Once subselecting access is obtained, the deflectable catheter, if used, can be removed and a lead advanced over the wire (see Video 11-1). The MCV drains the inferior aspect of the posterior left ventricle; the posterior vein provides a more direct access to the lateral region of the left ventricle. Nonetheless, these distinct venous systems exhibit a high occurrence of anastomoses, resulting in an interconnected venous system near the posterolateral wall of the left ventricle.[1] Thus it is useful to recognize these collaterals between the middle cardiac and posterior venous system to the lateral wall. This can be done with occlusion venography in the body of the coronary vein, coronary sinus, or subselective angiography of the MCV (Figure 11-5).

Effective cardiac resynchronization therapy changes the sequence of ventricular activation, to improve the cardiac efficiency measured in terms of LVEF (Figure 11-6). The left ventricular lead ideally should be at a maximum distance from the right ventricular lead to enhance the effects of biventricular pacing. Pacing site that is most delayed also can be an operational strategy to reduce dyssynchrony and decrease the QRS duration. It is also important that a pacing lead in the coronary vein does not stimulate the phrenic nerve, because this can cause painful stimulation of the diaphragm.[9] In this patient, the lead was advanced through such a collateral

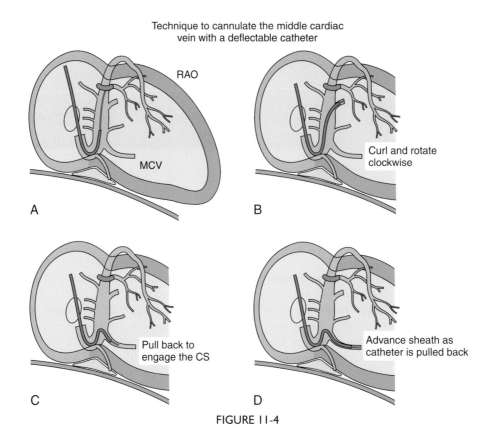

Technique to cannulate the middle cardiac vein with a deflectable catheter

A

B   Curl and rotate clockwise

C   Pull back to engage the CS

D   Advance sheath as catheter is pulled back

FIGURE 11-4

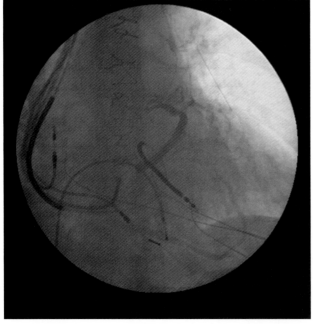

FIGURE 11-5

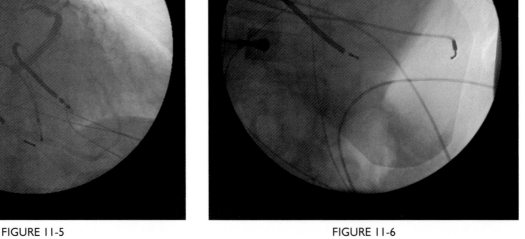

FIGURE 11-6

vein to the posterolateral wall of the left ventricle, an excellent pacing vector between the ICD lead and the lateral left ventricular lead pacing site obtained. The previous pacing lead was extracted, and the patient had symptomatic improvement and mild improvement in ventricular function (ejection fraction, 32%).

MCV pacing has proved useful in avoiding phrenic nerve stimulation in similar case studies. In a patient with class III to IV heart failure, a left ventricular pacing lead was placed in the posterolateral coronary sinus branch but biventricular pacing was unsuccessful because of phrenic nerve stimulation. Cannulation of the MCV and placement of a pacing lead in an optimal apical posterolateral position can be acheived, albeit with difficulty. A follow-up examination at 8 months revealed excellent pacing (<1 V, 0.5 ms), with considerable improvement in LVEF. The patient was able to avoid surgical trauma from the open thoracotomy necessary for epicardial lead placement.

FOCUSED CLINICAL QUESTIONS AND DISCUSSION POINTS

Question

Because the MCV is located posteriorly in the intraventricular groove and adjacent to the right ventricle, how does CRT with the left ventricular lead placed in the MCV benefit some patients?

Discussion

Figure 11-7 shows an inferior view of the autopsied heart and the course of the MCV. In most patients, beneficial left ventricular pacing therapy can be obtained despite the use of the MCV because lateral venous branches of this vein exist but drain the lateral wall of the left ventricle. These veins are analogous to the posterolateral branches of the coronary arterial system arising from the right coronary artery or the posterior descending artery. In these patients, placing a lead on the left ventricular free wall is equivalent to using, for example, a lateral vein or branch of an anterolateral vein. In other words, the pacing site is identical despite using a completely different branch of the coronary venous system to enter the ventricular veins—it is where you go that matters, not how you get there. For some patients, however, it is more difficult to understand why MCV pacing is beneficial. In these patients, as shown in the autopsied heart, there is a paucity of lateral branches and the lead is placed in the body of the MCV itself. No clear reason explains why these patients sometimes benefit, but possibilities include the following:

1. The epicardial surface myocardial fibers from the posterior wall are arranged in a radial fashion perpendicular to the long axis of the heart, whereas the endocardial fibers tend to be arranged along the long axis of the heart.[7] Thus even though a right ventricular apical lead and an MCV main lead may appear fairly close to each other radiographically, because of the differences in fiber orientation, the epicardial MCV lead will excite the lateral wall of the left ventricle sooner than will a right ventricular endocardial apical lead.

2. In some patients, standard pacing sites on the left ventricular free wall laterally or anterolaterally may not be the ideal site because of the location of the right ventricular pacing lead.

For example, as shown in Figures 11-8 and 11-9, the right ventricular lead has been placed in the high

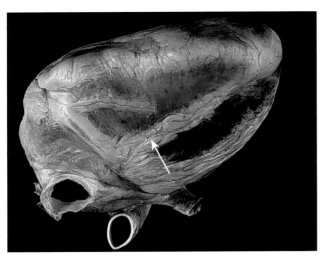

FIGURE 11-7

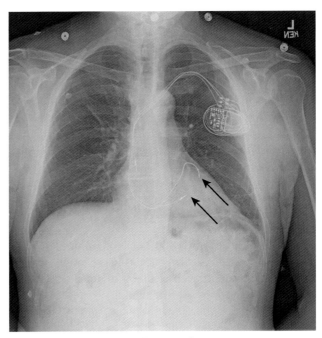

FIGURE 11-8

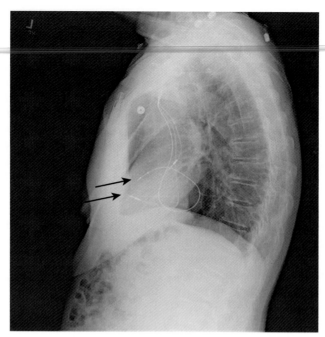

FIGURE 11-9

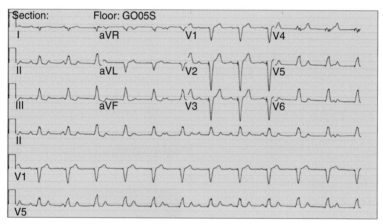

FIGURE 11-10

intraventricular septum quite anteriorly. Thus it is possible in these patients that biventricular stimulation from a site on the left ventricular high lateral wall would not be very dissimilar to the right ventricular lead site, as well.

Note in the 12-lead electrocardiogram obtained of this patient under biventricular pacing that although lead I shows a negative deflection (activation of the lateral wall), the QRS is wide, and a left bundle branch block pattern is seen (Figure 11-10). It is possible that such patients with right ventricular leads placed anteriorly and relatively leftward may benefit by a more posteriorly placed lead, such as through a posterior ventricular vein or MCV.

OUTCOME

MCV pacing with placement of the lead in a lateral branch to the lateral left ventricular wall was successfully done despite an occlusive Vieussens valve being present. The patient had significant symptomatic improvement and modest improvement in LVEF and continues to do well almost 2 years from the interventional procedure.

Selected References

1. Anderson SE, Lahm R, Iaizzo PA: The coronary vascular system and associated medical devices. In Iaizzo PA, editor: *Handbook of cardiac anatomy, physiology, and devices*, Totowa, NJ, 2005, Humana, pp 109-124.
2. Asirvatham SJ: Anatomy of the coronary sinus. In Yu CM, Hayes DL, Auricchio A, editors: *Cardiac resynchronization therapy*, Malden, 2008, Blackwell Futura, pp 211-238.
3. Bogaert J: Cardiac function. In Bogaert J, Dymarkowski S, Taylor AM, Muthurangu V, editors: *Clinical cardiac MRI*, Berlin, 2012, Springer-Verlag, pp 109-166.
4. Corcoran SJ, Lawrence C, McGuire MA: The valve of Vieussens: an important cause of difficulty in advancing catheters into the cardiac veins, *J Cardiovasc Electrophysiol* 10:804-808, 1999.
5. Hansky B, Lamp B, Minami K, et al: Coronary vein balloon angioplasty for left ventricular pacemaker lead implantation, *J Am Coll Cardiol* 40:2144-2149, 2002.
6. Hansky B, Schulte-Eistrup S, Vogt J, et al: Lead selection and implantation technique for biventricular pacing, *Eur Heart J Suppl* 6:D112-D116, 2004.
7. Lachman N, Syed FF, Habib A, et al: Correlative anatomy for the electrophysiologist. II. Cardiac ganglia, phrenic nerve, coronary venous system, *J Cardiovasc Electrophysiol* 22:104-110, 2011.
8. Leon AR, Delurgio DB, Mera F: Practical approach to implanting left ventricular pacing leads for cardiac resynchronization, *J Cardiovasc Electrophysiol* 16:100-105, 2005.
9. Manolis AS, Kappos K, Koulouris S, et al: Middle cardiac vein pacing avoids phrenic nerve stimulation, offers optimal resynchronization and obviates surgery for epicardial lead placement, *Hosp Chron* 2:44-45, 2007.

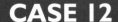

CASE 12

Mapping the Coronary Sinus Veins Using an Active Fixation Lead to Overcome Phrenic Nerve Stimulation

Azlan Hussin and Razali Omar

Age	Gender	Occupation	Working Diagnosis
69 Years	Male	Retired Government Clerk	Ischemic Cardiomyopathy and Ventricular Tachycardia

HISTORY

A 69-year-old man had underlying complete heart block and chronic atrial fibrillation, diabetes mellitus, and hypertension. He had a single-chamber pacemaker implanted in 2003 for complete heart block. He developed ventricular tachycardia 8 years previously, which required cardioversion. He was referred for further management.

CURRENT MEDICATIONS

The patient was taking bisoprolol 5 mg daily, atorvastatin 10 mg daily, perindopril 4 mg daily, warfarin 2 mg daily, and subcutaneous insulin injection. Mixtard 48 units in the morning and 20 units at night.

CURRENT SYMPTOMS

The patient was breathless on moderate exertion.

PHYSICAL EXAMINATION

BP/HR: 120/80 mm Hg/72 bpm
Height/weight: 160 cm/60 kg
Heart: Cardiomegaly

LABORATORY DATA

Hemoglobin: 11.3 g/dL
Hematocrit/packed cell volume: 34%

Mean corpuscular volume: 77.8 fL
Platelet count: $177 \times 10^3/\mu L$
Sodium: 143 mmol/L
Potassium: 4.2 mmol/L
Creatinine: 108 mmol/L
Blood urea nitrogen: 6.7 mmol/L

ELECTROCARDIOGRAM

Findings

Figure 12-1 shows the electrocardiogram (ECG) of the patient before admission to the casualty unit. Figure 12-2 shows the ECG of ventricular tachycardia on admission to the casualty unit.

CATHETERIZATION

Findings

The coronary angiogram showed mild coronary artery disease. A plan for conservative management was defined.

FOCUSED CLINICAL QUESTIONS AND DISCUSSION POINTS

Question

What is the anatomic basis of mapping the coronary sinus for location of a phrenic-free stimulation site?

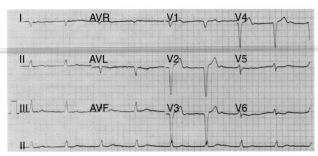

FIGURE 12-1

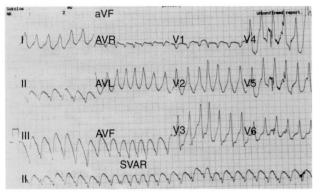

FIGURE 12-2

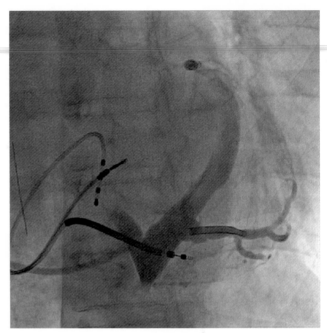

FIGURE 12-3

Discussion

Anatomic studies have shown that the distance between the left phrenic nerve and the target coronary sinus vein varies between 3.5 and 4.5 mm.[3] This variable relationship may be mapped to locate a phrenic-free point using the Medtronic 3830 lead (Medtronic, Minneapolis, Minn.), because the 3830 lead has a tip diameter of 1 mm.

Question

Can the screw tip of the Medtronic 3830 lead reach the myocardium through the coronary sinus wall?

Discussion

Histologic anatomy examination of the coronary sinus veins showed that the distance between the myocardium and the veins at mid and apical regions is approximately 1 to 1.42 mm.[1] This characteristic is well suited to the Medtronic 3830 lead because the helical structure, on four to five full turns, is 2.5 mm in length. Therefore the Medtronic 3830 lead needs to be rotated only two to three times to reach the myocardium.

Question

How can engagement of the screw tip be differentiated to be on the myocardial side of the coronary rather than the pericardial side?

Discussion

If the tip of the lead fixation mechanism engages the pericardial side of the coronary sinus, the pacing impedance will be excessively high, whereas pacing on the myocardial side of the pericardium will yield pacing impedance within the acceptable range.[2] Should engagement of the pericardium occur, the lead should be unscrewed and repositioned to another site.

Question

What is the risk for causing pericardial tamponade from multiple fixations within the coronary sinus?

Discussion

The fixation tip of the Medtronic 3830 lead is approximately 1 mm in diameter. Therefore, if the Medtronic 3830 lead must be repositioned, the breach in the coronary sinus wall also should measure 1 mm in diameter. A small breach such as this within a low-pressure system of the coronary sinus will not cause pericardial effusion or tamponade.

INTERVENTION

The patient underwent implantation of a cardiac resynchronization therapy device with a defibrillator. After the coronary sinus venogram was obtained (Figure 12-3), a conventional left ventricular lead was delivered to the target branch. However, pacing using the

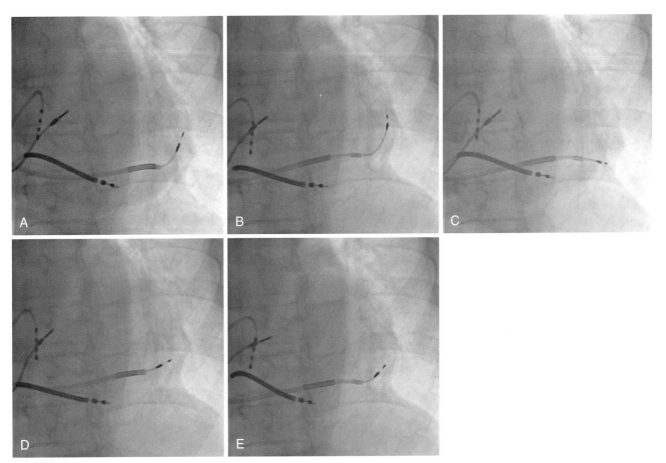

FIGURE 12-4

conventional lead caused phrenic nerve stimulation at different sites within the coronary branch.

An active fixation lead (SelectSecure 3830, Medtronic) was subsequently delivered into the target branch. Because the 3830 lead has a cable type of design that lacks over-the-wire capability, the lead was delivered to the targeted sites using an inner sheath (Attain Select II Sub-Selection Catheter, Medtronic) in a telescoping fashion.

The SelectSecure 3830 lead was actively secured at the targeted sites by twisting the lead body clockwise two to three rotations. Pacing parameters and lead stability were then tested. In the event the results were unsatisfactory, the lead was repositioned by twisting the lead body counterclockwise for two to three rotations and then actively securing it at another site.

OUTCOME

The lead was actively secured at five sites within the target coronary sinus branch. The initial two sites caused phrenic nerve stimulation (Figure 12-4, *A* and *B*). Failure to capture occurred at the third site (see Figure 12-4, *C*), and the fourth site had an unacceptably high capture threshold (Figure 12-4, *D*).

The site where pacing threshold was acceptable with no phrenic nerve stimulation was at the fifth site (see Figure 12-4, *D*). This spot was located only after careful mapping for its relation to the other site within the same target branch (Figure 12-5, *A*). The mapping process ensured that the tip of the lead was actively fixed to this spot, thus ensuring the stability of lead at this location (Figure 12-5, *B*).

FIGURE 12-5

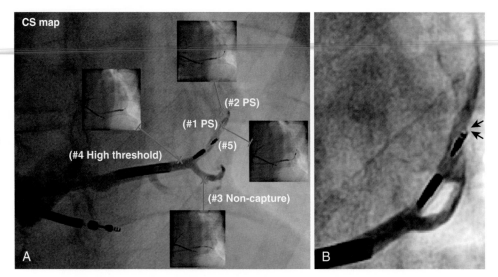

Selected References

1. Anderson SE, Hill AJ, Iaizzo PA: Microanatomy of human left ventricular coronary veins, *Anat Rec (Hoboken)* 292:23-28, 2009.
2. Hansky B, Vogt J, Gueldner H, et al: Implantation of active fixation lead in coronary veins for left ventricular stimulation: report of five cases, *Pacing Clin Electrophysiol* 30:44-49, 2007.
3. Sanchez-Quintana D, Cabrera JA, Climent V, et al: How close are the phrenic nerves to cardiac structures? Implications for the cardiac interventionalists, *J Cardiovasc Electrophysiol* 16:309-313, 2005.

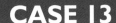

CASE 13

Utility of Active Fixation Lead in Unstable Left Ventricular Lead Positions in the Coronary Sinus for Left Ventricular Stimulation

Azlan Hussin and Razali Omar

Age	Gender	Occupation	Working Diagnosis
66 Years	Male	Retired Teacher	Ventricular Tachycardia and Recurrent Heart Failure

HISTORY

The patient had recurrent hospital admissions for heart failure despite optimal tolerable medical therapy. He had a left ventricular ejection fraction of 25% and mechanical dyssynchrony on tissue Doppler echocardiogram. He also had documented nonsustained ventricular tachycardia and paroxysmal atrial fibrillation on Holter monitoring.

CURRENT MEDICATIONS

The patient was taking warfarin 0.125 mcg/daily, furosemide 40 mg twice daily, carvedilol 12.5 mg twice daily, aldactone 25 mg daily, digoxin 0.125 mg daily, simvastatin 20 mg daily, and valsartan 80 mg daily.

CURRENT SYMPTOMS

Recurrent admissions for heart failure. Significantly breathless at mild exertion (New York Heart Association class III).

PHYSICAL EXAMINATION

BP/HR: 100/70 mm Hg/96 bpm
Height/weight: 167 cm/60 kg
Neck veins: Distended
Lungs/chest: Bilateral crepitations

Heart: Enlarged
Abdomen: Ascites

LABORATORY DATA

Hemoglobin: 11.1 g/dL
Hematocrit/packed cell volume: 32%
Mean corpuscular volume: 20.7 fL
Platelet count: 167 × 10^3/μL
Sodium: 141 mmol/L
Potassium: 4.3 mmol/L
Creatinine: 89 mmol/L
Blood urea nitrogen: 7.5 mmol/L

FOCUSED CLINICAL QUESTIONS AND DISCUSSION POINTS

Question

How frequently is a left ventricular lead with an active fixation mechanism required to pace the left ventricle?

Discussion

A left ventricular lead with some form of active fixation mechanism is required to overcome anatomic peculiarity, unstable lead position, and a circumscribed area of optimal pacing threshold without phrenic nerve stimulation in 12% of patients.[3]

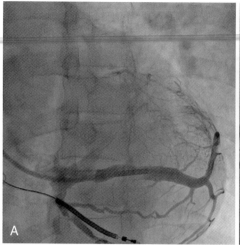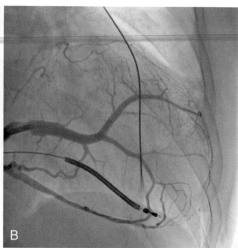

FIGURE 13-1 Subselective coronary sinus venogram in left anterior oblique **(A)** and right anterior oblique **(B)**. Note that the size of the distal coronary sinus branch is bigger than the size of the guiding catheter.

Question

Why was an active fixation lead chosen for this patient?

Discussion

The coronary sinus venogram (Figure 13-1) revealed a huge single posterolateral branch, the caliber of which exceeded even the biggest size of left-sided lead currently available. The trajectory of the posterolateral branch was straight and lacking in any degree of tortuosity that may help hold a conventional left ventricular lead in position after the support is removed. Therefore the chances of lead dislodgment if a standard left ventricular lead is used is relatively high.

Question

Why was a conventional left ventricular–specific active fixation lead not used in this patient?

Discussion

The currently available left ventricular–specific active fixation lead fixes itself indirectly by opposing the fixation lobes at the sides of the lead to the coronary sinus wall. This will promote tissue ingrowth from the coronary sinus side wall into the lead and therefore complicate future lead removal.[2,4] The size of the lead within the coronary sinus and tissue ingrowth also will lead to thrombosis of the coronary sinus branch,[3] a potential problem because the patient has a solitary coronary sinus branch if he is in need of left ventricular lead replacements in the future. Furthermore, this lead is a unipolar lead, thus limiting its use if electronic repositioning is required.

By using a 3830 lead, stability is achieved without compromising the coronary sinus if future use is required. Because the lead is bipolar, electronic repositioning can be performed easily if needed.

Question

How are the performances of the 3830 lead in the coronary sinus?

Discussion

The 3830 lead has an acceptable pacing threshold and impedance at implant and over a mean period of 8.1 months in 36 patients in whom it was implanted. No acute or long-term complications occurred. The pacing threshold and impedance remained stable at 8 months.[1]

Plan of Action

The patient was still symptomatic despite optimal medical therapy, with nonsustained ventricular tachycardia and evidence of mechanical dyssynchrony on a tissue Doppler echocardiogram; therefore the decision to implant a cardiac resynchronization therapy defibrillator was made.

INTERVENTION

The right ventricular lead was implanted conventionally. The coronary sinus was engaged with a standard coronary sinus conventional sheath. An inner catheter was used in a telescoping fashion to extend the reach of the sheath into the subselected coronary sinus branch. A venogram was then performed in two oblique views (Figure 13-2).

A Medtronic 3830 active fixation lead was then delivered to its target site via the telescoping sheath. At the target site, the lead is rotated clockwise two to three times to fix the lead to the underlying myocardium. Pacing parameters were then tested accordingly, and on completion, the telescoping and guiding sheaths were conventionally removed.

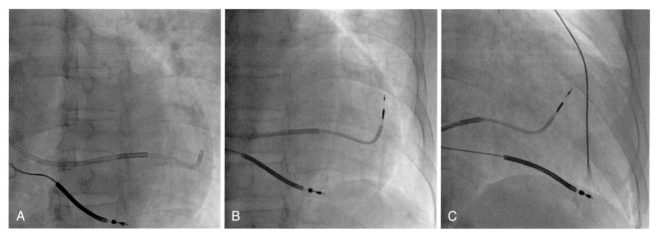

FIGURE 13-2 A 90-degree subselection catheter was used in telescoping fashion to guide the direction of the 3830 lead **(A).** Once the 3830 lead was in position, the lead was fixated by rotating the lead clockwise for two to three turns. The position of the lead was then checked in the left anterior oblique **(B)** and right anterior oblique views **(C).**

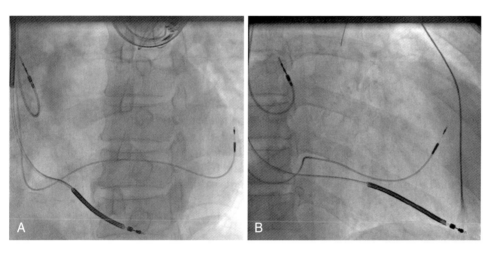

FIGURE 13-3 Final position of the leads in left anterior oblique **(A)** and right anterior oblique **(B)** views. Despite the size of the coronary sinus branch being bigger than the size of the lead, the lead retained its position at its fixed location.

OUTCOME

The implantation was completed successfully with acceptable pacing parameters without any complications (Figure 13-3). Follow-up at 1 month, 3 months, and 6 months did not show any significant parameter changes.

Selected References

1. Aziz AFA, Hussin A, Khelae SK, et al: Active fixation in the coronary sinus for left ventricular stimulation: an alternative method in improving left sided lead stability and overcoming phrenic nerve stimulation, *Heart Rhythm* 5(Suppl):S490, 2012.
2. Baranowski B, Yerkey M, Dresing T, et al: Fibrotic tissue growth into the extendable lobes of an active fixation coronary sinus lead can complicate extraction, *Pacing Clin Electrophysiol* 34:e64-e65, 2011.
3. Luedorff G, Kranig W, Grove R, et al: Improved success rate of cardiac resynchronization therapy implant by employing an active fixation coronary sinus lead, *Europace* 12:825-829, 2010.
4. Maytin M, Carrillo RG, Baltodano P, et al: Multicenter experience with transvenous lead extraction of active fixation coronary sinus leads, *Pacing Clin Electrophysiol* 35:641-647, 2012.

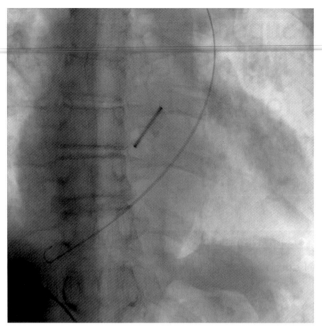

FIGURE 14-1 Posteroanterior view of a left-sided venous access with the J-wire tracking down the PLSVC into the coronary sinus and right atrium.

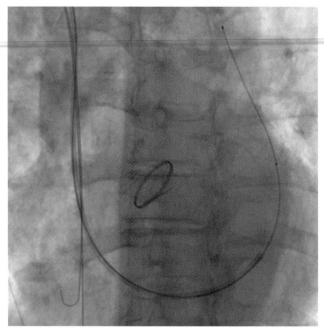

FIGURE 14-2 Posteroanterior fluoroscopic view after right-sided venous access and retrograde cannulation of the coronary sinus with a guiding catheter and 0.035-inch guide wire. Note that the guide wire may be mistaken to be in the pulmonary artery in this view (the cranial excursion of the guide wire and a left anterior oblique view showing a posterior course of the guide wire allow the operator to make the correct diagnosis).

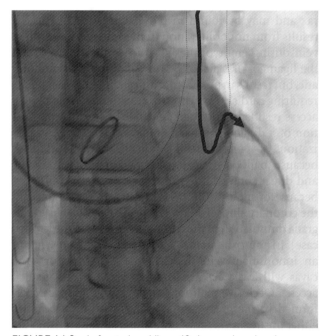

FIGURE 14-3 Left anterior oblique 40-degree view showing a balloon catheter subselecting a lateral branch. Note that access to this branch would be impossible via the left-sided persistent superior vena cava (PLSVC) (curved arrow). The dotted lines outline the contours of the coronary sinus and PLSVC.

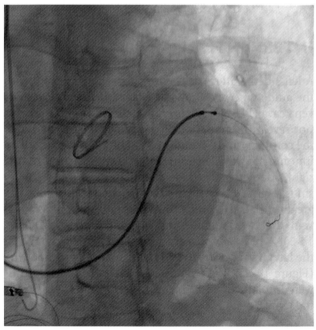

FIGURE 14-4 Positioning of the coronary sinus lead in the lateral vein over a 0.014-inch angioplasty guide wire.

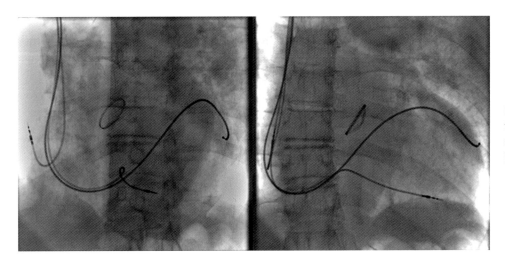

FIGURE 14-5 Final position of the leads in the 40-degree left anterior oblique *(left)* and posteroanterior *(right)* views.

Selected References

1. Biffi M, Bertini M, Ziacchi M, et al: Clinical implications of left superior vena cava persistence in candidates for pacemaker or cardioverter-defibrillator implantation, *Heart Vessels* 24:142-146, 2009.

2. Ratliff HL, Yousufuddin M, Lieving WR, et al: Persistent left superior vena cava: case reports and clinical implications, *Int J Cardiol* 113:242-246, 2006.

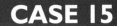

Persistent Left Superior Vena Cava: Cardiac Resynchronization Therapy with Left-Sided Venous Access

Haran Burri and Skand Kumar Trivedi

Age	Gender	Occupation	Working diagnosis
55 Years	Female	Housewife	Idiopathic Cardiomyopathy

HISTORY

This patient had complete heart block, with 30% left ventricular ejection fraction (LVEF) visualized on echocardiography. A temporary pacemaker wire was inserted into the right ventricle via femoral venous access. Coronary artery angiography was performed, ruling out coronary artery disease. The patient was scheduled for a biventricular pacemaker.

CURRENT MEDICATIONS

The patient was taking carvedilol 6.25 mg twice daily, digoxin (Lanoxin) 0.25 mg daily, furosemide plus spironolactone (Lasilactone) 25 mg twice daily, and enalapril 2.5 mg twice daily.

CURRENT SYMPTOMS

The patient was experiencing symptoms consistent with New York Heart Association (NYHA) class III symptoms.

PHYSICAL EXAMINATION

BP/HR: 110/70 mm Hg/78 bpm
Height/weight: 144 cm/62 kg
Neck veins: Engorged
Lungs/chest: Clear
Heart: Prominent third heart sound (S_3), no murmur

Abdomen: No organomegaly
Extremities: Normal

LABORATORY DATA

Hemoglobin: 13.9 g/dL
Sodium: 143 mmol/L
Potassium: 3.4 mmol/L
Creatinine: 73 mmol/L
Blood urea nitrogen: 22 mmol/L

Comments

The patient's hematologic and chemistry values were normal.

ELECTROCARDIOGRAM

Findings

The patient had a left bundle branch block and a QRS duration of 140 ms.

CHEST RADIOGRAPH

Findings

Chest radiography revealed cardiomegaly, with a cardiothoracic ratio of 60%.

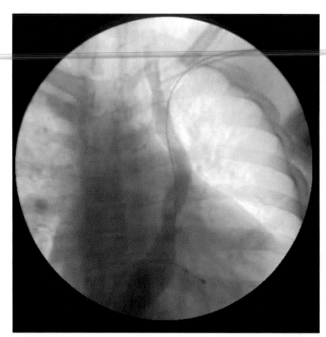

FIGURE 15-1   Posterior-anterior fluoroscopic view showing the guide wire in serted via left axillary vein puncture, tracking into the persistent left superior vena cava. Contrast injection did not show an innominate vein or posterior lateral tributaries suitable for coronary sinus lead implantation.

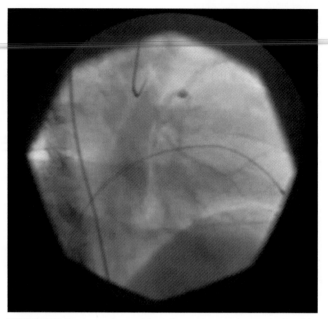

FIGURE 15-2   Levophase of the left coronary angiogram in the right anterior oblique 30-degree projection showing a dilated coronary sinus (the persistent left superior vena cava is also visible) and a posterior lateral vein.

ECHOCARDIOGRAM

Findings

Echocardiography revealed dysynergic septal motion with an LVEF of 30%.

FINAL DIAGNOSIS

The final diagnosis in this patient was idiopathic cardiomyopathy with persistent left superior vena cava and NYHA class III disease.

INTERVENTION

Left axillary vein access was obtained, revealing a persistent left superior vena cava (PLSVC). A venogram was performed via the introducer sheath, showing absence of an innominate vein; it did not show any posterolateral branches (Figure 15-1). The levophase of the coronary artery angiogram was then retrieved, revealing a posterolateral vein (Figure 15-2). A Judkins right 4 diagnostic catheter was inserted via an Attain MB2 coronary sinus guiding sheath (Medtronic, Minneapolis, Minn.) to subselect the posterolateral vein (Figure 15-3). A Medtronic Starfix lead was implanted over a

0.014-inch balanced middle-weight guide wire (Figure 15-4). This lead was chosen to ensure stability. A right atrial screw-in lead was placed in the right atrial appendage, and a right ventricular lead on the interventricular septum using a J-stylet that allowed easy positioning of the lead directly at the desired site (Figure 15-5).

OUTCOME

Comments

As mentioned in the case in Chapter 14, coronary sinus lead implantation is often easier via a right-sided venous access with retrograde cannulation of the coronary sinus. However, in rare cases, the right superior vena cava is absent[1] or coronary sinus atresia[2] may be present, with drainage to the subclavian vein. In these cases, the only option is to implant the coronary sinus lead via the PLSVC.

In our patient, the levophase of the coronary arteriogram was useful in revealing the presence of a lateral vein that was accessible via the PLSVC and allowed successful coronary sinus lead implantation without having to cross over to a right-sided venous access. Positioning of the right atrial lead is easy via the PLSVC, but the right ventricular lead may be challenging. A useful technique is to use a J-shaped stylet that allows positioning of the lead directly on the interventricular septum.

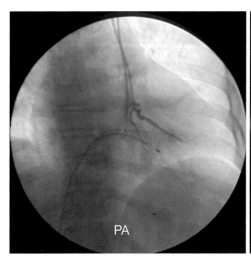
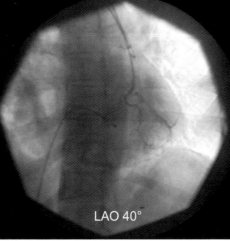

FIGURE 15-3 Subselection of the lateral vein with a Judkins right 4 diagnostic catheter in the posterior-anterior *(left)* and left anterior oblique 40-degree *(right)* views.

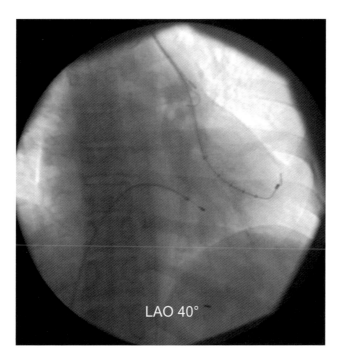

FIGURE 15-4 Positioning of the left ventricular lead in the lateral branch.

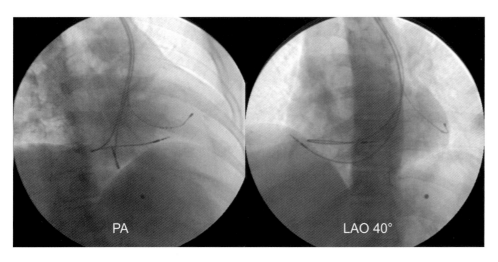

FIGURE 15-5 Final position of the lead in the posterior-anterior *(left)* and left anterior oblique 40-degree *(right)* views.

Selected References

1. Ratliff HL, Yousufuddin M, Lieving WR, et al: Persistent left superior vena cava: case reports and clinical implications, *Int J Cardiol* 113:242-246, 2006.

2. Gasparini M, Mantica M, Galimberti P, et al: Biventricular pacing via a persistent left superior vena cava: report of four cases, *Pacing Clin Electrophysiol* 26:192-196, 2003.

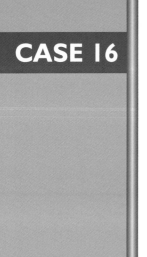

CASE 16

Video-Assisted Thoracotomy Surgery for Implantation of an Epicardial Left Ventricular Lead

Juan B. Grau, Christopher K. Johnson, Dan Musat, and Jonathan S. Steinberg

Age	Gender	Occupation	Working Diagnosis
80 Years	Female	Retired	Congestive Heart Failure

HISTORY

Nonischemic cardiomyopathy with a left ventricular ejection fraction of 15% to 20%, down from 30% in a span of 6 months, and New York Heart Association (NYHA) class III congestive systolic heart failure was diagnosed 5 months before the current admission. The patient also had a long history of chronic anemia that predates the decompensated heart failure. The patient was on optimal medical therapy. She underwent placement of an implantable cardioverter-defibrillator (ICD) 2 months earlier with the intent to place a cardiac resynchronization therapy device, but a left ventricular lead could not be placed through the coronary sinus. During the procedure, coronary sinus venography showed one high lateral branch with a proximal right-angle curve and a tight stenosis at the tip of the angle, a midcardiac vein with no posterior or lateral branches, and an anterior branch. The high lateral branch was cannulated with a Whisper wire, and using the over-the-wire technique an attempt was made to advance the lead into the branch. However, the lead could not be advanced beyond the stenosis. Repeat venography to better assess the severity of the stenosis demonstrated the vein to be occluded beyond the stenosis. Because no other vein suitable for transvenous left ventricular lead placement was available, the patient was referred for surgical epicardial lead implantation.

CURRENT MEDICATIONS

The patient was taking aspirin 81 mg daily, carvedilol 6.25 mg twice daily, furosemide 20 mg twice daily, potassium chloride 10 mEq daily, spironolactone 25 mg daily, and valsartan 40 mg daily.

CURRENT SYMPTOMS

The patient was experiencing shortness of breath when walking short distances (NYHA class III).

PHYSICAL EXAMINATION

BP/HR: 116/56 mm Hg/76 bpm
Height/weight: 157.48 cm/51.8 kg
Neck veins: Nondistended
Lungs/chest: Clear lungs, well-healed ICD incision
Heart: First heart sound (S_1) and second heart sound (S_2), regular rhythm with soft systolic murmur and no gallop
Abdomen: Soft and nontender, with no organomegaly
Extremities: Without edema

LABORATORY DATA

Hemoglobin: 7.0 g/dL
Hematocrit/packed cell volume: 22.4%
Mean corpuscular volume: 85.8 fL
Platelet count: 195×10^3 μL
Sodium: 138 mmol/L
Potassium: 4.4 mmol/L
Creatinine: 0.9 mmol/L
Blood urea nitrogen: 20 mmol/L

ELECTROCARDIOGRAM

Findings

The findings on the electrocardiogram were ventricular rate 81 bpm, atrial rate 81 bpm, pulse rate 146 ms, QRS

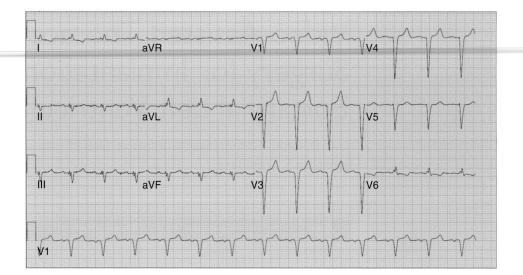

FIGURE 16-1 Electrocardiogram 3 days before surgery.

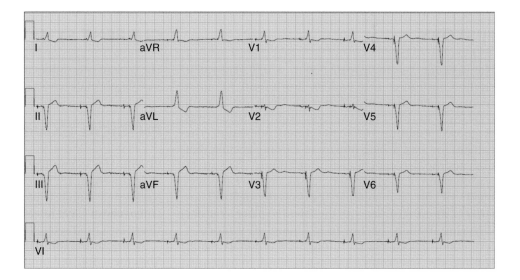

FIGURE 16-2 Electrocardiogram 20 days after surgery.

140 ms, QT 420 ms, QTc 487 ms, and P-R-T axes 039, –51, and 127 degrees (Figure 16-1).

Comments

Normal sinus rhythm, left axis deviation, anterior wall myocardial infarction (age indeterminate) were noted.

Findings

Repeat electrocardiogram findings were ventricular rate 60 bpm, atrial rate 60 bpm, pulse rate 128 ms, QRS 130 ms, QT 400 ms, QTc 400 ms, and P-R-T axes 0, –80, and 105 degrees (Figure 16-2).

Comments

Atrioventricular pacing with biventricular system.

CHEST RADIOGRAPHS FINDINGS

Figure 16-3 shows the heart is mildly enlarged, with left ventricular dominance. Calcification is seen within the aortic knob. An ICD is satisfactorily oriented with right atrial and ventricular leads. The hilar structures are mildly prominent. Small bilateral pleural effusions are seen.

In Figure 16-4, the cardiac silhouette is marginal in size, with intracardiac defibrillator leads directed into the right atrium and both ventricles. Also, a left chest tube had been placed. An abnormal pleural-based opacity is visible in the right lower thorax. Parenchymal consolidation or pleural fluid is not otherwise demonstrated.

Immediately postoperatively there was a patchy right basilar infiltrate and/or a right pleural effusion present with small residual left pneumothorax, see white arrows (see Figure 16-4).

On postoperative day 20 all the previous changes noted on Figure 16-5 have disappeared with no evidence

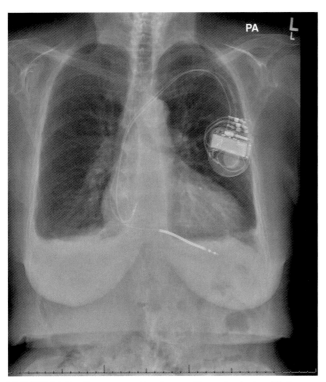

FIGURE 16-3   Anteroposterior chest radiograph obtained 3 days before surgery.

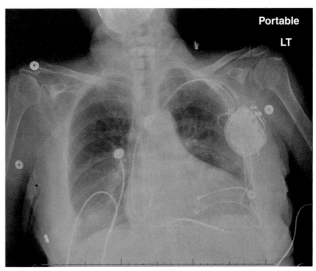

FIGURE 16-5   Anteroposterior chest radiograph obtained 3 days postoperatively. The small pneumothorax is no longer seen.

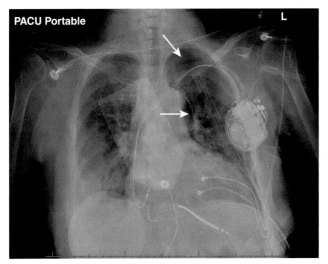

FIGURE 16-4   Postoperative anteroposterior chest radiograph. *Arrows* denote a very small postoperative pneumothorax.

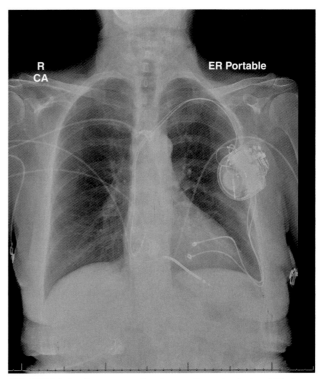

FIGURE 16-6   Anteroposterior chest radiograph obtained 20 days postoperatively.

of focal pulmonary consolidation, pleural effusion, or active vascular congestion (Figure 16-6).

ECHOCARDIOGRAM

5 Months Before Surgery

Findings

The echocardiogram revealed severely reduced systolic function of the left ventricle, with an ejection fraction of 15% to 20%. The left ventricular cavity was moderately increased. Both atria were moderately to severely dilated. Mild pulmonic regurgitation was seen, and the aortic valve was moderately calcified. Moderate-to-severe regurgitation was noted in both mitral and tricuspid valves. There was mitral valve sclerosis with a valve area of 1.36 cm^2 and the pulmonary artery systolic pressure was mildly elevated at 40 to 50 mm Hg.

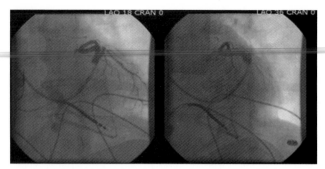

FIGURE 16-7   Venogram 2 months before surgery.

Postoperative Day 3

Findings

The postoperative echocardiogram revealed severely reduced systolic function of the left ventricle and ejection fraction increased to 20% to 25%. Moderate paradoxical motion of the septum was seen. The left ventricular cavity size was moderately increased and the left atrium mildly dilated. A pacemaker wire was identified in the right ventricle. Mild-to-moderate regurgitation was noted in both mitral and tricuspid valves. The pulmonary artery systolic pressure was mildly elevated, at 35 to 45 mm Hg.

VENOGRAM

Findings

Using the balloon occlusion technique a coronary sinus venogram was obtained in the left anterior oblique (LAO) projection using ioversol (Optiray) contrast agent (Figure 16-7). Venography showed one high lateral branch with a proximal right-angle curve and tight stenosis at the tip of the angle, a midcardiac vein with no posterior or lateral branches, and an anterior branch. A Whisper wire with extra distal support was used to cannulate the high lateral branch. Using an over-the-wire technique, a bipolar Attain Ability Plus steerable lead was advanced to the proximal portion of the lateral branch. However, the lead was unable to advance beyond the stenosis point and was removed so a smaller lead could be used. A repeat venogram in right anterior oblique and LAO projections to better assess the degree of stenosis showed that the vein was occluded beyond the stenosis. Left ventricular lead placement was abandoned because no other vein could accommodate a left ventricular lead on the lateral or posterior wall.

FOCUSED CLINICAL QUESTIONS AND DISCUSSION POINTS

Question

Why was this patient recommended for biventricular pacing?

Discussion

The patient had NYHA class III congestive heart failure and severely impaired left ventricular systolic function, as demonstrated by the extremely low ejection fraction. In addition, the patient had impairment despite traditional right atrial–right ventricular pacing. The lack of response is likely related to the nonspecific intraventricular block, indicating the potential benefit of the addition of left ventricular pacing.

Question

Why was this patient considered for surgical left ventricular lead placement?

Discussion

The surgical platform allows for direct epicardial access, thereby overcoming the limitations of coronary sinus anatomy in situations in which no branches or inadequate venous branches in the preferred target zone are available. In this patient, venography of the heart showed only one high lateral branch suitable for left ventricular lead placement, but it had a proximal right-angle curve and a tight stenosis at the tip of the angle that occluded beyond the stenosis during the lead placement attempt. The other coronary sinus branches, a midcardiac vein with no posterior or lateral branches, and an anterior branch were not desirable alternatives. Direct visualization of scar tissue and phrenic nerve position avoids left ventricular lead placement at sites of a previous myocardial infarction and diaphragmatic capture, respectively. Transvenous left ventricular placement should be the first option, but epicardial lead placement should be considered in cases of aberrant coronary sinus anatomy, venous branching that precludes stable lead placement or placement in a suitable target zone (as in this patient), phrenic nerve stimulation, or excessive pacing thresholds via transvenous route.

Question

What are the advantages and disadvantages of performing video-assisted thoracotomy surgery over other surgical platforms?

Discussion

Video-assisted thoracotomy surgery is a minimally invasive technique that produces less pain and has a shorter recovery time while still allowing for visualization of the epicardium. However, because the procedure is minimally invasive, the operating field is smaller than that with a limited thoracotomy. In addition, the lack of tactile feedback can make the operation difficult for an inexperienced surgeon. However, these obstacles can be overcome as the surgeon gains more experience with the procedure.

FINAL DIAGNOSIS

The final diagnosis was severe congestive heart failure after placement of an ICD.

PLAN OF ACTION

The plan of action for this patient was video-assisted thoracotomy for implantation of an epicardial left ventricular lead.

INTERVENTION

The patient was positioned in the supine position on the operating room table. Intravenous cefazolin was given less than 1 hour before skin incision (discontinued within 24 hours). The patient was then intubated with a double-lumen endotracheal tube. The lines were placed by the anesthesia team. She was then prepped and draped in the usual sterile manner, and a beanbag was used to keep her in the right lateral decubitus position. To avoid interfering with the procedure, the left arm was supported and retracted to allow access to the pacemaker pocket.

Three small incisions were made in the third, fifth, and eighth intercostal spaces, and three ports were inserted. A camera was passed through the middle port, and the pericardium was visualized. The pericardium was opened and the first marginal branch of the circumflex artery visualized. The left atrial appendage was also visualized. At this time, an attempt to deploy one of the leads through the superior port failed; the lead would not deploy properly from its holder because of the small intercostal space. A small, 2-cm incision was made at the level of the camera and the leads deployed through the opening. Two leads were placed at the base of the heart in between the obtuse marginal branch and branches of the circumflex artery.

The proximal ends of the pacing wires were then guided submuscularly through the third intercostal space to the pacemaker pocket. One of the leads was connected to the ICD generator, and the backup lead was capped and placed posterior to the ICD generator. At this time, a Blake drain was placed in the pericardial sac and the pericardium was closed. A posterior chest tube was placed in the pleural space. The working port, generator pocket, and port site incisions were all closed in the usual manner. The patient was then extubated in the operating room and taken to the recovery room in stable condition. No complications occurred during the operation.

The new leads were tested and were found to be working very well. The left ventricular lead connected to the generator had a pacing threshold of 0.5 V with an impedance of 532 Ω, and the backup left ventricular lead had a threshold of 2.5 V with an impedance of 794 Ω. The pacemaker was programmed to DDD and set to an atrioventricular delay of 130 msec and a V-V delay of 20 ms, with left ventricular stimulation preceding right ventricular stimulation by 20 ms.

OUTCOME

Left ventricular lead implantation carries a small failure rate because of variant coronary sinus and venous anatomy, as demonstrated in this patient.[1,2] Furthermore, lead dislodgement can result in an additional 5% to 10% late failure rate of left ventricular lead capture and sensing.[2,7] In cases in which transvenous left ventricular lead insertion is not feasible, the patient should be considered for surgical implantation of an epicardial lead. Surgical left ventricular lead placement has been shown to be highly successful in nearly 100% of attempts and offers the additional advantage of direct access to the left ventricular surface, leading to the possibility of detailed left ventricular mapping and precise site-directed resynchronization.[10]

The development of video-assisted thoracotomy surgery began with the thoracotomy, which was an attempt to avoid the complications associated with a full sternotomy while still allowing for excellent exposure of the posterolateral wall. However, the traditional thoracotomy involved a large incision and formal rib spreading and therefore was quite invasive; thus the limited thoracotomy was created. The limited thoracotomy approach allows for minimally invasive access to the anterior or lateral walls without rib spreading. In both cases, the incisions are kept to a minimum and rib spreading is avoided. Surgeons have gained significant experience in using these methods because they are commonly used in coronary revascularization procedures such as in minimally invasive direct coronary artery bypass in which the left internal mammary artery is anastomosed to the left anterior descending artery by a small anterior thoracotomy. Reports on the outcomes of limited left thoracotomy are positive, showing an average length of stay in the intensive care unit of 2.1 days, with no reports of significant complications, morbidity, or mortality rates[7-9] with a 5-day hospital stay.[8]

Video-assisted thoracotomy developed as an extension of the limited thoracotomy. Videoscopic guidance enhances exposure to the posterolateral surface of the left ventricle, limiting incision size and the need for rib spreading. Postoperative pain and discomfort are decreased with these approaches, and significant improvement of visualization of the entire area of interest allows more precise left ventricular lead placement. The proper site of lead implantation is paramount to the success of complete resynchronization.[3] More specifically, posterolateral pacing on the left ventricle has been shown to result in optimal resynchronization, whereas some evidence suggests that more anterior sites may actually hinder resynchronization.[3] The ideal lead for this approach is the screw-in lead. The introduction of new tools for the secure and controlled deployment of the lead has made minimally invasive approaches for left ventricular lead placement more feasible. Video-assisted thoracotomy has been shown to be comparable to the limited thoracotomy in terms of complication and mortality rates.[4-6]

The average length of hospital stay for a patient who has undergone video-assisted thoracotomy is approximately 4 days.[4,5] In the patient with prior cardiac surgery, fine and careful dissection of all surrounding structures can be difficult because the surgeon works without tactile feedback. Nonetheless, enhanced left ventricular access and left ventricular mapping have been facilitated by the aid of the videoscope and can be easily accomplished in most cases.

Selected References

1. Abraham WT: Cardiac resynchronization therapy for heart failure: biventricular pacing and beyond, *Curr Opin Cardiol* 17:346-352, 2002.
2. Alonso C, Leclercq C, d'Allonnes FR, et al: Six year experience of transvenous left ventricular lead implantation for permanent biventricular pacing in patients with advanced heart failure: technical aspects, *Heart* 86:405-410, 2001.
3. Ansalone G, Giannantoni P, Ricci R, et al: Doppler myocardial imaging to evaluate the effectiveness of pacing sites in patients receiving biventricular pacing, *J Am Coll Cardiol* 39:489-499, 2002.
4. Fernandez AL, Garcia-Bengochea JB, Ledo R, et al: Minimally invasive surgical implantation of left ventricular epicardial leads for ventricular resynchronization using video-assisted thoracoscopy, *Rev Esp Cardiol* 57:313-319, 2004.
5. Gabor S, Prenner G, Wasler A, et al: A simplified technique for implantation of left ventricular epicardial leads for biventricular re-synchronization using video-assisted thoracoscopy (VATS), *Eur J Cardiothorac Surg* 28:797-800, 2005.
6. Mair H, Jansens JL, Lattouf OM, et al: Epicardial lead implantation techniques for biventricular pacing via left lateral minithoracotomy, video-assisted thoracoscopy, and robotic approach, *Heart Surg Forum* 6:412-417, 2003.
7. Mair H, Sachweh J, Meuris B, et al: Surgical epicardial left ventricular lead versus coronary sinus lead placement in biventricular pacing, *Eur J Cardiothorac Surg* 27:235-242, 2005.
8. Puglisi A, Lunati M, Marullo AG, et al: Limited thoracotomy as a second choice alternative to transvenous implant for cardiac resynchronisation therapy delivery, *Eur Heart J* 25:1063-1069, 2004.
9. Shah RV, Lewis EF, Givertz MM: Epicardial left ventricular lead placement for cardiac resynchronization therapy following failed coronary sinus approach, *Congest Heart Fail* 12:312-316, 2006.
10. Steinberg JS, Derose JJ: The rationale for nontransvenous leads and cardiac resynchronization devices, *Pacing Clin Electrophysiol* 26:2211-2212, 2003.

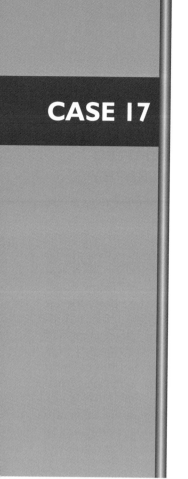

CASE 17

Role of Cardiac Computed Tomography Before Implant: Diagnosis of a Prominent Thebesian Valve as an Obstacle to Left Ventricular Lead Deployment in Cardiac Resynchronization Therapy

Jerold S. Shinbane, Farhood Saremi, Antereas Hindoyan, Gregory Rivas, and David Cesario

Age	Gender	Occupation	Working Diagnosis
54 Years	Female	Business	Prominent Thebesian Valve

HISTORY

The patient had a medical history of hypertrophic cardiomyopathy with progression to the dilated phase of cardiomyopathy (New York Heart Association class III) and conduction abnormalities, including a prolonged QRS duration of 154 msec with right bundle branch block (RBBB) and left anterior fascicular block. Her family history was positive for hypertrophic cardiomyopathy in her father and one brother. Genetic testing revealed a mutation in the *TNNI3* gene, resulting in replacement of the normal glutamic acid codon with a glutamine codon at position 124 in the *troponin I* gene. She had no history of hypertension, dyslipidemia, diabetes mellitus, or tobacco use. An echocardiogram demonstrated an ejection fraction of 20% to 25%. She underwent attempted cardiac resynchronization therapy defibrillator (CRT-D) implantation at a different institution, but the coronary sinus could not be cannulated. In addition, concern existed about possible coronary sinus dissection. Therefore a CRT-D device was implanted, with the left ventricular lead port capped. The patient was referred for evaluation for potential upgrade to a CRT-D via the implantation of the left ventricular lead. Cardiac computed tomography angiography (CCTA) was ordered for further evaluation of anatomic abnormalities impeding coronary venous lead placement.

CURRENT MEDICATIONS

The patient was taking carvedilol 6.25 mg in the morning and 12.5 mg at night, enalapril 7.5 mg daily, spironolactone 25 mg daily, furosemide 10 mg daily, and potassium chloride 10 mEq daily.

PHYSICAL EXAMINATION

BP/HR: 90/56 mm Hg/60 bpm
Height/weight: 165 cm/58 kg
Neck veins: Jugular venous pressure 5 cm H_2O
Lungs/chest: Lungs are clear to auscultation and percussion bilaterally; implantable cadioverter-defibrillator incision well healed
Heart: Left ventricular impulse was laterally displaced; regular heart rate and rhythm; normal first heart sound (S_1) and second heart sound (S_2), without third heart sound (S_3) or fourth heart sound (S_4); 1/6 holosystolic murmur at the left lower sternal border radiating to the axilla

Abdomen: Soft, nontender, nondistended; no evidence of hepatosplenomegaly, pulsatile abdominal masses, or abdominal bruits

Extremities: Without clubbing, cyanosis, or edema

LABORATORY DATA

Hemoglobin: 12.8 g/dL
Hematocrit: 37.6%
Mean corpuscular volume: 94 fL
Platelet count: 119 cells/µL
Sodium: 139 mmol/L
Potassium: 3.9 mmol/L
Creatinine: 0.9 mg/dL
Blood urea nitrogen: 22 mg/dL

Comments

Renal insufficiency is a factor that must be taken into account with iodinated contrast studies, such as CCTA. This is an issue for the heart failure patient population who require CRT.

ELECTROCARDIOGRAM

Findings

The electrogram demonstrated an atrial paced rhythm and ventricular sensed rhythm at 60 bpm. The PR interval was 198 msec; QRS duration was 156 msec, with RBBB and left anterior fascicular block; and corrected QT interval was 450 msec. Left ventricular hypertrophy was present.

ECHOCARDIOGRAM

A transthoracic echocardiogram showed mild left ventricular enlargement with wall thickness at the upper limits of normal and severe global hypokinesis with akinesis of the midinferior wall, inferior septum, and apex. The left ventricular ejection fraction was 22%, with a left ventricular end-diastolic dimension of 54 mm, a posterior wall thickness of 11 mm, and an interventricular septal thickness of 12 mm. Mildly decreased right ventricular systolic function was noted, as well as biatrial enlargement, with a left atrial volume index of 43 mL/m². The aortic valve was trileaflet, without aortic regurgitation or aortic stenosis. The mitral valve morphology was normal, with no evidence of mitral stenosis or regurgitation. No evidence of pulmonary regurgitation was seen. Trace tricuspid regurgitation was present, with an estimated right ventricular systolic pressure of 28 mm Hg. The right atrial pressure was estimated to be 5 mm Hg. The inferior vena cava size and respiratory variation were normal. No evidence of pericardial effusion was observed.

CARDIOVASCULAR COMPUTED TOMOGRAPHIC ANGIOGRAPHY

Findings

Coronary Venous Findings

The coronary sinus ostium was patent, with an ostial diameter of 1.2 cm. A prominent Thebesian valve was noted covering the coronary sinus ostium (Figure 17-1). The middle cardiac vein was followed by a posterior cardiac vein branching off 1.5 cm after the coronary sinus ostium with a gentle angulation of 146 degrees and coursed posterolaterally (Figures 17-2 to 17-4). At 6 cm distal to the takeoff of the posterior vein (mid to apical ventricular level), the vein bifurcated, with one branch coursing posteriorly and the other laterally. No evidence of a branch vein in the lateral territory of the left ventricle was seen. An anterior interventricular vein was present. No evidence of coronary sinus dissection was noted.

OTHER CARDIOVASCULAR FINDINGS

The coronary artery system was right dominant, with normal location of the coronary artery origins. Evidence of calcified and noncalcified plaques was present, without evidence of severe coronary artery stenosis

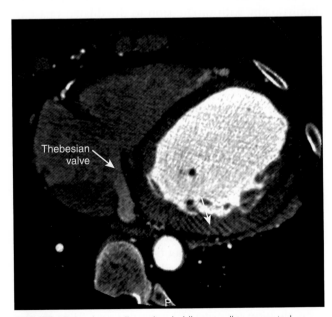

FIGURE 17-1   A two-dimensional oblique cardiac computed tomography angiography image demonstrates a prominent Thebesian valve (*white arrows*) covering the coronary sinus ostium.

(Figure 17-5). The left ventricle was moderately dilated, with thinning and aneurysmal dilation of the apex. A thin layer of mural thrombus was seen in the region of the apical aneurysm (Figure 17-6). The left atrium was severely enlarged. The right ventricle demonstrated normal morphology. The right atrium was normal in size. A dual-chamber implantable cardiac defibrillator (ICD) was present with leads in the right atrial appendage and right ventricular apex. The aorta and pulmonary arteries appeared unremarkable.

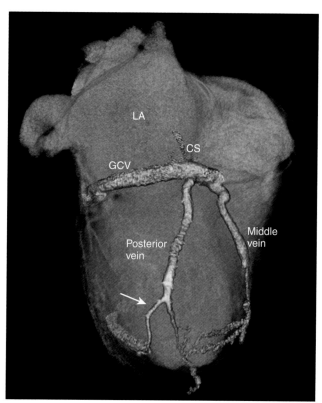

FIGURE 17-2 A three-dimensional cardiac computed tomography angiography reconstruction shows the coronary venous system. A posterior cardiac vein was present branching off 1.5 cm after the coronary sinus ostium coursing posterolaterally. At 6 cm distal to the takeoff of the posterior vein, the vein bifurcated, with one branch coursing posteriorly while the other branch coursed laterally. There was no evidence of a branch vein in the lateral territory of the left ventricle. The vein targeted for implant is shown (white arrow). CS, Coronary sinus; GCV, great cardiac vein; LA, left atrium.

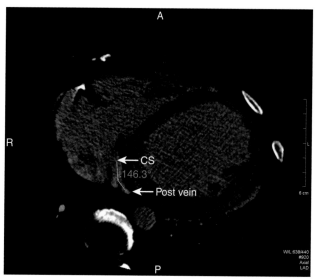

FIGURE 17-4 A two-dimensional oblique cardiac computed tomography angiography image shows the gentle angulation of 146 degrees of the posterior vein off of the coronary sinus. CS, Coronary sinus; Post vein, posterior vein.

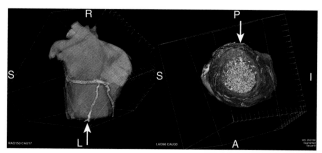

FIGURE 17-3 A three-dimensional cardiac computed tomography angiography reconstruction demonstrates localization of the myocardial segments associated with the posterior vein. The arrows demonstrate the myocardial location of the bifurcation of the vein at the mid to apical ventricular level.

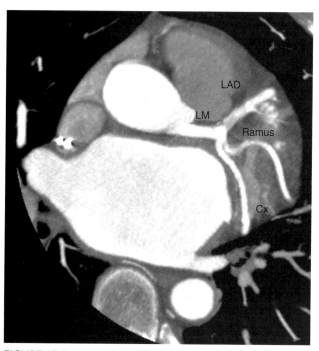

FIGURE 17-5 A two-dimensional oblique cardiac computed tomography angiography image showing the left coronary artery circulation without significant coronary artery disease. Cx, Circumflex coronary artery; LAD, left anterior descending coronary artery; LM, left main coronary artery; Ramus, ramus intermedius coronary artery.

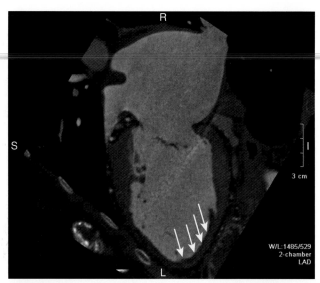

FIGURE 17-6   A two-dimensional chamber cardiac computed tomography angiography image demonstrates the left ventricle to be moderately dilated with thinning and aneurysmal dilatation of the apex. A thin layer of mural thrombus was seen in the region of the apical aneurysm *(white arrows)*. The left atrium was severely enlarged.

FOCUSED CLINICAL QUESTIONS AND DISCUSSION POINTS

Question

What are the potential anatomic limitations and challenges to left ventricular lead placement?

Discussion

Impediments to coronary venous lead placement are multiple and include (1) coronary venous valves or valve remnants, such as the Thebesian valve covering the coronary sinus ostium or Vieussen's valve at the ostium of the great cardiac vein; (2) an unroofed coronary sinus; (3) coronary venous diverticulum, aneurysm, stenosis, or occlusion; (4) coronary sinus atresia; (5) absent or underdeveloped coronary veins in the target area for left ventricular lead placement; (6) procedural complications, such as coronary sinus dissection; (7) thoracic venous anomalies, such as a persistent left-sided superior vena cava draining into a dilated coronary sinus with or without a right-sided superior vena cava; (8) close proximity of the phrenic nerve to a coronary venous branch target site causing diaphragmatic pacing; and (9) presence of significant myocardial scar at the target coronary venous branch site.

Question

What information important to CRT can be gleaned from a CCTA relevant to CRT lead placement?

Discussion

CCTA can provide anatomic characterization for CRT implant, including right atrial size, coronary sinus ostial characteristics, presence and location of coronary sinus branch veins, angulation of the branch vein off of the the coronary sinus or great cardiac vein, course of the target vein, and assessment for anomalies that may limit lead placement (see previous question).[1-7]

Question

What are the current guidelines for coronary venous CT imaging?

Discussion

Based on the American College of Cardiology Foundation, Society of Cardiovascular Computed Tomography, American College of Radiology, American Heart Association, American Society of Echocardiology, American Society of Nuclear Cardiology, North American Society of Cardiovascular Imaging, Society for Cardiovascular Angiography and Interventions, and Society for Cardiovascular Magnetic Resonance 2010 Appropriate Use Criteria for Cardiac Computed Tomography, noninvasive coronary vein mapping before placement of a biventricular system was deemed appropriate with a score of 8/9.[8] Preliminary data suggest that review of CT coronary venous angiography findings before CRT can facilitate placement of CRT devices.[5]

Question

What are the special considerations for coronary venous CT angiography in patients undergoing evaluation for CRT?

Discussion

Because patients undergoing evaluation for CRT have significant ventricular dysfunction, special considerations and potential limitations apply to coronary venous imaging. Patients must be able to lie in the supine position and follow breathing instructions for an appropriately timed breath-hold during imaging. Heart rate control can be challenging because some patients cannot be acutely beta-blocked to a heart rate of 60 bpm for imaging. Atrial or ventricular ectopy and arrhythmias such as atrial fibrillation can decrease study quality. Issues can relate to the volume load of contrast agent and iodinated contrast-induced nephrotoxicity.

The optimal timing of image acquisition in relation to administration of the contrast bolus may be delayed in patients with significant ventricular dysfunction as a result of prolonged circulation time of contrast to target structures. In addition, visualization of the coronary venous system requires a delay in triggering of image acquisition because contrast must course through coronary arteries to the myocardium and back through the coronary venous system. Coronary venous imaging can be achieved by performing a test bolus at the region of interest to assess timing before the study injection, with triggering based on a surrogate region of interest such as the descending aorta at the lowest slice of the study, adding several seconds to the timing based on a standard coronary artery study or using the timing of a standard coronary artery study with the trigger set at a higher Hounsfield unit threshold.

Question

What is the relevance of the Thebesian valve to cardiovascular procedures?

Discussion

The Thebesian valve is a remnant structure of the embryonic right valve, which commonly exists as a minimal remnant but can occur as fenestrated partial valve remnant, or fully formed valve. Thebesian valves can make coronary sinus cannulation more challenging for procedures such as coronary sinus catheter placement for electrophysiology studies, retrograde cardioplegia for cardiothoracic surgical procedures and CRT procedures. CCTA can allow visualization of prominent Thebesian valves, which may impede placement of left ventricular leads.[9]

FINAL DIAGNOSIS

CCTA demonstrated a prominent Thebesian valve covering the coronary sinus ostium as the impediment to placement of the left ventricular lead via the coronary venous system.

PLAN OF ACTION

Some Thebesian valves are challenging to cross with standard approaches and require other methods, including (1) use of alternative guide wires and sheaths from a standard subclavian or cephalic approach; (2) a double cannulation technique in which the valve is opened using a catheter from a different approach via a femoral vein, subsequently allowing the guide wire, sheath, and left ventricular lead to be placed from a subclavian or cephalic approach;[10] or (3) rarely an epicardial approach to left ventricular lead placement, which can be achieved through a minimally invasive surgical approach. In this case, the CCTA can help identify the

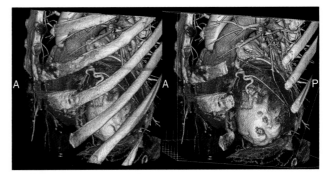

FIGURE 17-7   A three-dimensional cardiac computed tomography angiography reconstruction demonstrates the relationship of the left ventricle to the skeletal structures. These views could potentially be useful to planning an epicardial approach to left ventricular lead placement.

target site in relation to the three-dimensional thoracic anatomy and skeletal structures for decisions as to the optimal incision site (Figure 17-7).

INTERVENTION

An upgrade procedure was performed with addition of a left ventricular lead through the coronary venous system to the CRT-D device. The device pocket was exposed through an incision at the site of the generator incision, and the generator was disconnected. Left subclavian venous access was obtained. A multipurpose curved catheter was advanced under fluoroscopic guidance over a Wholey wire (Coviden, Mansfield, Mass.) into the mid–right atrium, rotated septally, and advanced across the tricuspid annulus into the right ventricle. The catheter and wire were slowly pulled back with counterclockwise torque into the right atrium, rotating the catheter posteriorly. Once in the right atrium, the Wholey wire was advanced to gain access to the coronary sinus through the Thebesian valve. Because of the difficulty in advancing the multipurpose sheath into the coronary sinus, a flexible Terumo catheter (Terumo Medical, Somerset, N.J.) was advanced over the Wholey wire into the main coronary sinus body. Then the multipurpose sheath was advanced over the transit catheter and the Wholey wire into the main coronary sinus and great cardiac vein. A contrast injection was performed that identified the posterolateral branch vein. The Wholey wire and transit catheter were removed. The sheath was flushed, and the coronary venous lead was advanced over a PT2 wire (Boston Scientific, Natick, Mass.) and positioned in the posterolateral branch vein (Figure 17-8). Excellent sensing and capture thresholds were confirmed. Diaphragmatic stimulation was absent during a test pulse at 10 V and 2 ms.

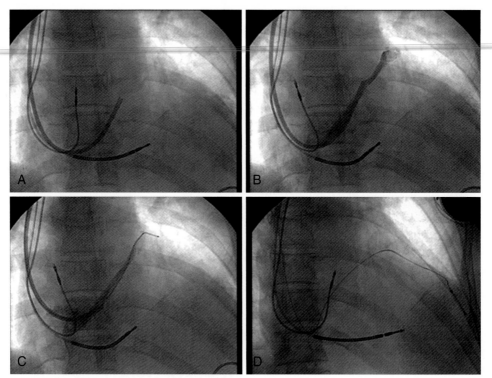

FIGURE 17-8   Fluoroscopy images show the multipurpose catheter that has been advanced beyond the Thebesian valve into the main body of the great cardiac vein, with subsequent deployment of the left ventricular endovascular lead.

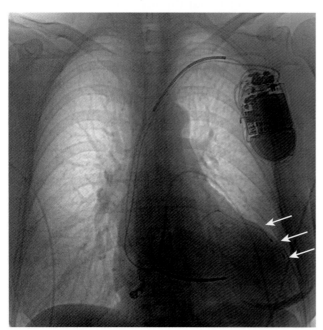

FIGURE 17-9   A chest radiograph demonstrates the final left ventricular lead position *(white arrows).*

OUTCOME

The patient had successful deployment of a coronary venous lead with a normally functioning CRT-D device (Figure 17-9).

Selected References

1. Auricchio A, Sorgente A, Soubelet E, et al: Accuracy and usefulness of fusion imaging between three-dimensional coronary sinus and coronary veins computed tomographic images with projection images obtained using fluoroscopy, *Europace* 11:1483-1490, 2009.
2. Cao M, Chang P, Garon B, et al: Cardiac resynchronization therapy: double cannulation approach to coronary venous lead placement via a prominent Thebesian valve. pacing and clinical electrophysiology, *Pacing Clin Electrophysiol*, 2012. in press.
3. Girsky MJ, Shinbane JS, Ahmadi N, et al: Prospective randomized trial of venous cardiac computed tomographic angiography for facilitation of cardiac resynchronization therapy, *Pacing Clin Electrophysiol* 33:1182-1187, 2010.
4. Jongbloed MR, Lamb HJ, Bax JJ, et al: Noninvasive visualization of the cardiac venous system using multislice computed tomography, *J Am Coll Cardiol* 45:749-753, 2005.
5. Mao S, Shinbane JS, Girsky MJ, et al: Coronary venous imaging with electron beam computed tomographic angiography: three-dimensional mapping and relationship with coronary arteries, *Am Heart J* 150:315-322, 2005.
6. Mark DB, Berman DS, Budoff MJ, et al: ACCF/ACR/AHA/NASCI/SAIP/SCAI/SCCT 2010 expert consensus document on coronary computed tomographic angiography: a report of the American College of Cardiology Foundation Task Force on Expert Consensus Documents, *Circulation* 121:2509-2543, 2010.
7. Mlynarski R, Mlynarska A, Sosnowski M: Anatomical variants of coronary venous system on cardiac computed tomography, *Circulation* 75:613-618, 2011.
8. Shinbane JS, Girsky MJ, Mao S, et al: Thebesian valve imaging with electron beam CT angiography: implications for resynchronization therapy, *Pacing Clin Electrophysiol* 27:1331-1332, 2004.

9. Taylor AJ, Cerqueira M, Hodgson JM, et al: ACCF/SCCT/ACR/ AHA/ASE/ASNC/NASCI/SCAI/SCMR 2010 appropriate use criteria for cardiac computed tomography: a report of the American College of Cardiology Foundation Appropriate Use Criteria Task Force, the Society of Cardiovascular Computed Tomography, the American College of Radiology, the American Heart Association, the American Society of Echocardiography, the American Society of Nuclear Cardiology, the North American Society for Cardiovascular Imaging, the Society for Cardiovascular Angiography and Interventions, and the Society for Cardiovascular Magnetic Resonance, *Circulation* 122:e525-e555, 2010.

10. Van de Veire NR, Marsan NA, Schuijf JD, et al: Noninvasive imaging of cardiac venous anatomy with 64-slice multi-slice computed tomography and noninvasive assessment of left ventricular dyssynchrony by 3-dimensional tissue synchronization imaging in patients with heart failure scheduled for cardiac resynchronization therapy, *Am J Cardiol* 101:1023-1029, 2008.

SECTION 4

New Cardiac Resynchronization Therapy Implantation Techniques

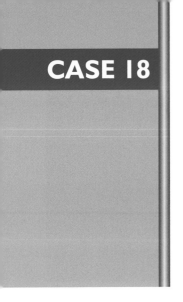

Endocardial Left Ventricular Lead: High Approach

Philippe Ritter, Pierre Jaïs, and Pierre Bordachar

Age	Gender	Occupation	Working Diagnosis
65 Years	Male	Retired	Heart Failure

HISTORY

The patient was a 65-year-old retired man seeking treatment for dilated cardiomyopathy with normal coronary arteries for about 10 years. Risk factors are dyslipidemia and obesity (91 kg, 173 cm). Two procedures of ablation for atrial fibrillation and atrial tachycardia were performed 6 and 2 years earlier. One year previously, a new episode of atrial fibrillation was treated with direct current shock and amiodarone. The patient is currently in sinus rhythm and remains in New York Heart Association (NYHA) class III under medical therapy. The patient has no pulmonary disease, and respiratory tests are normal.

Comments

This is a long history of heart failure in a patient being followed adequately and benefiting from currently available therapeutic techniques. The cardiomyopathy is considered idiopathic, and atrial arrhythmias are events that do not fully explain the current heart failure status of the patient.

MEDICATIONS

The patient was taking bisoprolol 2.5 mg daily, ramipril 5 mg daily, rosuvastatin 20 mg daily, furosemide 40 mg daily, warfarin with international normalized ratio (INR) between 2 and 3, amiodarone 200 mg daily.

Comments

The patient could not tolerate the recommended dosages of beta blockers and angiotensin-converting enzyme (ACE) inhibitors because of symptomatic hypotension. The spironolactone that was given previously had to be stopped for occurrence of hyperkalemia. Thus medical

treatment is not optimal, because patient ideally should require 10 mg daily each of bisoprolol and ramipril. The statin is given for the hypercholesterolemia. Amiodarone and warfarin are for rhythm control and prevention of thromboembolism, respectively. The furosemide dosage is sufficient for controlling the heart failure symptoms.

CURRENT SYMPTOMS

The patient is in NYHA class III, with predominant dyspnea on exertion, accompanied with palpitations, fatigue, and mild peripheral edema.

Comments

The patient never experienced symptoms of acute heart failure even during the occurrence of atrial tachyarrhythmias. Increasing the dosage of furosemide did not minimize symptoms.

PHYSICAL EXAMINATION

BP/HR: 98/71 mm Hg/95 bpm at rest
Height/weight: 173 cm/91 kg
Neck veins: Not dilated
Lungs/chest: No crackle at auscultation
Heart: No murmur, no abnormal heart sound
Abdomen: No ascites
Extremities: Mild limb edema

Comments

Although the patient had symptoms of heart failure, no objective sign can be observed except from sinus tachycardia and hypotension. This may occur in patients with chronic heart failure.

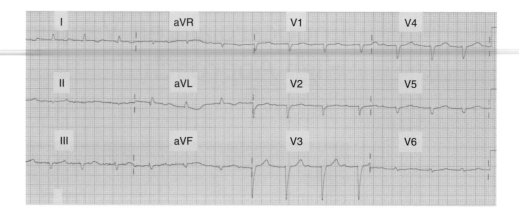

FIGURE 18-1   Baseline electrocardiogram.

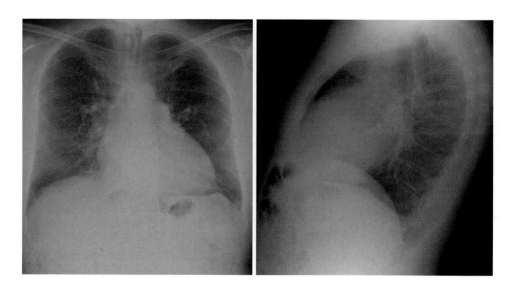

FIGURE 18-2   The cardiothoracic ratio is over 50%. Some pulmonary overloading can be observed.

LABORATORY DATA

Hemoglobin: 12.7 g%
Hematocrit/packed cell volume: 37.6%
Platelet count: 184 g/L
Sodium: 139 mmol/L
Potassium: 4.2 mmol/L
Creatinine: 109 mmol/L
Urea nitrogen: 8.4 mmol/L
B-type natriuretic peptide: 1287 pg/mL

Comments

The patient has mild impairment of renal function, and B-type natriuretic peptide (BNP) is elevated.

ELECTROCARDIOGRAM

Findings

The electrocardiogram (ECG) showed sinus rhythm 82 bpm, P duration 80 ms, P axis 40 degrees, PR interval 320 ms, QRS 120 ms, and QRS axis −30 degrees; QTc 489 ms (Figure 18-1).

Comments

The ECG showed first-degree atrioventricular block, and the QRS was not prolonged. QRS morphology could correspond to left anterior hemiblock, although left axis deviation is not that important. This ECG tracing does not fit a cardiac resynchronization therapy (CRT) indication.

ECHOCARDIOGRAM

Findings

The echocardiogram revealed left ventricular ejection fraction (LVEF) 25%; moderate left ventricular dilation, with end-diastolic volume 87 mL/m² and end systolic volume 65 mL/m²; global hypokinesia; left ventricular filling time less than 40% of the RR duration; left ventricular preejection time 160 ms; normal right ventricular

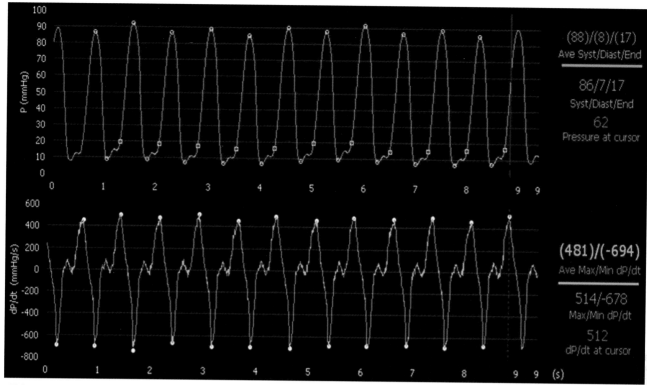

FIGURE 18-3   In spontaneous rhythm, dP/dt_{max} is very low (481 mm Hg/sec) with a low left ventricular systolic pressure found at 88 mm Hg.

function; dilation of the atria; no valvular abnormality; and increased filling pressures (Figure 18-2).

Comments

A discrepancy was seen between low LVEF and moderate left ventricular dilation, although the patient's heart failure history is 10 years. The short left ventricular filling time is related to the prolonged PR interval. The prolonged preejection time may be related to left ventricular dyssynchrony. Increased filling pressure is compatible with the high BNP level.

CATHETERIZATION

A coronary angiogram was performed again (the first since 2006) to exclude coronary artery disease. The examination provides an opportunity to assess the coronary sinus network during venous-phase recording. This examination shows a huge distribution of very small and tortuous veins that predict major difficulties in case of a decision for a CRT implantation.

Analysis of the effects of atriobiventricular pacing with an endocardial left ventricular lead placed at different sites within the left ventricle is performed, and three temporary leads are introduced: one at the atrial appendage and one at the right ventricular apex via the right femoral vein and one left ventricular lead introduced via

the right femoral artery from the groin. A radial approach was used for the coronary angiogram, to introduce a pressure wire to record left ventricular pressure, and to calculate left ventricular dP/dt. All pacing configurations are applied in the VDD mode, with the AVD set at 100 ms. Three left ventricular lead positions are tested in biventricular pacing: apical, anterolateral, and posterior. Each pacing is applied for 2 minutes before a 10-second recording to measure mean dP/dt_{max} and dP/dt_{min}. Between each pacing configuration, the baseline intrinsic rhythm is restored (Figures 18-3, 18-4, 18-5, and 18-6).

In conclusion, both dP/dt_{max} and dP/dt_{min} increase during biventricular pacing at all left ventricular sites in contrast to baseline spontaneous rhythm. However, the left ventricular pacing site does influence the result—when the left ventricular lead is placed at the left ventricular apex, the improvement in dP/dt_{max} is 7% (not significant), whereas it is 45% at the anterolateral left ventricular site, and 67% at the midposterior left ventricular site.

Comments

Left ventricular dP/dt_{max} is considered a hemodynamic reference parameter to assess cardiac function. However, the methodology of measurement is quite important, especially when differences in the effect of two therapies are small. Each measurement done under each pacing configuration must be compared to baseline applied between each pacing configuration. The

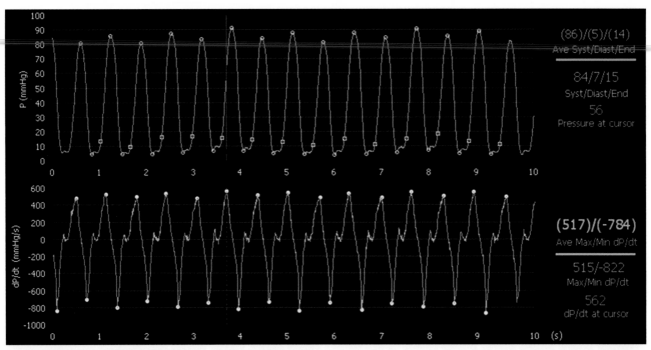

FIGURE 18-4   During atriobiventricular pacing with the endocardial left ventricular lead placed at the apex, dP/dt$_{max}$ rises to 517 mm Hg/sec, without change in the left ventricular systolic pressure, but the difference is not significant.

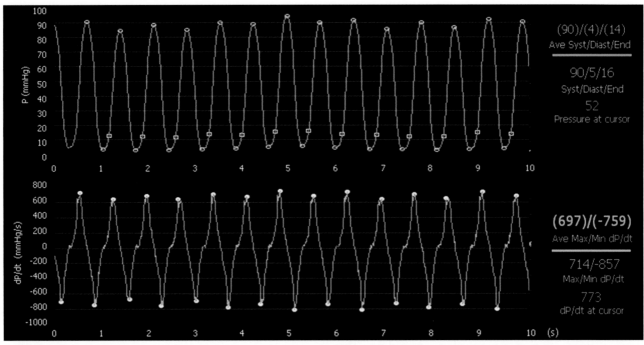

FIGURE 18-5   During atriobiventricular pacing with the endocardial left ventricular lead placed at the anterior and lateral site, dP/dt$_{max}$ rises significantly to 697 mm Hg/sec, with a slight increase in left ventricular systolic pressure.

different methods of measurement are not standardized. Measurements can be done after 30 seconds to 2 minutes in each pacing mode. Plateaus of several seconds or cycles are then compared, with the condition that no extrasystole occurs that would induce a drop in dP/dt$_{max}$. Another technique is to record a few

cycles before and after the pacing configuration transition at a moment when the direct mechanical effect of the pacing configuration change is observed without peripheral adaptation. In any case, repetition of measurements should be performed to minimize the effects of artifacts, such as respiration, especially when

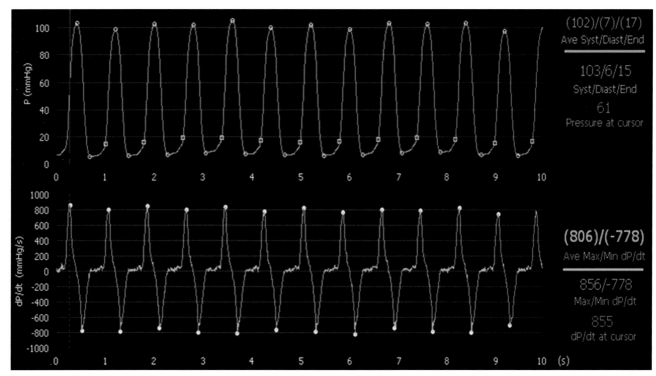

FIGURE 18-6   During atriobiventricular pacing with the left ventricular lead placed at the posterior site, left ventricular dP/dt$_{max}$ rises further to 806 mm Hg and systolic pressure to 102 mm Hg. dP/dt$_{min}$ is also higher than in the spontaneous condition, demonstrating faster left ventricular relaxation.

observed differences between pacing modes are small. In the example, the biventricular pacing configuration with the left ventricular lead placed at the apex does not provide a significant difference in contrast to baseline AAI mode. However, the two other left ventricular locations did provide a significant improvement in dP/dt well above two times the standard deviation. A limitation in this case is the absence of repetition of dP/dt measurements in each pacing mode.

IMPLANTATION

Implantation of the atriobiventricular system is performed under general anesthesia. The atrial lead is placed at the right atrial appendage, the right ventricular lead (a single-coil implantable cardioversion defibrillator lead) at the apex (rather than at the right ventricular free wall close to the apex, as suggested by the postprocedure chest radiographic examination). The left ventricular lead is placed through a transseptal puncture, from the left subclavian vein, to the location designated by the temporary preoperative hemodynamic test, which provided the maximal dP/dt$_{max}$ increase, that is, the posterior endocardial site. The lead being used was the Select Secure (Medtronic, Northridge, Calif.). This implantation is currently done in the context of the ALternate Site Cardiac ReSYNChronization (ALSYNC)

feasibility trial, assessing the feasibility and safety of the left ventricular endocardial pacing through an atrial transseptal approach.

POSTOPERATIVE RADIOGRAPH

The postoperative radiographic examination includes four views: anteroposterior, lateral, right anterior oblique, and left anterior oblique. It confirms that the location of the left ventricular lead is close to the site of pacing applied during the preoperative hemodynamic study. See Figure 18-7.

POSTOPERATIVE ELECTROCARDIOGRAM

The recorded ECG under biventricular pacing shows right deviation of the QRS axis. QRS duration (~130 ms) does not really differ from the intrinsic QRS complex (120 ms). Atrioventricular delay is set at its nominal value (120 ms) and VV interval at 0 ms (Figure 18-8).

When left ventricular pacing alone is programmed, the ECG shows the classic QRS pattern of left posterior pacing with large QRS (160 ms) (Figure 18-9).

Electrical performance of the left ventricular lead is excellent—650 Ω impedance and 0.5-V pacing threshold at 0.4-ms pulse width.

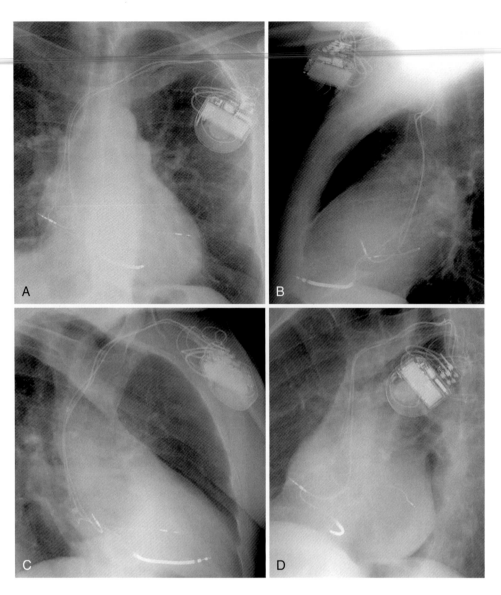

FIGURE 18-7 Postoperative chest radiographic examination showing the location of the three leads: atrial lead at the lateral wall of the right atrium, right ventricular lead at the right ventricular paraapical site, and left ventricular lead at the midposterior wall of the left ventricular endocardium. **A,** Anteroposterior view. **B,** Lateral view. **C,** right anterior oblique view. **D,** Left anterior oblique view.

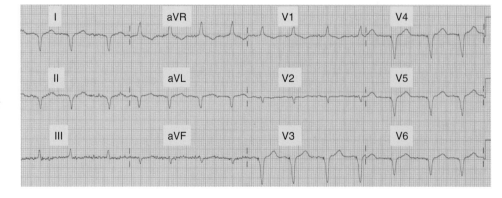

FIGURE 18-8 Postoperative electrogram recorded in DDD mode during atrio–left ventriciular pacing.

ELECTRICAL ACTIVATION PATTERN

A new system (EcVUE, CardioInsight, Cleveland, Ohio) that noninvasively generates maps of the electrical activity of the heart, has been developed. A vest consisting of 252 electrodes is placed on the patient's thorax. One beat is recorded, and an electrocardiographic map can be obtained that is plotted on a three-dimensional anatomic image of the patient's heart obtained with computed tomography. This map allows

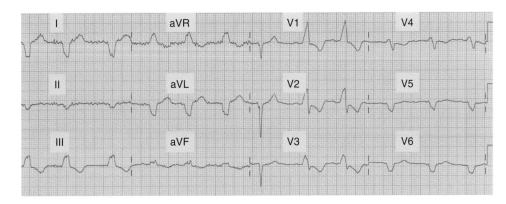

FIGURE 18-9 Postoperative electrogram recorded in DDD mode during atrial left ventricular pacing.

analysis of the electrical activation of the atria and ventricles.

Left ventricular pacing elicits variable electrical activation patterns affecting electrical synchrony. Electrocardiographic mapping produces noninvasive, biventricular electrical activation maps that can be acquired during different pacing configurations. The red color indicates the zone of primary activation, and the dark blue indicates the zone of latest activation. Isochrones delineate the zones of equal activation time. Narrowing of the zones indicates slower conduction. These activation maps can be used in the context of CRT to evaluate electrical synchrony—visual inspection of activation maps at baseline and during pacing, interventricular, and intraventricular quantitative assessments.

In this patient, the intrinsic QRS complex is measured by the system at 118 ms. Left lateral and posterior wall depolarization is delayed in contrast to right ventricular activation. The difference between mean right ventricular and mean left ventricular activations is –64 ms. The pattern of activation is similar to a left bundle branch block pattern. Note also that the midseptal activation cannot be observed.

During biventricular pacing, the activation pattern looks more homogeneous. The paced QRS duration is 126 ms. The posterior and inferior left ventricular wall remains slightly delayed. The difference between mean right ventricular and mean left ventricular activations is –20 ms (Figures 18-10, 18-11, and 18-12).

In conclusion, this technique helps in understanding the ventricular activation patterns according to the lead locations.

OUTCOMES

During the 3-month follow-up period, the medical treatment has not been changed, but the anticoagulant dosage was reduced. The patient is in NYHA class I, and fatigability is less frequent. He has no symptom of heart failure, and peripheral edema has disappeared. He lost 10 kg of weight. Blood pressure is 106/70 mm Hg.

Laboratory data showed an increase in creatinine level up to 164 mmol/L, with a potassium level of 5.1 mmol/L and urea 15 mmol/L. BNP is 405 pg/mL.

Echocardiographic data improved. The ejection fraction increased to 44%, left ventricular end-diastolic volume to 64 mL/m², and left ventricular end-systolic volume to 43 mL/m². LV preejection time is 120 ms. Right ventricular function is normal, and no mitral regurgitation was seen. Filling pressures are normal. The ECG pattern is the same as at hospital discharge. The left ventricular threshold is 0.5 V at 0.4 ms, and the left ventricular pacing impedance is 560 Ohm. Device memories are free from atrial or ventricular arrhythmias. The patient demonstrated 100% biventricular pacing.

Comments

The patient is a responder to CRT. His NYHA class improved by two grades, ejection fraction had increased, left ventricular end-systolic volume had decreased more than 15%. BNP was reduced, although not totally restored to normal.

Drug dosages were later increased (for beta blocker and ACE inhibitor) in the future as his BP has increased. Furosemide was withheld as filling pressures are normal while urea, creatinine, and potassium levels were increasing. These latter changes could be explained by dehydration. This phenomenon is not infrequent in responders to CRT. In this patient, the drug dosages, including diuretics, are not changed after implantation of the CRT device until the first follow-up visit. As cardiac function improves rapidly with evidence of left ventricular reverse remodeling, the need for diuretics diminishes rapidly, so they can be stopped earlier. The patient no longer reports dyspnea, although he has symptoms of fatigue.

FOCUSED CLINICAL QUESTIONS AND DISCUSSION POINTS

Question

Was the patient recommended for CRT?

FIGURE 18-10 **A,** Left anterior oblique view. The right ventricle activates first, and this activation is homogeneous. The left anterior wall is rapidly activated, whereas the lateral wall is much delayed. **B,** Posteroanterior view. The atrioventricular valves are on the right, and the left ventricular apex is on the left. This view demonstrates the delay in activation of the lateral and posterior wall. **C,** A posterior and inferior view of the left ventricle (atrioventricular valves on the right, apex on the left). This view confirms the late activation of the posterior wall. The inferior wall is less delayed and activation goes fast **(D).**

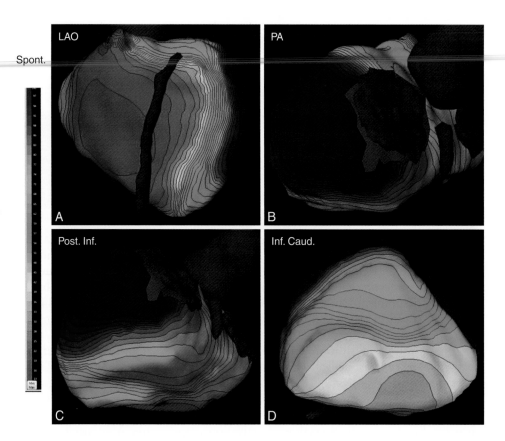

FIGURE 18-11 The same views as in intrinsic rhythm and same time scale. During biventricular pacing, the activation pattern is quite altered. Depolarization clearly starts from the spots of lead locations—apical right ventricular and posterior left ventricular walls. As a result, the right ventricular free wall and anterior, posterior, and some inferior left ventricular walls appear to be electrically synchronized. The posterior and inferior left ventricular wall is slightly delayed, and basal segments are the most delayed, but the concerned region is small.

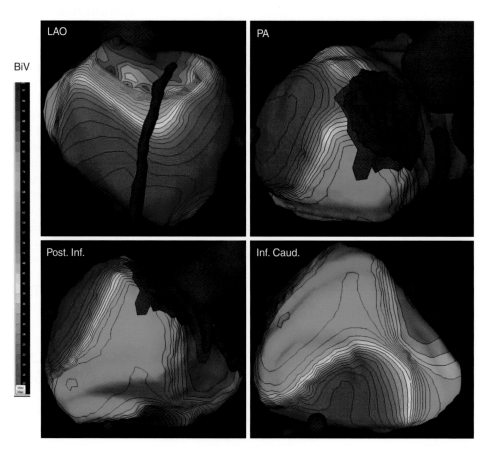

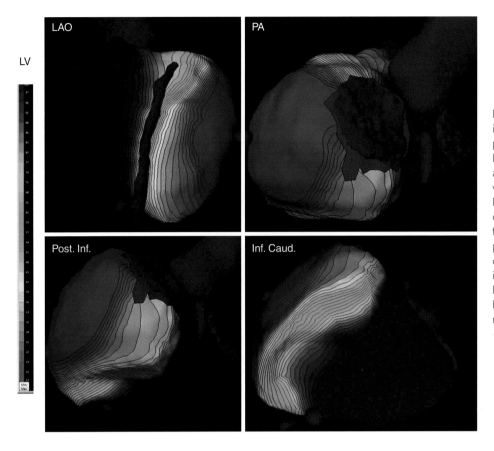

FIGURE 18-12   The same views as in intrinsic rhythm and biventricular pacing and same time scale. During left ventricular pacing only, the activation pattern is totally reversed with primodepolarization at the lateral left ventricular wall. Two lines of block appear at the anterior wall facing the septum and at the posterior and lateral wall. As a consequence, right ventricular and inferior left ventricular walls are largely delayed. The difference between mean right ventricular and mean left ventricular activations is +110 ms.

Discussion

This patient has most of the criteria for an indication for a CRT device, except a borderline ECG criteria (i.e., QRS 120 msec and a non–left bundle branch block [LBBB] pattern). According to the latest ESC guideline, however, he is not a candidate for CRT.[4]

Initially, CRT has been proposed to patients with LBBB with QRS longer than 150 ms, to resynchronize a delayed activated left ventricle to the right ventricle, the gross concept being that systolic dyssynchrony is the primary reason for the further decline of cardiac function. Later, recommendations were extended to patients with shorter QRS complex, but still longer than 120 ms, and earlier clinical stages of heart failure. However, as a matter of fact, patients with non-LBBB ECG morphologies are not good responders to CRT. Today, the ESC recommendations rank patients with LBBB and QRS of 120 ms or greater as class IA candidates, whereas patients with non-LBBB morphology with QRS of 150 ms or greater are ranked class IIA candidates.[4]

Question

What were the reasons for indicating CRT in this patient?

Discussion

In some countries (including France), if a patient does not fit recommendations but objective arguments are found that indicate the patient may benefit from a given therapy, it will be allowed by the administration. This is the reason why a temporary hemodynamic assessment was performed to determine the possible acute benefit over intrinsic rhythm that could be measured during atriobiventricular pacing from endocardial sites, including the left ventricle (a previous coronary artery angiogram with venous return timing demonstrated the prediction of a difficult access to the veins of the coronary sinus network). In addition, the left ventricular endocardial approach provides much more flexibility for moving a catheter inside the left ventricular cavity, thus allowing determination of the optimal site of pacing. Previous studies showed that optimal pacing sites are individualized.[2] The designated site can then be used again during the implantation procedure.

The dP/dt_{max} value is a hemodynamic reference parameter for assessing left ventricular function and has been used during the last decade for atrioventricular and VV-interval optimizations during acute CRT implantation and has been suggested as an option to guide the choice of pacing sites. In this patient, a huge difference was found between intrinsic rhythm condition and biventricular pacing with the left ventricular endocardial lead placed at the midposterior wall. Currently, the use of preoperative acute hemodynamic assessment to predict a good left ventricular reverse remodeling or clinical response to CRT remains controversial.[3,6] From what we have observed in the current case, it is conceivable that more studies are needed for the role of using acute hemodynamic-guided placement of left ventricular leads for patients in whom the use of CRT may have less-than-expected benefits, such as those with a borderline QRS duration (e.g., 120 to 150 ms) or non-LBBB pattern of ECG.

Question

Why was this patient implanted with an endocardial left ventricular lead, a technique that is not currently recommended? Why was a surgical epicardial approach not preferred?

Discussion

The surgical epicardial approach is an accepted option in the case of failure or expected major difficulties of the coronary sinus approach. However, the acute hemodynamic evaluation before implantation was performed with an endocardial left ventricular lead, and it cannot be certain that similar effects of epicardial and endocardial pacing would be found at the same spot. Although the patient had no coronary artery disease or scar zone, local conduction disorders might arise, leading to inhomogeneity in the hemodynamic results between the two pacing modalities. The patient was already on anticoagulation therapy for paroxysmal atrial fibrillation, so acceptance of long-term anticoagulation was not an issue even at a higher dosage (with INR between 2.5 and 3.5).

However, this technique is currently under investigation and may have severe drawbacks.[5,10] It requires an atrial transseptal puncture, which can be a tricky exercise when sheaths are coming from the upper part of the body. The lead is crossing the mitral valve, and long-term mitral leaflet movement disturbance might be an issue. Clotting must be cautiously prevented. In case of infection, vegetation embolism might occur, and the removal of the lead will probably be done in the cardiac surgical room. Currently, this technique is still investigational, and the ALSYNC trial will address the issues of safety and efficacy of the endocardial approach for left ventricular lead implantation and whether it is superior to the conventional transvenous approach.

Question

What is the usefulness of cardiac activation maps?

Discussion

The new ESC guidelines that restrict the class IA indications to patients with LBBB morphology were discussed earlier. However, some patients exhibit a non-LBBB morphology at ECG, but invasive endocardial and epicardial maps demonstrate a left ventricular activation delay. This delay seems essential to obtain a favorable response after CRT.[1,7-9] This is the situation in the patient in this case, who did not show a prolonged QRS complex but had delayed electrical activation of the left ventricle. After CRT, the effect of left ventricular pacing on the activation pattern is clearly shown—inversion of the activation pattern when left ventricular pacing only is applied and significant electrical resynchronization when both left ventricular and right ventricular leads are paced. These noninvasive maps are obtained in nearly real time and require only one heart beat to be displayed. Consequently, this technique can theoretically be useful not only for the diagnosis of electrical dyssynchrony before implantation but also during implantation because it provides fast and reproducible information of the electrical resynchronization. Thus the choice of the optimal pacing site is foreseeable, with the condition that electrical activation resynchronization and mechanical improvement occur in parallel. Finally, this tool potentially can be used for optimization of atrioventricular and VV intervals during follow-up, especially in nonresponders to CRT to better understand the possible mechanism of lack of efficacy and plan ahead the various options of device programming and implantation revision.

Currently, this technique remains investigational and needs the scientific proof to be demonstrated in the clinical setting.

Selected References

1. Bourassa MG, Khairy P, Roy D: An early proof-of-concept of cardiac resynchronization therapy, *World J Cardiol* 3:374-376, 2011.
2. Derval N, Steendijk P, Gula LJ, et al: Optimizing hemodynamics in heart failure patients by systematic screening of left ventricular pacing sites: the lateral left ventricular wall and the coronary sinus are rarely the best sites, *J Am Coll Cardiol* 55:566-575, 2010.
3. Duckett SG, Ginks M, Shetty AK, et al: Invasive acute hemodynamic response to guide left ventricular lead implantation predicts chronic remodeling in patients undergoing cardiac resynchronization therapy, *J Am Coll Cardiol* 58:1128-1136, 2011.
4. McMurray JJ, Adamopoulos S, Anker SD, et al: ESC guidelines for the diagnosis and treatment of acute and chronic heart failure 2012: The Task Force for the Diagnosis and Treatment of Acute and Chronic Heart Failure 2012 of the European Society of Cardiology. Developed in collaboration with the Heart Failure Association (HFA) of the ESC, *Eur J Heart Fail* 14:803-869, 2012.
5. Ploux S, Whinnett Z, Bordachar P: Left ventricular endocardial pacing and multisite pacing to improve CRT response, *J Cardiovasc Transl Res* 5:213-218, 2012.
6. Prinzen FW, Houthuizen P, Bogaard MD, et al: Is acute hemodynamic response a predictor of long-term outcome in cardiac resynchronization therapy? *J Am Coll Cardiol* 59:1198, 2012.
7. Rickard J, Kumbhani DJ, Gorodeski EZ, et al: Cardiac resynchronization therapy in non-left bundle branch block morphologies, *Pacing Clin Electrophysiol* 33:590-595, 2010.
8. Strik M, Ploux S, Vernooy K, et al: Cardiac resynchronization therapy: refocus on the electrical substrate, *Circ J* 75:1297-1304, 2011.
9. Strik M, Regoli F, Auricchio A, et al: Electrical and mechanical ventricular activation during left bundle branch block and resynchronization, *J Cardiovasc Transl Res* 5:117-126, 2012.
10. Whinnett Z, Bordachar P: The risks and benefits of transseptal endocardial pacing, *Curr Opin Cardiol* 27:19-23, 2012.

Left Ventricular Endocardial Pacing in a Patient with an Anomalous Left-Sided Superior Vena Cava

John Mark Morgan

Age	Gender	Occupation	Working Diagnosis
67 Years	Male	Builder	Heart Failure (Ischaemic Cardiomyopathy) and Pacemaker Dependence After Atrioventricular Node Ablation

HISTORY

The patient had a complex past medical history. He underwent bioprosthetic aortic valve replacement in 2006 related to infective endocarditis with consequent severe aortic regurgitation and had moderately impaired left ventricular systolic function (left ventricular ejection fraction [LVEF] 45%-50%). Coronary angiography did not show significant coronary artery disease, and therefore surgical revascularization was not necessary at the time of aortic valve replacement.

The patient then developed persistent (cardioversion on two occasions in 2007) and then permanent atrial fibrillation with fast ventricular rate response despite the use of digoxin, verapamil, and beta blockade (all in maximum tolerated or appropriate doses). He underwent atrioventricular nodal ablation in 2007 with implantation of a single-chamber rate-responsive right ventricular pacemaker.

Over the subsequent 2 years, he developed worsening systolic heart failure (New York Heart Association [NYHA] class III) that was refractory to medical therapy at maximal tolerated dosages (including an angiotensin-converting enzyme [ACE] inhibitor, beta blocker, nitrate, hydralazine, and loop diuretic). His ejection fraction was reduced to 35%. He therefore received an upgrade to a biventricular pacemaker.[1] Because of the presence of an anomalous left-sided superior vena cava, left ventricular pacing via an epicardial coronary sinus branch was challenging. Nevertheless pacing was achieved at an anatomically appropriate site, although only one target coronary sinus tributary was available.

The patient responded well to biventricular pacing with improvement in ejection fraction (LVEF 45%) and NYHA status to class II.

Thirty-six months after implantation of the left ventricular pacing lead, he had late infection of the pacing pocket, with raised inflammatory markers and positive blood cultures for *Staphylococcus*.

FOCUSED CLINICAL QUESTIONS AND DISCUSSION POINTS

Question

What is the indication for device and lead extraction?

Discussion

With evidence for both local and systemic infection, no other option is available but to perform system extraction.

Question

What is the reason for delay between extraction and reimplantation?

Discussion

This patient is pacing-dependent and requires temporary pacing before reimplantation of a new pacing system.

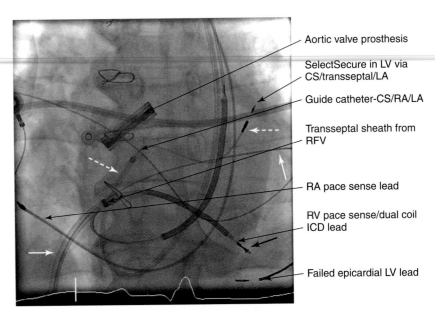

FIGURE 19-1 Left ventricular *(LV)* endocardial lead on anteroposterior projection. A transseptal sheath was passed from the right femoral vein *(RFV)* and has dilated the puncture site. Then a steerable guide catheter was passed via the anomalous left superior vena cava, through the enlarged coronary sinus to the right atrium *(RA)* and maneuvered across the transseptal puncture site into left atrium *(LA)*. Then a Select Secure pacing lead has been passed to the LV via the guide catheter. *CS,* Coronary sinus; *ICD,* implantable cardioversion defibrillator.

Aortic valve prosthesis

SelectSecure in LV via CS/transseptal/LA

Guide catheter-CS/RA/LA

Transseptal sheath from RFV

RA pace sense lead

RV pace sense/dual coil ICD lead

Failed epicardial LV lead

Question

What are the challenges of pacing via an anomalous left-sided superior vena cava draining into an enlarged coronary sinus.

Discussion

Access is difficult, and manipulation of leads to achieve entry to the appropriate cardiac chamber requires expert handling. However, it is possible to gain access to the right ventricle and right atrium.

Question

Can transseptal access be gained from a superior approach?

Discussion

Transseptal access can be achieved using modified catheters.[4] Studies are ongoing to understand the clinical value of this approach and of left ventricular endocardial pacing,[2,3] although several studies supported the approach in terms of feasibility, safety, and patient response.

FINAL DIAGNOSIS

The infected pacing system with all three pacing leads was extracted. A temporary pacing lead was inserted to provide pacing during a period of prolonged intravenous and subsequent oral antibiotic treatment. The patient received vancomycin and intravenous flucloxacillin followed by oral flucloxacillin.

PLAN OF ACTION

The decision was made to continue with antibiotic treatment for 6 weeks before reimplantation of a new, permanent biventricular pacing system. An attempt was made to establish LV epicardial pacing[5] but the implanted pacing lead failed two days after the surgical procedure and the decision was made to attempt LV endocardial pacing.

INTERVENTION

A new biventricular pacing system was implanted. Patency of the left subclavian vein was confirmed by venography before commencement of the procedure. Access then was gained to the left subclavian vein using a cutdown and after creation of a new pacemaker pocket in the left prepectoral region.

Anterograde coronary sinus angiography via the anomalous left superior vena cava showed occlusion of the previously targeted coronary sinus branch and no alternative target. A permanent right ventricular pacing lead was implanted via the left subclavian vein, coronary sinus, and right atrium.

Right femoral venous access was gained, and a transseptal catheter passed to the right atrium via the inferior vena cava. The procedure's catheter and lead manipulations are summarized in the fluoroscopic images (Figures 19-1 and 19-2). Transseptal access to left atrium was achieved using a radiofrequency needle. The transseptal puncture site was dilated using a 12-French transseptal guide catheter and an extra support guide wire passed to left atrium. Intravenous heparin was administered to maintain an activated clotting time at greater than 300 seconds. Via the left subclavian vein and coronary sinus access route, a steerable guide

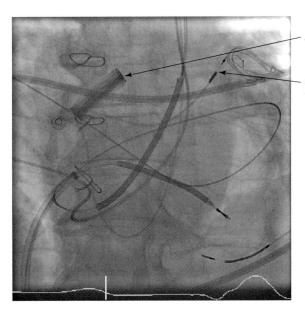

Aortic valve prosthesis

SelectSecure in LV via
CS/RA - transseptal/LA

FIGURE 19-2   Anteroposterior projection. The transseptal guide catheter has now been withdrawn, leaving the Select Secure lead in place after fixation. The transseptal catheter remains in place until the end of the procedure to allow for reentry to the left atrium *(LA)* should there be displacement of the pacing lead as its delivery system is withdrawn. *CS,* Coronary sinus; *LV,* left ventricle; *RA,* right atrium; *RV,* right ventricle.

catheter was passed to right atrium. Then, using a dilator inserted into this guide catheter and with the inferior approach guide wire as reference, the steerable guide was introduced to the left atrium and orientated to left ventricle. Using this steerable orientated catheter, a polyurethane 4.1-French pacing lead was passed to the left ventricle and secured by an active fixation screw to the lateral left ventricular endocardial wall, just beneath the mitral ring. Pacing assessment demonstrated a pacing impedance of 980 Ω at 0.2 mV amplitude and 0.04 msec pulse width. When the pacing leads were secured, the delivery systems were removed and a biventricular pacemaker (atrial port capped) was attached to the respective leads. The pacemaker was secured in the prepectoral pouch, and the wound was closed in a standard fashion (Figure 19-3).

Postprocedure assessment demonstrated appropriate pacing parameters and a narrow paced QRS. The patient was established on an anticoagulation regimen using warfarin and maintaining an international normalized ratio between 2 and 3. The patient experienced remarkable clinical improvement within 1 month, with an LVEF of 50% and improvement to NYHA I.

OUTCOME

The patient received biventricular pacing using left ventricular endocardial pacing[4,6] in a clinical situation in which alternative mechanisms for achieving biventricular pacing were not possible. The patient has experienced remarkable clinical benefit from the procedure.

Findings

No periprocedural or postprocedural complications occurred, and to date the patient has received significant clinical benefit from left ventricular endocardial pacing.

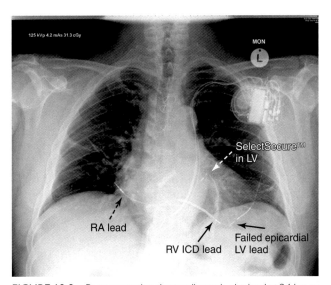

FIGURE 19-3   Posteroanterior chest radiograph obtained at 24 hours after implantation of the left ventricular *(LV)* lead. Permanent pacing lead positions are indicated. *CS,* Coronary sinus; *LA,* left atrium; *RA,* right atrium.

Selected References

1. Cazeau S, Alonso C, Jauvert G, et al: Cardiac resynchronization therapy, *Europace* 5(Suppl 1):S42-S48, 2004.
2. Fish JM, Brugada J, Antzelevitch C: Potential proarrhythmic effects of biventricular pacing, *J Am Coll Cardiol* 46:2340-2347, 2005.
3. Garrigue S, Jaïs P, Espil G, et al: Comparison of chronic biventricular pacing between epicardial and endocardial left ventricular stimulation using Doppler tissue imaging in patients with heart failure, *Am J Cardiol* 88:858-862, 2001.
4. Morgan JM, Scott PA, Turner NG, et al: Targeted left ventricular endocardial pacing using a steerable introducing guide catheter and active fixation pacing lead, *Europace* 11:502-506, 2009.
5. Puglisi A, Lunati M, Marullo AG, et al: Limited thoracotomy as a second choice alternative to transvenous implant for cardiac resynchronisation therapy delivery, *Eur Heart J* 25:1063-1069, 2004.
6. van Gelder BM, Scheffer MG, Meijer A, et al: Transseptal endocardial left ventricular pacing: an alternative technique for coronary sinus lead placement in cardiac resynchronization therapy, *Heart Rhythm* 4:454-460, 2007.

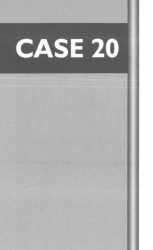

Novel Wireless Technologies for Endocardial Cardiac Resynchronization Therapy

François Regoli, Marta Acena, Tiziano Moccetti, and Angelo Auricchio

Age	Gender	Occupation	Working Diagnosis
68 Years	Male	Retired	Nonresponder to Cardiac Resynchronization Therapy Evaluated for Wireless Left Ventricular Endocardial Cardiac Stimulation to Deliver Cardiac Resynchronization Therapy

HISTORY

A 68-year-old man previously underwent implantation of a cardiac resynchronization therapy defibrillator (CRT-D) device (February 2007) after a class I indication for CRT at the time—symptomatic drug-refractory ischemic-based heart failure disease, New York Heart Association (NYHA) class III, severe left ventricular dysfunction, and left bundle branch block (LBBB) ventricular conduction delay, with a 130-msec duration QRS complex. Despite CRT, clinical follow-up of the patient was characterized by gradually worsening heart failure progression with further reduction of left ventricular function (left ventricular ejection fraction [LVEF] <20%), dilation of the left ventricle, and, as a result of dilation of the mitral annulus, progression of mitral regurgitation to grade III. Therefore the patient underwent successful positioning of a MitraClip (Abbott Vascular, Abbott Park, Ill.) device in September 2009, thus achieving mitral regurgitation reduction to grade I or II. Paroxysmal atrial fibrillation gradually progressed to become permanent, and ablation of the atrioventricular node was performed to achieve adequate CRT delivery. Other comorbidities included chronic renal insufficiency (reduced glomerular filtration rate of 40 to 50 mL/min/1.73 m²), previous nephrectomy for renal papillary carcinoma, and hyperuricemia.

Because of persistent severe heart failure symptoms (NYHA class IIII to IV), in May 2011 the patient consented to participate in a prospective multicenter safety and feasibility study evaluating a wireless cardiac stimulation system of the left ventricular endocardium (wireless cardiac stimulation cardiac resynchronization therapy [WiCS-CRT]).

CURRENT MEDICATIONS

At presentation, the patient's therapeutic scheme included maximally tolerated dosages of beta blocker, an angiotensin-converting enzyme [ACE] inhibitor, and other relevant drugs: clopidogrel 75 mg daily, acenodecumerol 1 mg to maintain international normalized ratio between 2 and 3, carvedilol 12.5 mg daily, enalapril 40 mg daily, spironolactone 25 mg daily, atorvastatin 40 mg daily, and aspirin 100 mg daily.

CURRENT SYMPTOMS

The patient exhibited breathlessness at mild exertion and had NYHA class III to IV heart disease.

PHYSICAL EXAMINATION

BP/HR: 105/70 mm Hg/70 bpm
Height/weight: 175 cm/70.3 kg
Neck veins: Normal
Lungs/chest: Normal
Heart: Normal
Abdomen: Normal
Extremities: Normal

LABORATORY DATA

Hemoglobin: 14.1 g/dL
Hematocrit/packed cell volume: 38.1%

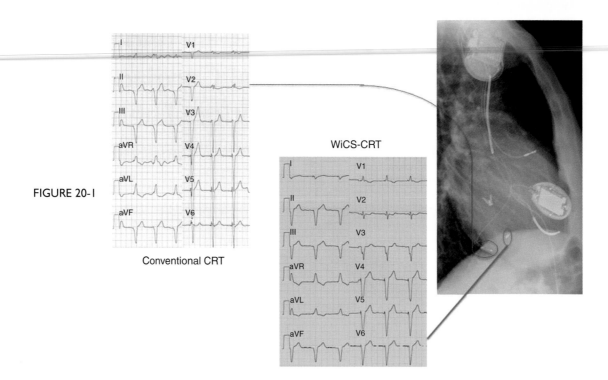

FIGURE 20-1

Conventional CRT

WiCS-CRT

Platelet count: 191 × 1000 μL
Sodium: 145 mmol/L
Potassium: 4.6 mmol/L
Creatinine: 166 mmol/L
Blood urea nitrogen: 19.3 mmol/L

ELECTROCARDIOGRAM

Findings

The electrocardiogram of conventionally delivered CRT is shown in Figure 20-1 *(left panel)*. Vertical QRS axis (160 msec) coupled with R wave in V_1 indicates regular epicardial biventricular pacing in VVI modality at 70 bpm. Left ventricular stimulation from a bipolar left ventricular tip positioned in a postero-lateral branch of the coronary sinus *(red circle)* confers a vertical axis to the QRS complex and QS morphology in the inferior leads.

CHEST RADIOGRAPH

Findings

Anteroposterior and right lateral (Figure 20-2, *upper panels*) show the positioning of the three leads with the transvenous left ventricular lead positioned in a posterolateral branch of the cornoary sinus *(red circle)* and reaching a posterolateral apical position.

ECHOCARDIOGRAM

Findings

At baseline, echocardiographic examination revealed a severely dilated left ventricle with diffuse hypokinesia and highly compromised left ventricular function (LVEF 19%). Despite MitraClip implantation, residual moderate mitral insufficiency was present; moderate tricuspid insufficiency was also present (Figure 20-3, *left panel*, and video *left panel*). Pulmonary pressures were increased, with an estimated arterial pulmonary pressure of 40 mm Hg (see video baseline).

FOCUSED CLINICAL QUESTIONS AND DISCUSSION POINTS

Question

What is the pathophysiologic basis for considering left ventricular endocardial pacing to deliver CRT?

Discussion

Impulse propagation physiologically travels from the endocardium to the epicardium. Most of the evidence in animal models has been supplied by the Maastricht group.[1-3] The experimental data have demonstrated that CRT delivered from the left ventricular endocardium allows quicker propagation of the electrical impulse

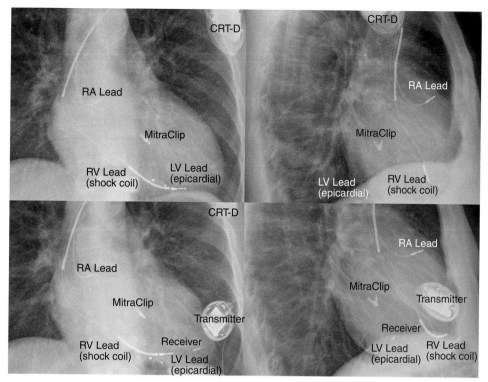

FIGURE 20-2

through the myocardium in contrast to epicardium.[1] Better impulse propagation translates to greater mechanical and hemodynamic effect, in terms of both systolic and diastolic functions.[2] These data have been further substantiated by favorable hemodynamic effects in animal models with induced ischemic heart failure and the presence of electrical dyssynchrony.[3] This study concluded that endocardial CRT improved, to a greater extent, electrical synchrony of activation and left ventricular pump function in contrast to conventional epicardial CRT in compromised canine hearts with LBBB. This benefit was explained by a shorter path length along the endocardium and faster circumferential and transmural impulse conduction during endocardial left ventricular pacing.

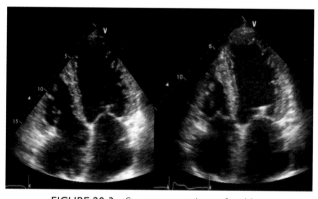

FIGURE 20-3   See *expertconsult.com* for video.

Question

Has clinical evidence shown that left ventricular endocardially delivered CRT can confer clinical benefits?

Discussion

Some evidence is available from isolated case-based reports or small patient series on the clinical benefits of left ventricular endocardially delivered CRT.[4-6] Access to the left ventricular endocardium is achieved through transseptal catheterization of an active fixation lead into the left ventricle. Besides being technically challenging

because transseptal catheterization is required, higher risk for thromboembolic complications and the likelihood of lead dislocation are possible issues that may arise. These potential risks have discouraged the diffusion of this approach.

Spragg and colleagues[5] performed an acute study in heart failure patients with LBBB. Comparison between endocardial and conventional epicardial CRT revealed a greater hemodynamic response for the former modality of cardiac stimulation. Hemodynamic response during endocardial pacing was typically superior when the lead was placed remotely from an infarct zone. This study advocates that endocardial lead position may require individual patient tailoring for clinical response.

Question

What are the most important aspects that should be evaluated when planning to treat a patient with WiCS-CRT?

Discussion

Several factors contributed to achieving the clinical response. Assessment of global and regional left ventricular contractility represents key information derived form transthoracic echocardiography. In the present case, preprocedural transthoracic echocardiogram allowed detection of diffuse hypokinesia in the absence of akinetic segments, particularly in the lateral and posterolateral regions of the left ventricle. Preserved kinetics indicated myocardial vitality, thus suggesting that functional recruitment of myocardial tissue through cardiac stimulation was possible.

Preprocedural ultrasound examination using a vascular probe is indispensable to precisely define the intercostal acoustic window in which the transmitter pulse generator should be fixed during the implant procedure.[7] The transmitter pulse should be fixed within this predefined acoustic window during the implantation procedure.

Anchoring of the receiver electrode of the WiCS-CRT system to the endocardial left ventricular lateral wall represents the most important part of the procedure and is technically challenging. Competence to perform this part of the procedure requires both interventional cardiologic skills (for dye contrast injection in the left ventricle) and electrophysiologic skills (for manipulation of long sheath and interpretation of electrical measures and signals) for procedural success.

FINAL DIAGNOSIS

This patient was a CRT nonresponder considered eligible for wireless left ventricular endocardial cardiac stimulation for CRT.

PLAN OF ACTION

The plan for this patient was implantation of a WiCS.

INTERVENTION

Under general anesthesia, using a retrograde transaortic approach, a long steerable sheath was placed into the left ventricle and gently brought against the endocardial wall. Then, another internal delivery catheter at the tip of which the receiver electrode was mounted was carefully advanced to the distal portion of the outer sheath. Before injecting and releasing the receiver electrode, sensing and pacing were repeatedly measured and the receiver electrode position was monitored using conventional transthoracic echocardiography; contrast dye was injected to ensure good and perpendicular contact (Figure 20-4). The receiver electrode was then released and the delivery system removed. A pocket for the pulse generator was surgically created in the left lateral abdominal wall, and another pocket was made in the anterolateral part of the chest (at approximately the fifth and sixth intercostal spaces) in a position that was within the acoustic window mentioned previously; this position should allow for the best communication and interaction between the transmitter and the endocardial

FIGURE 20-4

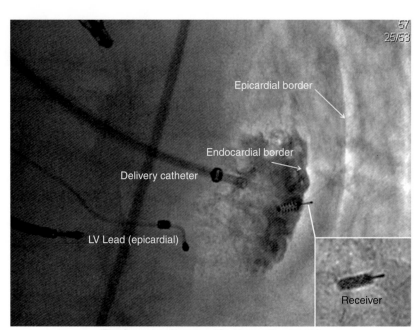

Epicardial border

Endocardial border

Delivery catheter

LV Lead (epicardial)

Receiver

(The figure has been modified from reference 8.)

receiver electrode. Finally, the transmitter and the pulse generator were connected and the electrical and pacing integrity of the entire system was tested. Device control performed the next day confirmed adequate functioning of the entire system and ECG showed effective and continuous biventicular capture (Figure 20-1). Post-implantation chest radiograph (Figure 20-2, *lower panels*) show the wireless endocardial electrode, implanted subendocardially in the lateral apical region of the left ventricle and the transmitter pulse generator fixed subcutaneously in the sixth intercostal space. The battery is implanted subcutaneously in the upper left abdominal quadrant (not visible on the chest radiograph).

OUTCOME

The outcome was clinically favorable. During the month of September, 16 months after WiCS positioning, hospitalization was planned for device change.

Findings

In the clinical follow-up of more than 1 year the patient's global clinical status gradually improved. Although the patient was hospitalized two times over 1 year for non-cardiac reasons (gastric bleeding and worsening renal insufficiency), he was not hospitalized for heart failure. NYHA functional class gradually improved to II. Device controls as well as serial ECGs confirmed effective and continuous biventricular pacing. On the ECG (Figure 20-1, *center panel*) greater right axis deviation coupled with low-amplitude negative QS in D_1 and greater R wave in V_1 lead are suggestive of greater (and quicker) electrical depolarization of the left ventricle in contrast to conventional CRT. Transthoracic echocardiogram revealed effective reversal of maladaptive remodeling, with reduction of both left ventricular systolic and diastolic volumes, clear recovery of left ventricular lateral wall movement and kinetics, and overall increase of global left ventricular contractile function, with the LVEF increasing from 19% to 35% (see Figure 20-3, *right panel* and video loop 1 B).

Comments

The WiCS system determined mechanical recovery of previously hypokinetic lateral wall, thus conferring clinical benefit.

WIRELESS CARDIAC STIMULATION TECHNOLOGY FOR CARDIAC RESYNCHRONIZATION THERAPY

WiCS-CRT is a novel cardiac stimulation system that converts ultrasound energy to electrical energy to stimulate the myocardium.[8] For cardiac resynchronization this system functions in parallel to a conventional coimplanted device, either a pacemaker or an implantable cardioverter-defibrillator. The system is composed of three components: (1) a target wireless endocardial electrode, which is implanted endocardially and receives ultrasound impulses converting these to electrical energy; (2) the impulse transmitter, localized and fixed in the intercostal space (usually fifth or sixth), which produces ultrasound pulses that are triggered through sensing of the right ventricular pacing activity of the coimplanted device; and (3) the battery component, which is implanted subcutaneously in the upper abdominal quadrant.

At present, the feasibility and safety of the WiCS-CRT system are being evaluated in the scheme of a multicenter, prospective, longitudinal study (the WISE-CRT study).[8] The study has been momentarily halted because of technical issues with the delivery system of the endocardial receiver electrode.

Selected References

1. Van Deursen C, Van Geldrop I, Van Hunnik A, et al: Improved myocardial repolarization and left ventricular systolic and diastolic function during endocardial cardiac resynchronization, *Heart Rhythm* 5:S188, 2008.
2. Van Deursen C, van Geldorp IE, Rademakers LM, et al: Left ventricular endocardial pacing improves resynchronization therapy in canine left bundle-branch hearts, *Circ Arrhythm Electrophysiol* 2:580-587, 2009.
3. Strik M, Rademakers LM, van Deursen CJ, et al. *Circ Arrhythm Electrophysiol* 5:191-200, 2012.
4. Garrigue S, Jaïs P, Espil G, et al: Comparison of chronic biventricular pacing between epicardial and endocardial left ventricular stimulation using Doppler tissue imaging in patients with heart failure, *Am J Cardiol* 88:858-862, 2001.
5. Spragg DD, Dong J, Fetics BJ, et al: Effective LV endocardial pacing sites for cardiac resynchronization in patients with ischemic cardiomyopathy, *Heart Rhythm* 7:S75-S76, 2010.
6. Kutyifa V, Merkely B, Szilágyi S, et al: Usefulness of electroanatomical mapping during transseptal endocardial left ventricular lead implantation, *Europace* 14:599-604, 2012.
7. DeFaria Yeh D, Lonergan KL, et al: Clinical factors and echocardiographic techniques related to the presence, size, and location of acoustic windows for leadless cardiac pacing, *Europace* 13:1760-1765, 2011.
8. Auricchio A, Delnoy PP, Regoli F, et al. First-in-man implantation of leadless ultrasound-based cardiac stimulation pacing system: novel endocardial left ventricular resynchronization therapy in heart failure patients, *Europace* 15:1191-1197, 2013.

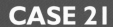
Robotically Assisted Lead Implantation for Cardiac Resynchronization Therapy in a Reoperative Patient

Juan B. Grau, Christopher K. Johnson, and Jonathan S. Steinberg

Age	Gender	Occupation	Working Diagnosis
79 Years	Male	Retired	Chronic Right Ventricular Pacing with Falling Left Ventricular Ejection Fraction and Progressive Heart Failure

HISTORY

The patient has an extensive cardiac history, beginning with a myocardial infarction and subsequent coronary artery bypass and three grafts in 1988. In 2002, he underwent a reoperative three-vessel bypass. He was diagnosed with sick sinus syndrome in 2001 that required the implantation of a dual-chamber pacemaker. The device was updated to an implantable cardioversion defibrillator (ICD) in 2002 after he experienced cardiac arrest. He was successfully resuscitated without neurologic sequelae. The prior right ventricular lead was abandoned and capped, and the patient received a dual-coil high-voltage lead. The generator was replaced in 2005 and again in late 2011. On the current admission, the patient had poorly controlled hypertension and worsening heart failure in the setting of chronic right ventricular pacing. Left ventricular ejection fraction had fallen from greater than 55%, 1 year previously, to 31%. The patient experienced progressive dyspnea on exertion.

CURRENT MEDICATIONS

The patient was taking aspirin 81 mg daily, atorvastatin 80 mg daily, candesartan 16 mg daily, carvedilol 12.5 mg twice daily, dutasteride 0.5 mg daily, niacin 500 mg daily, and spironolactone 25 mg daily.

PHYSICAL EXAMINATION

BP/HR: 138/80 mm Hg/70 bpm, regular
Height/weight: 172.7 cm/82.5 kg

Neck veins: Not distended
Lungs/chest: Clear, well-healed sternotomy scar
Heart: Fourth heart sound (S_4) gallop without murmur
Abdomen: Soft, without hepatic distention
Extremities: No edema, well-healed scar from radial artery harvest

LABORATORY DATA

Hemoglobin: 14.5 g/dL
Hematocrit/packed cell volume: 42.5%
Mean corpuscular volume: 92 fL
Platelet count: $152 \times 10^3/\mu L$
Sodium: 139 mmol/L
Potassium: 3.7 mmol/L
Creatinine: 0.9 mg/dL
Blood urea nitrogen: 17 mmol/L

ELECTROCARDIOGRAM

Findings

The electrocardiogram revealed atrial-sensed ventricular-paced rhythm (Figure 21-1), with a heart rate of 62 bpm and QRS duration of 192 msec.

Sinus bradycardia with underlying left bundle branch block also was seen (Figure 21-2). The heart rate was 59 bpm and QRS duration 132 msec.

Atrial sensing and biventricular pacing were demonstrated on the electrogram (Figure 21-3), with a heart rate of 66 bpm and QRS duration of 138 msec.

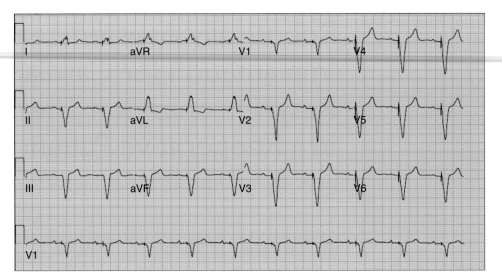

FIGURE 21-1   Electrocardiogram before the battery change. *SVG-OM,* Saphenous vein graft–obtuse margin.

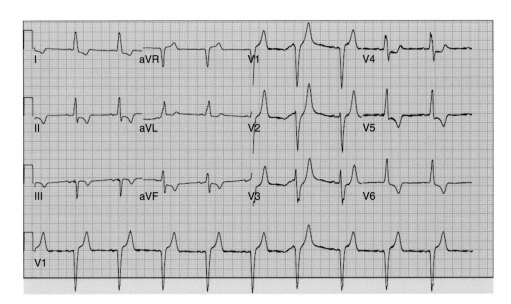

FIGURE 21-2   Unpaced postoperative electrocardiogram.

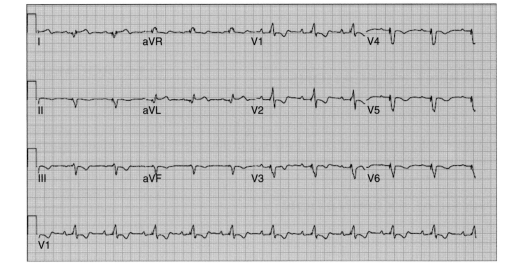

FIGURE 21-3   Postoperative paced electrocardiogram.

CHEST RADIOGRAPH

Findings

A frontal view of the chest demonstrates the heart to be normal in size and configuration (Figure 21-4). Median sternotomy sutures are present in the midline. A right-sided pocket is seen with an ICD and three leads: right atrial lead in the appendage, abandoned right ventricular pacing lead, and ICD lead in the right ventricular apex. The hilar and pulmonary vascular markings are normal, with no parenchymal infiltrates visualized.

The right ventricle appears normal in size and contractility (Figure 21-5). The intraventricular septum moves paradoxically toward the right in systole. The images demonstrate the left ventricle to be moderately dilated, with moderate diffuse hypokinesis. The left ventricular ejection fraction is 31%.

COMPUTED TOMOGRAPHY

Findings

Computed tomography (Figure 21-6) with intravenous contrast was performed to visualize the status and location of previous grafts. The right atrial to left anterior descending, SV OM, and saphenous vein to right coronary artery grafts appear patent. The trajectory of the saphenous vein to obtuse margin graft was such that it allowed for consideration of placement of an epicardial lead on the basilar aspect of the posterolateral wall of the

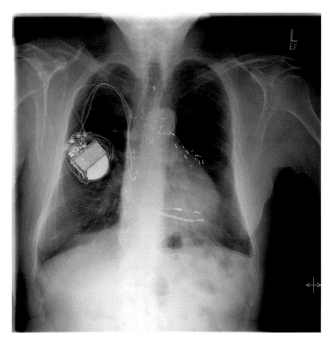

FIGURE 21-4   Chest radiograph on admission.

left ventricle. The proximal native coronary arteries are heavily calcified and occluded. There is mild cardiomegaly, with remodeling of the anterior wall of the left ventricle, presumably resulting from previous myocardial infarction.

FOCUSED CLINICAL QUESTIONS AND DISCUSSION POINTS

Question

What potential advantages does direct epicardial access offer in contrast to a transvenous lead?

Discussion

Direct epicardial access overcomes the limitations of coronary sinus anatomy in situations in which no veins can be found in the preferred target zone or only inadequate venous branches are found. Visualization of scar tissue and phrenic nerve position avoids left ventricular lead placement at sites of prior myocardial infarction and diaphragmatic capture, respectively.

Question

What is the impact of the patient's extensive surgical history on left ventricular lead placement?

Discussion

As with any reoperative surgery, adhesions will form between the tissues in the chest cavity. These adhesions can affect visualization of and access to the heart, as well as increase the technical demands of the procedure.

Question

What must be considered when deciding the location for placement of an epicardial lead?

Discussion

A previous graft, areas of previous infarction, and the location of the phrenic nerve should be noted because they can affect the successful implantation of an epicardial left ventricular lead.

FINAL DIAGNOSIS

The final diagnosis in this patient was decreasing left ventricular ejection fraction in the setting of chronic right ventricular pacing, underlying left bundle branch block, and unstable heart failure symptoms.

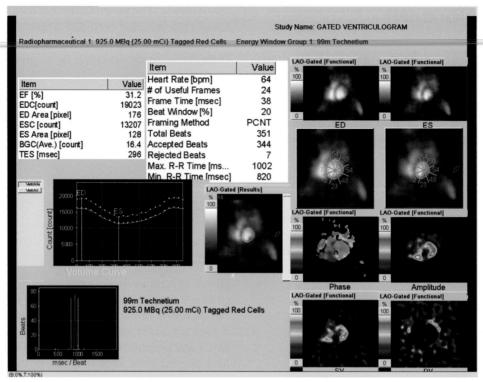

FIGURE 21-5 Gated cardiac ventriculogram.

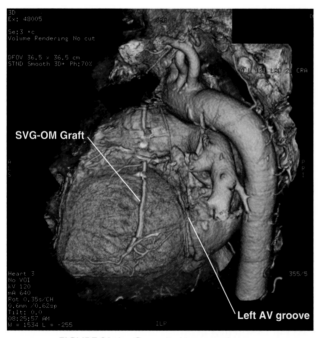

FIGURE 21-6 Computed tomography scan.

PLAN OF ACTION

The plan for this patient consisted of robotically assisted left thorax approach for placement of left ventricular epicardial leads, lysis of adhesions from previous cardiac surgeries, and tunneling and routing of the two new epicardial leads to the ICD generator located in right chest pocket.

INTERVENTION

Typically, left ventricular lead implantation would be attempted through a transvenous approach; however, a venogram demonstrated very tight stenoses of the subclavian and innominate veins in this patient. This prevented transvenous access for left ventricular lead placement without an extensive revision procedure. Thus a robotic approach was determined to be the optimal platform for left ventricular lead placement. The patient was placed in the right lateral decubitus position with retraction of the left arm cephalad to expose the posterolateral aspect of the left chest. The patient was intubated with a double-lumen endotracheal tube for single-lung ventilation. This allows for a more accurate location of the optimal site for lead placement and mapping.

The lead implantation was achieved through three ports in this case; however, recent advances in technology have shown a single-port approach could potentially be technically feasible.[1] Ports for the robotic arms were placed in the fifth (right robotic arm) and ninth intercostal spaces (left robotic arm) between the left-mid or posterior axillary line via a 1-cm incision. An additional 1-cm port in the seventh intercostal space was made at the same level for the robotic three-dimensional HD camera. In traditional left ventricular lead placement, a lateral 8-mm incision in the pacemaker pocket would have been created; however, this was not performed in this patient because his ICD generator was located on the right chest wall and the leads required extensions and tunneling toward the generator pocket from the left side. At the conclusion of the robotic part of the procedure, the patient was repositioned, redraped, and prepped for tunneling of the new left ventricular leads to the right-sided generator.

Through fine, deliberate movement, the robotic arm easily dissected the tenacious adhesions between the left lung and chest wall and from the lung to the pericardium and mediastinum. Lysis of adhesions was achieved using a combination of the robotic spatula and Debakey and Endo scissors.

After all adhesions had been lysed, both the saphenous vein to obtuse marginal graft and the phrenic nerve were visualized and protected throughout the procedure. In reoperative cases, obtaining information regarding the location of previous coronary bypass grafts becomes paramount when planning a minimally invasive approach for left ventricular lead placement. Identifying the trajectory of previous bypass grafts helps avoid intraoperative complications that could potentially become catastrophic. The pericardium was opened lateral to the vein graft and anterior to the phrenic nerve. At this time, adhesions were cleared between the pericardium and the graft, as well as from the pericardium and the posterolateral and basal wall of the heart. The spatula, robotic Debakey forceps, and Endo scissors attachments were used to lyse these adhesions. Two screw-in epicardial leads were placed between the saphenous vein to obtuse margin graft and the second obtuse margin branch over the base of the left ventricle. Pacing thresholds were tested and found to be excellent. The right atrial lead had an intrinsic amplitude of 3.1 mV, impedance of 515 Ω, and a pacing threshold of 2.2 V at 0.5 msec. The right ventricular lead had an impedance of 463 Ω with a pacing threshold of 0.6 V at 0.5 msec. The left ventricular lead had an impedance of 548 Ω with a pacing threshold of 0.6 V at 1 msec and a shock impedance of 46 Ω. The right ventricular lead had an intrinsic R-wave of 17 mV. Because the patient's generator was in the right chest, the pacing wires were passed through the eighth intercostal space and routed inferiorly toward the costal margin and anterior to the posterior fascia of the abdominal wall and temporarily left in a submuscular plane. At this time, the robotic arms and camera were removed and their respective ports closed in layers.

The patient was then reprepped, draped, and placed in the supine position. The leads were extended and tunneled following a submuscular plane toward the right-sided generator. Once again, the leads tested excellently when reaching the pocket. A second left ventricular lead was placed posterior to the generator to be used as a backup should the primary lead fail. The generator was placed back in its pocket after the new leads had been connected, and the incisions were closed in layers. A chest tube was placed in the left pleural cavity. The patient was extubated in the operating room, and no complications occurred during the surgery or in the perioperative period.

OUTCOME

Findings

The patient had the chest tube removed on postoperative day 1 and was discharged on postoperative day 2. The pacemaker was set to DDD, with a rate limit of 60 bpm, atrioventricular delay of 160 ms, and left ventricular offset of 0 ms. At early follow-up, the patient described a significant improvement in exercise tolerance and had no heart failure symptoms.

Comments

Patients undergoing robotic left ventricular lead implantation have been shown to have a reduced rate of heart failure, improved quality of life, higher ejection fraction, and reverse ventricular remodeling.[3,4] The robotic approach has a high success rate (98%), and reports indicate the leads perform well over the long term, making routine replacements unnecessary.[5] The minimally invasive robotic approach has been shown to be successful even in patients who have previously undergone open-heart surgery.[5]

Robotically assisted surgeries combine the benefits of open and minimally invasive surgery. The DaVinci robotic system (Intuitive Surgical Incorporated, Sunnyvale, Calif.) uses the EndoWrist microinstrument system and three-dimensional images created by the use of two side-by-side videoscopes, providing excellent depth perception. This system is able to mimic the full seven planes of motion of a surgeon's wrist, thereby merging the unrestricted movement afforded by a sternotomy with the minimally invasive nature of thoracoscopic surgery. The surgeon controls the instruments through a control console away from the surgical field, viewing the surgery through a double eye-piece that provides a real-time, high-definition, magnified endoscopic video feed in real three-dimensional view. The extreme accuracy and precision of the robotic system in such a small space can be attributed to the computer interface, which allows for scaled motion and eliminates tremor. In addition, the three-dimensional endoscopic view makes left ventricular mapping possible.[2]

Traditionally, left ventricular lead placement has been done using either a minimally invasive thoracotomy or a videoscopic-assisted approach with good results. In our experience, and particularly in reoperative cases, the robotic approach adds a new dimension with regard to ease of instrument manipulation, especially when significant adhesions are present. The addition of three-dimensional imaging, permitting excellent depth perception, is another of the improvements provided by the robotic approach. With an average stay of 48 hours it compares favorably to nonsurgical efforts when those either fail or cannot be attempted in patients in need of chronic resynchronization therapy. After the procedure, the patients enjoy quick return to normal life activities with minimal discomfort. Complications in these cases are avoided by careful patient selection and adequate preoperative imaging studies.

Selected References

1. Choset H, Zenati M, Ota T, et al: Enabling medical robotics for the next generation of minimally invasive procedures: minimally invasive cardiac surgery with single port access. In Rosen J, Hannaford B, Satava RM, editors: *Surgical robotics*, New York, 2011, Springer, pp 257-270.
2. DeRose JJ, Steinberg JS: Surgical approaches to epicardial left ventricular lead implantation for biventricular pacing. In Yu C, Hayes DL, Auricchio A, editors: *Cardiac resynchronization therapy*, Blackwell, 2006, Malden, Massachusetts, pp 227-236.
3. Derose Jr JJ, Balaram S, Ro C, et al: Midterm follow-up of robotic biventricular pacing demonstrates excellent lead stability and improved response rates, *Innovations (Phila)* 1:105-110, 2006.
4. Joshi S, Steinberg JS, Ashton Jr RC, et al: Follow-up of robotically assisted left ventricular epicardial leads for cardiac resynchronization therapy, *J Am Coll Cardiol* 46:2358-2359, 2005.
5. Kamath GS, Balaram S, Choi A, et al: Long-term outcome of leads and patients following robotic epicardial left ventricular lead placement for cardiac resynchronization therapy, *Pacing Clin Electrophysiol* 34:235-240, 2011.

SECTION 5

Optimization of Cardiac Resynchronization Therapy Device

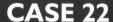
Atrioventricular Optimization by Transthoracic Echocardiography in a Patient with Interatrial Delay

Fang Fang and Yat-Sun Chan

Age	Gender	Occupation	Working Diagnosis
71 Years	Male	Retired	Congestive Heart Failure and Post–Cardiac Resynchronization Therapy Status

HISTORY

The patient had a history of acute myocardial infarction with triple vessel disease and underwent coronary artery bypass surgery.

Comments

This patient had congestive heart failure with an ischemic cause.

CURRENT MEDICATIONS

The patient was taking aspirin 80 mg daily, candesartan 8 mg daily, furosemide 40 mg daily, metoprolol 50 mg twice daily, and simvastatin 20 mg daily.

Comments

This patient was on optimal medical therapy.

CURRENT SYMPTOMS

The patient exhibited mild shortness of breath on exertion.

Comments

This patient was in New York Health Association class II.

PHYSICAL EXAMINATION

BP/HR: 157/80 mm Hg/82 bpm
Height/weight: 160 cm/56 kg
Neck veins: Normal
Lungs/chest: Clear
Heart: Jugular venous pressure not elevated, apex beat at anterior axillary line of the sixth intercostal space, heart sounds normal, no murmur detected
Abdomen: Soft, nontender
Extremities: No edema

Comments

The patient had a dilated left ventricle.

LABORATORY DATA

Hemoglobin: 13 g/dL
Hematocrit/packed cell volume: 0.462
Mean corpuscular volume: 89.3 fL
Platelet count: $142 \times 10^3/\mu L$
Sodium: 141 mmol/L
Potassium: 4.1 mmol/L
Creatinine: 119 μmol/L
Blood urea nitrogen: 6.9 mmol/L

Comments

The patient's laboratory tests were normal.

ELECTROCARDIOGRAM

Findings

Bifid P wave was shown on the electrocardiogram (Figure 22-1) and nearly disappeared after AV optimization (Figure 22-2)

Comments

The electrocardiogram showed an enlarged atrium and interatrial delay before atrioventricular optimization and improvement after atrioventricular optimization.

ECHOCARDIOGRAM

Findings

When atrioventricular delay was set up as 30 ms, a truncated mitral valve A wave, with QA of 50 ms, was seen. (Figure 22-3)

```
Rate      69
RR        870
PR        208
QRSD      128
QT        416
QTcB      446
QTcF      436
  —Axis—
P         55
QRS       42
T         257
```

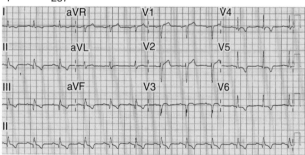

Dev. EDU-1004   Speed: 25 mm/sec   Limb: 10 mm/mV
Chest: 10.0 mm/mV   F 50~ 0.50–100 Hz W   PH09 CL P?

FIGURE 22-1

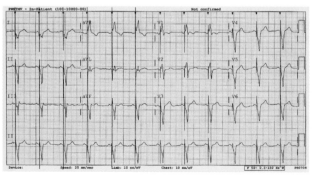

FIGURE 22-2

Comments

The atrioventricular delay was too short.

Findings

When atrioventricular delay was set up as 270 ms, mitral inflow E and A waves were merged, with QA of –20 ms. (Figure 22-4)

Comments

The atrioventricular delay was too long.

Findings

In this patient, the optomized atrioventricular delay was 200 ms with the Ritter Method. (Figure 22-5)

Comments

Atrioventricular delay in this patient was longer than in most other patients.

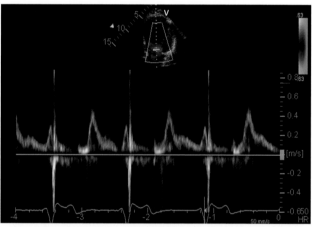

FIGURE 22-3

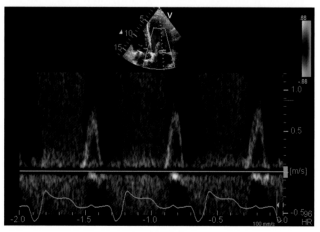

FIGURE 22-4

Findings

The mitral regurgitation method showed that when atrioventricular delay is set to a very long value, there is a time interval between the end of the mitral inflow A wave and onset of the systolic component of mitral regurgitation (δt). The optimized AV delay is AVlong – δt. (Figure 22-6)

Comments

With this method, we can use a single beat to perform atrioventricular optimization. However, it can be used only in patients with significant mitral regurgitation.

FOCUSED CLINICAL QUESTIONS AND DISCUSSION POINTS

Question

Why should we optimize atrioventricular delay even in patients with successful implantation of CRT?

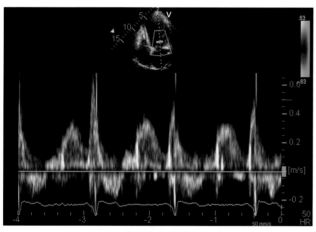

FIGURE 22-5

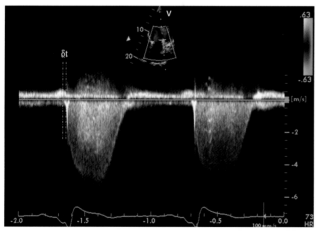

FIGURE 22-6

Discussion

Although out-of-box setting is possible for atrioventricular delay, in the real world the optimal atrioventricular delay differs widely and optimization should be performed individually. Optimization of the atrioventricular interval will ensure atrioventricular synchrony, maintaining the coordination between atria and ventricles. If the delay is too short, the mitral inflow A wave will be truncated. On the other hand, when delay is programmed too long, even with biventricular capture, diastolic mitral regurgitation may be present. Therefore atrioventricular optimization after CRT will decrease presystolic time, eliminate presystolic mitral regurgitation, improve left ventricular filling, and increase cardiac output.[2,6]

Question

What methods are usually used for atrioventricular optimization with transthoracic echocardiography?

Discussion

Several methods are used to optimize atrioventricular delay in CRT, usually based on the pulse wave mitral inflow acquired with transthoracic echocardiography.

Ritter Method

With the Ritter Method, the atrioventricular interval should be programmed short first and QA short is measured in the interval between the ventricular contraction spike and the end of the A wave.[4] Then the atrioventricular interval is programmed long and the QA long is determined. Optimized AV delay = AVshort + ([AVlong + QAlong] – [AVshort + QAshort]).

Mitral Regurgitation Method

Atrioventricular delay is programmed longest with biventricular capture, and the interval between the end of the A wave and onset of the systolic component of mitral regurgitation can be obtained subsequently (δ t).[5] Optimized AV delay = AVlong – δt.

The Iterative Method

Atrioventricular delay is programmed slightly shorter than the intrinsic atrioventricular interval.[1] Then atrioventricular delay is gradually shortened by 20 ms every time until the mitral A wave is truncated. The next step is to prolong 10 ms until the truncated A wave disappears and the optimal AV delay is determined.

Question

What is the effect of interatrial delay on atrioventricular interval?

Discussion

When the patient has significant intraatrial conduction delay before implantation, the optimal atrioventricular delay will be longer than those without to allow adequate time for the electrical signal to travel to the left atrium. To ensure optimization of CRT, the atrial lead should be implanted in the atrial septum.

In this case, we showed that in a patient with inter-atrial delay, as detected with ECG, the optimized atrioventricular delay was approximately 200 ms, as assessed by Ritter Method, which was longer than the 100 to 130 ms in most patients. Published data also have demonstrated that patients with interatrial conduction delays benefit most by prolonging the delays during atrioventricular optimization.[3]

FINAL DIAGNOSIS

The final diagnosis in this patient is CRT implantation with interatrial delay.

PLAN OF ACTION

The plan for this patient was to prolonged atrioventricular delay during the optimization.

INTERVENTION

The atrioventricular delay was programmed to be longer.

Selected References

1. Cleland JG, Daubert JC, Erdmann E, et al: The CARE-HF study (CArdiac REsynchronisation in Heart Failure study): rationale, design and end-points, *Eur J Heart Fail.* 3:481-489, 2001.
2. Heydari B, Jerosch-Herold M, Kwong RY, et al: Imaging for planning of cardiac resynchronization therapy, *JACC Cardiovasc Imaging* 5:93-110, 2012.
3. Gorcsan 3rd J, Abraham T, Agler DA, et al: Echocardiography for cardiac resynchronization therapy: recommendations for performance and reporting. Report from the American Society of Echocardiography Dyssynchrony Writing Group endorsed by the Heart Rhythm Society, *J Am Soc Echocardiogr* 21:191-213, 2008.
4. Ritter P, Dib JC, Lelievre T, et al: Quick determination of the optimal AV delay at rest in patients paced in DDD mode for complete AV block. (abstract), *Eur J CPE* 4:A163, 1994.
5. Meluzín J, Spinarová L, Bakala J, et al: Pulsed Doppler tissue imaging of the velocity of tricuspid annular systolic motion: a new, rapid, and non-invasive method of evaluating right ventricular systolic function, *Eur Heart J* 22:340-348, 2001.
6. Zhang Q, Fung JW, Chan YS, et al: The role of repeating optimization of atrioventricular interval during interim and long-term follow-up after cardiac resynchronization therapy, *Int J Cardiol* 124:211-217, 2008.

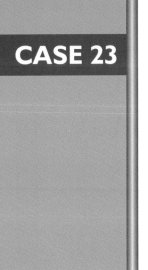

CASE 23

Left Ventricular Quadripolar Lead in Phrenic Nerve Stimulation: It Is Better to Prevent Than to Treat

Christophe Leclercq

Age	Gender	Occupation	Working Diagnosis
59 Years	Male	Electrician	Dilated Cardiomyopathy and Heart Failure

HISTORY

In 2010 the patient reported dyspnea with New York Heart Association (NYHA) class II, then class III. A nonischemic dilated cardiomyopathy was diagnosed. The surface electrocardiogram (ECG) showed a complete left bundle branch block (LBBB) and the echocardiography a left ventricular ejection fraction (LVEF) of 25% and a left ventricular end-diastolic diameter of 63 mm. A medical treatment including angiotensin-converting enzyme inhibitors, beta blockers, and diuretics was prescribed with a significant improvement in symptoms and echocardiographic parameters over 1 year. A NYHA class II to III dyspnea occurred in 2012, as well as a deterioration in LVEF (25%). The implantation of a cardiac resynchronization therapy defibrillator (CRT-D) was attempted in another center, but the left ventricular lead could not be implanted because of a coronary sinus dissection. A CRT-D device was implanted, with a plug into the left ventricular port. The patient was referred to our center 2 months later for a new attempt of left ventricular lead implantation. Computed tomography (CT) was performed to assess the patency of the coronary sinus. A Medtronic 4194 (Minneapolis, Minn.) left ventricular lead was implanted into a lateral vein. The lead must be positioned at the proximal part of the lateral vein because of a permanent phrenic nerve simulation at the distal and medial part of the vein despite the electrical repositioning. The following day the chest radiograph showed the dislodgement of the left ventricle lead into the body of the coronary sinus.

CURRENT MEDICATIONS

The patient was taking bisoprolol 10 mg daily, ramipril 10 mg daily, eplerenone 50 mg daily, and furosemide 40 mg daily.

Comments

The patient was on optimal drug treatment according to the new European Society of Cardiology 2012 guidelines.

CURRENT SYMPTOMS

The patient was experiencing dyspnea with NYHA class III and no signs of right heart failure.

PHYSICAL EXAMINATION

BP/HR: 115/75 mm Hg/60 bpm
Height/weight: 1.83 m/97 kg
Neck veins: Not distended
Lungs/chest: No heart failure
Heart: Mild mitral regurgitation
Abdomen: Normal
Extremities: Normal

Comments

The patient had symptoms of left heart failure but no signs of heart failure decompensation.

LABORATORY DATA

Hemoglobin: 13.6 g/dL
Hematocrit/packed cell volume: 42%
Platelet count: 230 × 10^3/μL
Sodium: 137 mmol/L
Potassium: 4.4 mmol/L
Creatinine: 88 μmol/L
Blood urea nitrogen: 5.9 mmol/L

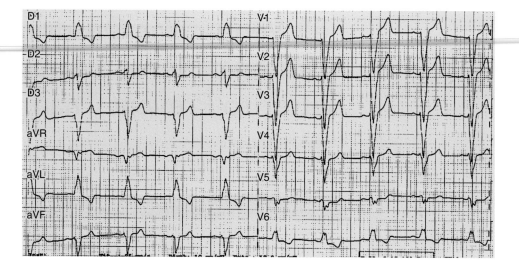

FIGURE 23-1 Baseline electrocardiogram with sinus rhythm and left bundle branch block.

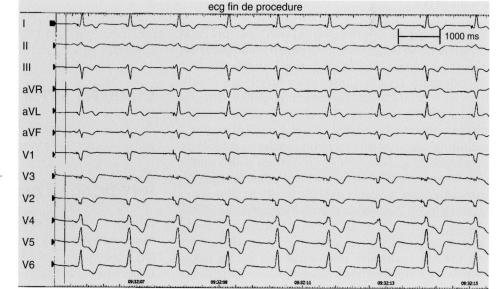

FIGURE 23-2 Surface electrocardiogram with biventricular pacing, with the bipolar lead positioned at the proximal portion of the lateral vein (see Figure 23-1).

Comments

The N-terminal pro-brain natriuretic peptide was 450 pg/mL.

ELECTROCARDIOGRAM

Findings

The electrocardiogram revealed sinus rhythm and complete LBBB (Figure 23-1), biventricular pacing with the bipolar lead (Figure 23-2), and biventricular pacing with final quadripolar lead (Figure 23-3).

CHEST RADIOGRAPH

Findings

Figure 23-4 shows dislodgement of the Attain 4194 left ventricular lead (Medtronic) into the body of the cornonary sinus *(arrow 2)*. Arrow 1 shows the initial location of the tip of the left ventricular lead in the operating room. Figure 23-5 shows the left ventricular lead with four poles positioned into the lateral vein.

Comments

Dislodgement lead can be seen in Figure 23-4. A quartet lead (St. Jude Medical) can be seen in the lateral vein in Figure 23-5.

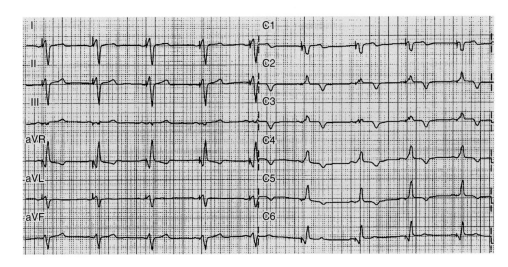

FIGURE 23-3 Final surface electrocardiogram with biventricular pacing with left ventricular pacing configuration M4 (proximal pole) to right ventricular coil.

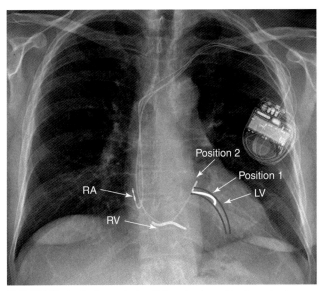

FIGURE 23-4 Left ventricular *(LV)* projection of the lateral vein. *Position 1:* Position of the LV lead at the end of the implantation. *Position 2:* Position of the LV lead the day after into the body of the coronary sinus. *RA,* Right atrial; *RV,* right ventricular.

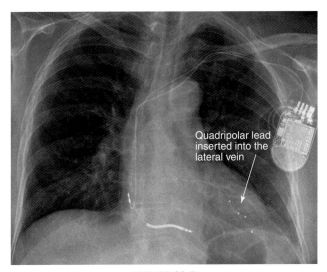

FIGURE 23-5

FOCUSED CLINICAL QUESTIONS AND DISCUSSION POINTS

Question

What should be done if a complete coronary sinus dissection occurred during the implantation of a left ventricular lead into the coronary sinus?

Discussion

The recommendation is to stop the left ventricular lead implantation and monitor the patient in the intensive care unit with repeated echocardiographic examinations to diagnose a potential pericardial effusion or tamponade.

Question

Is the coronary sinus dissection definitive?

Discussion

In clinical follow-up, after 1 month, the coronary sinus was patent without dissection.

Question

How should one deal with phrenic nerve stimulation?

Discussion

The first possibility is to decrease the left ventricular output to avoid phrenic nerve stimulation (PNS) by providing left ventricular pacing if the left ventricular threshold is really inferior to the PNS threshold. The second possibility—more reliable—is to use the electrical

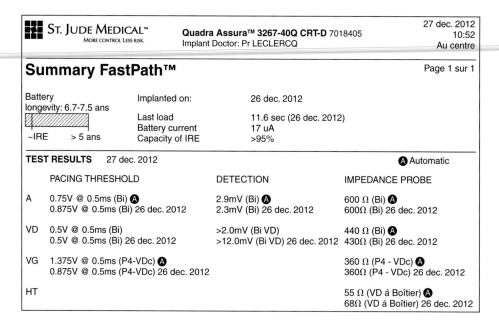

FIGURE 23-6 Summary of the pacing threshold, sensing, and impedances.

repositioning (different pacing configurations) according to the capabilities of the devices. The third solution is reoperation to reposition the lead or to implant a new lead, such a quadripolar lead, to offer more pacing configurations.

The first solution may be hazardous, with risk for losing the left ventricular capture. The second is usually efficient but in some cases is not sufficient, as in our case, in which activation of the proximal or distal pole enhanced PNS even with low output when the lead was stable, that is, inserted at the distal part of the vein. The systematic use of a quadripolar lead may be an interesting option to offer more pacing configurations and thus more solutions.

FINAL DIAGNOSIS

In this patient the final diagnosis was left ventricular lead dislodgement related to the need for positioning the bipolar left ventricular lead at the entry of the coronary sinus lateral vein.

PLAN OF ACTION

A repeat operation was peformed. The bipolar left ventricular lead was removed and a new quadripolar left ventricular lead (Quartet, St. Jude Medical) implanted.

INTERVENTION

The quadripolar left ventricular lead was inserted more distally in the same vein. Pacing at the distal pole and pole 2 enhanced PNS in all of the pacing configurations. Only pacing with pole 3 and 4 in pseudo-bipolar mode with the right ventricular lead provided an acceptable pacing threshold without PNS.

OUTCOME

After 4 months of follow-up the left ventricular pacing theshold is stable at approximately 1.3 V without PNS (see Figures 23-3 and 23-6), with permanent biventricular capture and improvement in symptoms and exercise capacity.

Selected References

1. Forleo GB, Della Rocca DG, Papavasileiou LP, et al: Left ventricular pacing with a new quadripolar transvenous lead for CRT: early results of a prospective comparison with conventional implant outcomes, *Heart Rhythm* 8:31-37, 2011.
2. Landolina M, Gasparini M, Lunati M, et al: Long-term complications related to biventricular defibrillator implantation: rate of surgical revisions and impact on survival: insights from the Italian Clinical Service Database, *Circulation* 123:2526-2535, 2011.
3. Thibault B, et al: Posters PO 04-117 to 04-183, *Heart Rhythm* 8, 2011, S291.

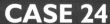

Loss of Left Ventricular Pacing Capture Detected by Remote Monitoring

Laura Perrotta, Giuseppe Ricciardi, Paolo Pieragnoli, Emanuele Lebrun, and Luigi Padeletti

Age	Gender	Occupation	Working Diagnosis
76 Years	Male	Retired High School Teacher	Dilated Cardiomyopathy

HISTORY

The patient was a 76-year-old man with heart failure, left bundle branch block (LBBB), and paroxysmal atrial fibrillation.

Comments

The patient with symptomatic heart failure (New York Health Association [NYHA] III) was referred for cardiac resynchronization therapy defibrillator (CRT-D) implantation. He had a dilated cardiomyopathy with left ventricular disfunction (ejection fraction <35% documented by echocardiography) and prolonged QRS duration (>120 ms) with LBBB morphology. He was on optimal medical therapy for heart failure, including angiotensin-converting enzyme (ACE) inhibitors and beta blockers. In addition, the patient was on oral anticoagulation therapy with warfarin because of recurrent episodes of atrial fibrillation. A coronary angiography was performed and ruled out an ischemic cause of the cardiomyopathy.

On May 5, 2010, he was implanted with a CRT-D device; the left ventricular lead was positioned into the midlateral vein through the coronary sinus. The best left ventricular capture threshold was 1.5 V at 0.4 ms with left ventricular tip to left ventricular ring vector polarity. No phrenic nerve stimulation was observed, and no complications occurred during and soon after the procedure.

The CRT-D was programmed with left ventricular tip to left ventricular ring polarity, and an algorithm to measure the left ventricular threshold and adapt left ventricular output was activated (LV Capture Management, Medtronic, Minneapolis, Minn.).

A CareLink monitor (Medtronic) for remote monitoring was given to the patient because he lived alone, far from the clinic, and was not able to attend all of the scheduled follow-up visits.

CURRENT MEDICATIONS

The patient was taking warfarin, optimal medical therapy for heart failure.

CURRENT SYMPTOMS

Exacerbation of cardiac heart failure symptoms with worsening of NHYA class (II to III).

ELECTROCARDIOGRAM

The CareLink monitor transmission for July 3, 2010 was as follows:

- CareLink alert for burden atrial fibrillation (>6 hours) and for increased left ventricular pacing threshold
- Left ventricular pacing threshold 4.0 V at 0.4 ms (+1.75 V compared to that on June 25, 2010)
- Percent V pacing 99.1%
- Leadless electrogram (ECG) shows a changed axis compared to May 2012, 2010 recording
- Left ventricular lead is still pacing (but probably moved back a little)

FINDINGS

Two months after the CRT device implant (July 3, 2010), an automatic CareLink transmission was generated by two different alerts (burden atrial fibrillation longer than 6 hours and increased left ventricular pacing threshold [+1.75 V vs. that on June 25, 2010]) (Figures 24-1 and 24-2). The patient had a history of paroxysmal atrial fibrillation and was already on anticoagulant therapy, so the single atrial fibrillation event was not unexpected. On the leadless ECG transmitted (three electrograms plus high-resolution digital leadless ECG and Active Can-superior vena cava (SVC) Coil [Medtronic] corresponding to lead DI surface ECG), a variation of paced QRS was noted in contrast to the transmission on May 12, 2010 (Figure 24-3, *black arrows*). The patient was contacted by telephone. He was completely asymptomatic but unable to reach the medical center for clinical follow-up.

The CareLink monitor transmission for October 9, 2010 was as follows:

- CareLink alert for burden FA, OptiVol, and for high left ventricular pacing threshold on October 8, 2010
- Left ventricular pacing threshold 6.0 V at 0.4 ms, device unable to maintain an appropriate safety margin (more than 1 V of the pacing threshold)
- Three episodes of nonsustained ventricular tachycardia
- Leadless ECG shows same axis but larger than on July 7, 2010 (queried partial capture)
- Patient asked to go to the clinic the next day

Findings

On October 9, 2010 an automatic CareLink transmission was generated by three alerts (burden AF, OptiVol, and high pacing threshold, with the Automatic Capture Management algorithm unable to mantain the programmed +1 V safety margin) (Figures 24-4 and 24-5). A further increase in left ventricular pacing threshold was observed associated with an increased QRS paced width, and the axis was unchanged in contrast to that from July 3, 2010; see Figure 24-5). The OptiVol alert suggested an initial accumulation of interstitial liquid, probably as a result of an intermittent capture of biventricular pacing.

The patient was contacted for a follow-up visit on the next day (October 10, 2010). Changing the polarity from tipLV/ringLV to tipLV/coilRV obtained a lower left ventricular pacing threshold (3.5 V at 1.0 ms), left ventricular pacing output was set to 5.0 V at 1.0 ms, programming off (monitoring only) the Automatic Capture Management function to ensure continuous biventricular pacing at higher output.

The CareLink monitor transmission for December 10, 2010 was as follows:

- Reprogrammed polarity from tipLV/ringLV to tipLV/coilRV (left ventricular pacing threshold 3.5 V at 1.0 ms) on October 10, 2010 patient ambulatory visit

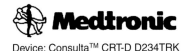
Medtronic

Quick Look II

Date of Interrogation: 03-Jul-2010 23:42:27

Physician: Dr. Ricciardi - - -

Device: Consulta™ CRT-D D234TRK

Device Status (Implanted: 05-May-2010)

Battery Voltage (RRT=2.63V)	3.19 V	(03-Jul-2010)	
Last Full Charge	8.1 sec	(05-May-2010)	
	Atrial(4574)	RV(6944) SVC	LV(4196)
Pacing Impedance Defibrillation Impedance	475 ohms	893 ohms RV=42 ohms SVC=52 ohms	646 ohms
Capture Threshold Measured on Programmed Amplitude/Pulse Width	1.000 V @ 0.40 ms 03-Jul-2010 3.50 V/0.40 ms	0.500 V @ 0.40 ms 03-Jul-2010 3.50 V/0.40 ms	- - - 5.00 V/0.40 ms
Measured P/R Wave Programmed Sensitivity	1.9 mV 0.30 mV	9.6 mV 0.30 mV	

OBSERVATIONS (7)
- Alert: 1 day with more than 6 hr AT/AF.
- Possible high LV threshold on 03-Jul-2010.
- LV Capture Management determined that threshold increased by 1.75 V from 25-Jun-2010 to 26-Jun-2010. This increase was greater than Amplitude Safety Margin (+1 V) and may have compromised capture.

- Patient Activity less than 1 hr/day for 5 weeks.
- Longest ventricular sensing episode since the last session is greater than 60 seconds.
- Ventricular sensing episodes averaged 5.1 min/day since the last session.
- VF detection may be delayed: VF Detection Interval is faster than 300 ms (200 bpm).

FIGURE 24-1

- Increased left ventricular pulse width from 0.4 ms to 1.0 ms
- Automatic Capture Management programmed off (monitoring only) to have continuous left ventricular pacing at 5.0 V at 1.0 ms output.

Findings

On December 10, 2010 (Figure 24-6), we received a programmed CareLink transmission with data indicating a satisfactory situation. The patient activity level was considerably increased, with only a few episodes of paroxysmal atrial fibrillation, as was usual for the patient.

On May 7, 2011, we received another programmed CareLink Transmission with a good clinical situation and a stable biventricular pacing (Figure 24-7). The patient did not experience any worsening heart failure episodes.

FOCUSED CLINICAL QUESTIONS AND DISCUSSION POINTS

Question

The first CareLink automatic transmission (July 3, 2010; see Figures 24-1 to 24-3) reported an increased left ventricular pacing threshold. Should it be considered a "normal" consequence of the chronic phase of the lead maturation process?

Discussion

Elevated thresholds that occur during the first several weeks after implantation were common, although the introduction of steroid eluting electrodes and other electrode materials and designs has markedly decreased this problem.

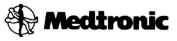

Lead Performance Trends

Device: Consulta™ CRT-D D234TRK

Date of Interrogation: 12-May-2010 23:42:27

Physician: Dr. Ricciardi - - -

LV Pace Polarity — LVtip to LVring
Lead Model — 4196

LV Impedance
(LVtip to LVring)
Last Measured 646 ohms

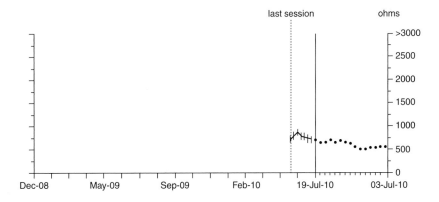

LV Threshold
Capture — Adaptive
Amplitude — 5.00 V
Pulse Width — 0.40 ms
Max. Adapted — 6.00 V
Last Measured — 4.000 V @ 0.40 ms
Measured on — 26-Jun-2010

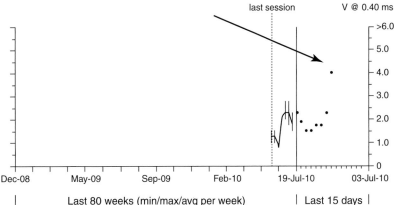

| Last 80 weeks (min/max/avg per week) | Last 15 days |

FIGURE 24-2

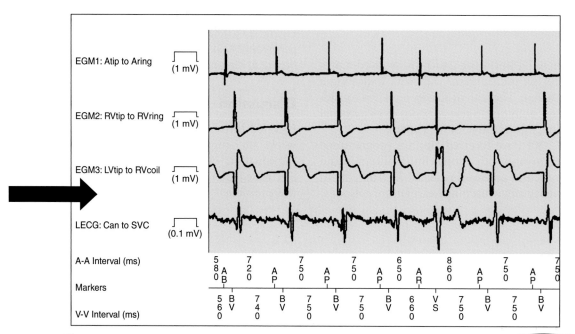

Medtronic

Device: Consulta™ CRT-D D234TRK

Current EGM

Date of Interrogation: 12-Jul-2010 11:43:23

Chart speed: 25.0 mm/sec

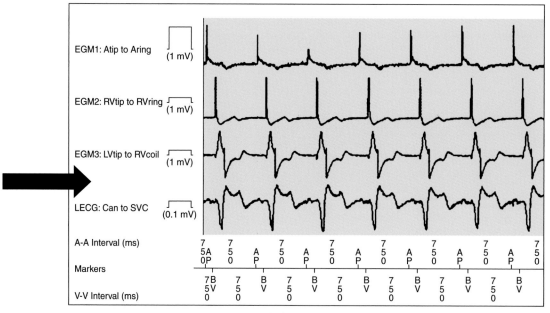

Medtronic

Device: Consulta™ CRT-D D234TRK

Current EGM

Date of Interrogation: 03-Jul-2010 23:42:27

Chart speed: 25.0 mm/sec

FIGURE 24-3

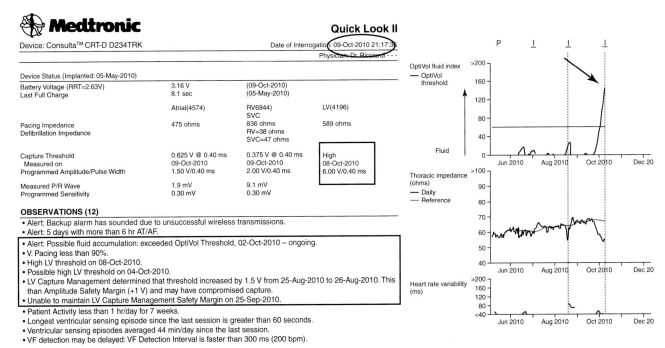

FIGURE 24-4

The rise in capture threshold usually has a peak between 2 and 6 weeks after implantation and may be attributed to an inflammatory reaction around the electrode. An elevation observed more than 6 weeks after implantation, as in this case, usually is considered to be in the chronic phase of the lead maturation process. It was also noted that biventricular pacing was still effective but with a different left ventricular activation and consequently a different QRS paced axis, probably as a result of a minimal left ventricular lead backdown. However, the CareLink System provided the opportunity to detect the increased pacing threshold and further monitor the evolution of the clinical situation without unscheduled follow-up visits.

Question

On October 9, 2010 a new automatic CareLink transmission was generated by three different alerts: burden atrial fibrillation, OptiVol, and high pacing threshold. Should the OptiVol alert be considered a consequence of atrial fibrillation and reduced biventricular pacing or of intermittent loss of left ventricular capture?

Discussion

The OptiVol alert suggested an initial accumulation of interstitial liquids and worsening of the heart failure condition, probably as a result of an intermittent loss of biventricular pacing.

The percentage of biventricular pacing was reduced because of an increased ventricular rate during atrial fibrillation. Moreover, likely there was not constant left ventricular capture because the Automatic Capture Management algorithm was unable to maintain the programmed safety margin for left ventricular output. Therefore the patient was contacted for a clinical follow-up visit.

Question

Was the rise in left ventricular pacing threshold the result of a gross dislodgment of the left ventricular lead or of chronic pacing threshold elevation?

Discussion

Changing the polarity from tipLV/ringLV to tipLV/coilRV restored left ventricular capture, ensuring continuous biventricular pacing at higher output. Thus the rise in the left ventricular pacing threshold until the loss of capture was not due to a gross dislodgment of the left ventricular lead.

FINAL DIAGNOSIS

The final diagnosis for this patient was the necessity for an increased left ventricular pacing threshold, as identified by monitoring with the CareLink system.

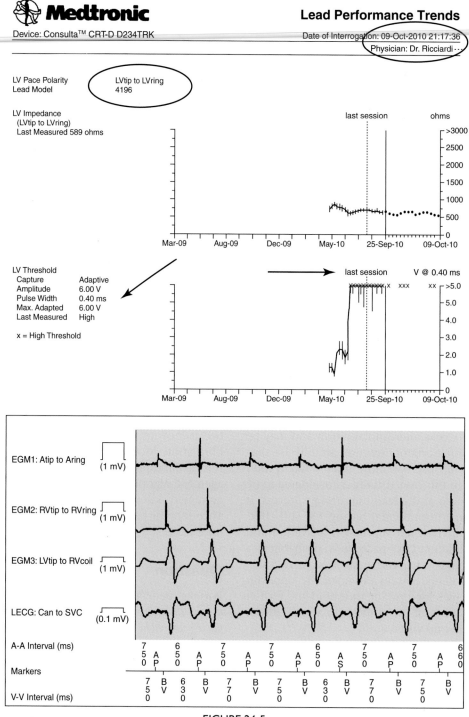

FIGURE 24-5

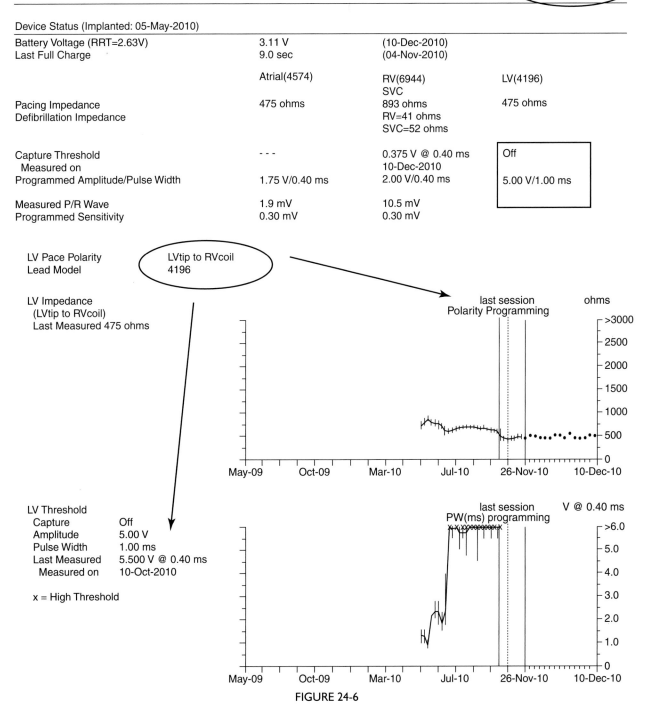

Figure 24-6

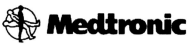

Quick Look II

Device: Consulta™ CRT-D D234TRK

Date of Interrogation: 10-Oct-2010 16:43:09

Physician: Dr. Ricciardi

Device Status (Implanted: 05-May-2010)

Battery Voltage (RRT=2.63V)	3.11 V	(10-Dec-2010)	
Last Full Charge	9.0 sec	(04-Nov-2010)	
	Atrial(4574)	RV(6944) SVC	LV(4196)
Pacing Impedance	475 ohms	893 ohms	475 ohms
Defibrillation Impedance		RV=41 ohms SVC=52 ohms	
Capture Threshold	- - -	0.375 V @ 0.40 ms	Off
Measured on		10-Dec-2010	
Programmed Amplitude/Pulse Width	1.75 V/0.40 ms	2.00 V/0.40 ms	5.00 V/1.00 ms
Measured P/R Wave	1.9 mV	10.5 mV	
Programmed Sensitivity	0.30 mV	0.30 mV	

LV Pace Polarity   LVtip to RVcoil
Lead Model   4196

LV Impedance
  (LVtip to RVcoil)
  Last Measured 475 ohms

last session
Polarity Programming   ohms

LV Threshold
  Capture   Off
  Amplitude   5.00 V
  Pulse Width   1.00 ms
  Last Measured 5.500 V @ 0.40 ms
  Measured on   10-Oct-2010

x = High Threshold

last session
PW(ms) programming   V @ 0.40 ms

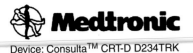**Medtronic**

Lead Performance Trends

Device: Consulta™ CRT-D D234TRK

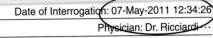Date of Interrogation: 07-May-2011 12:34:26

Physician: Dr. Ricciardi

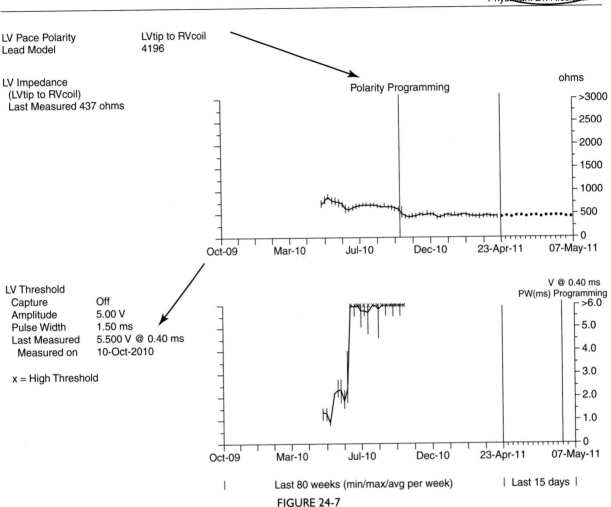

FIGURE 24-7

PLAN OF ACTION

The plan of action was monitoring of the increasing left ventricular pacing threshold using the CareLink system without unscheduled follow-up visits.

OUTCOME

The intervention resulted in restoration of effective biventricular pacing.

INTERVENTION

Left ventricular output and pacing configuration were reprogrammed only when loss of capture had been detected by the monitoring system.

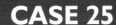

CASE 25

The Importance of Maintaining a High Percentage of Biventricular Pacing

Christopher J. McLeod

Age	Gender	Occupation	Working Diagnosis
54 Years	Male	Farmer	Nonischemic Cardiomyopathy

HISTORY

The patient is a 54-year-old man with a history of a nonischemic dilated cardiomyopathy. He was initially referred for consideration of a third procedure for atrial fibrillation. He had undergone pulmonary vein isolation procedures 1 year and 3 months previously. In addition to pulmonary vein isolation, linear ablation of both the left and right atria had been performed, as well as targeting of complex fractionated atrial electrograms. Despite this, the patient experienced early recurrences of atrial fibrillation and atypical atrial flutter soon after each ablation. In addition, amiodarone, digoxin, and beta blockade were used as adjunctive therapy, yet rate control remained poor. Heart rates during waking hours averaged approximately 110 bpm. Left ventricular systolic function was globally reduced, and the ejection fraction was estimated to be approximately 20%. His symptom was New York Heart Association (NYHA) class II to III dyspnea, yet he had no history of hospital admissions for heart failure, no palpitations, and no presyncopal symptoms.

The patient had failed an antiarrhythmic strategy using a combination of medication and ablation. Furthermore, he was failing a rate control strategy using three different atrioventricular nodal blocking agents. He remained tachycardic and symptomatic, and therefore the following therapeutic options were discussed with him and his family: (1) a third catheter ablation for atrial fibrillation, (2) permanent pacemaker implantation with adjunctive atrioventricular nodal ablation, and (3) open surgical cut-and-sew maze procedure. The patient elected to proceed with atrioventricular nodal ablation and permanent pacemaker implantation.

CURRENT MEDICATIONS

The patient was taking digoxin 250 mcg daily, furosemide 20 mg daily, losartan 50 mg daily, amiodarone 300 mg daily, metoprolol 100 mg twice daily, spironolactone 25 mg daily, and warfarin to maintain international normalized ratio between 2 and 3.

CURRENT SYMPTOMS

The patient's predominant symptom was dyspnea on exertion. His exercise tolerance was limited to flat surfaces. In addition, he was frequently becoming dyspneic with simple activities of daily living while working on his farm. He had not had any syncopal episodes and was not aware of any palpitations.

PHYSICAL EXAMINATION

BP/HR: 101/67 mm Hg/97 bpm
Height/weight: 180 cm/105 kg
Neck veins: No jugular vein distention, no carotid bruits
Lungs/chest: Clear
Heart: Rapid irregular heart rate with normal first heart sound (S_1) and second heart sound (S_2), no murmur
Abdomen: Soft, nontender with no organomegaly
Extremities: Minimal edema, normal volume pulses

LABORATORY DATA

Hemoglobin: 15.1 g/dL
Mean corpuscular volume: 88 fL

Platelet count: $351 \times 10^3/\mu L$
Sodium: 140 mmol/L
Potassium: 5.0 mmol/L
Creatinine: $1.2 \times 10^9/L$
Blood urea nitrogen: 30 mmol/L

ELECTROCARDIOGRAM

Findings

Figure 25-1 shows the electrocardiogram (ECG) obtained before device implantation. The rhythm is atrial fibrillation with a fairly rapid ventricular response. The QRS duration is less than 100 ms, and no evidence of acute ischemia is present.

Figure 25-2 shows the ECG obtained after atrioventricular node ablation and device implantation. The rhythm is atrial fibrillation, with evidence of biventricular pacing. Frequent premature ventricular contractions occurred, with varying degrees of fusion.

CHEST RADIOGRAPH

Findings

The chest radiograph showed the heart size to be normal. Mild pulmonary venous hypertension was noted (Figure 25-3).

ECHOCARDIOGRAM

Findings

The electrogram revealed mild-to-moderate left ventricular enlargement with severe decrease in systolic

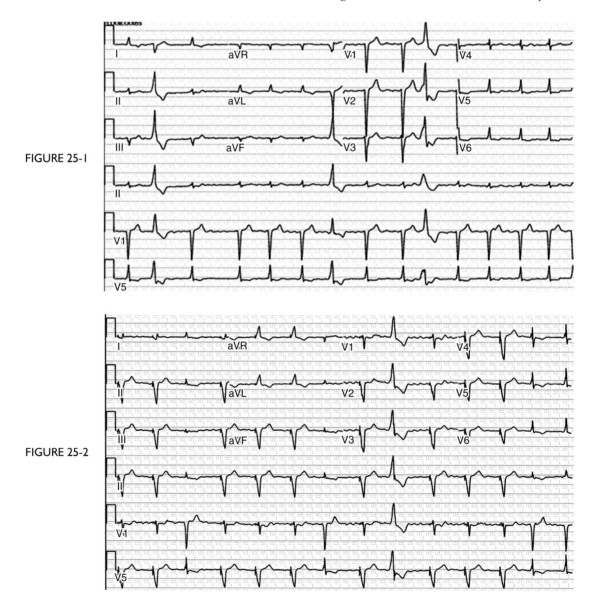

FIGURE 25-1

FIGURE 25-2

function. The left ventricular ejection fraction was estimated to be 20%. Severe generalized left ventricular hypokinesis was evident. Mild right ventricular enlargement with a mild decrease in systolic function was noted. The estimated right ventricular systolic pressure was 44 mm Hg. No significant valvular heart disease was seen. No pericardial effusion was present. The left atrial volume index was 52 mL/m^2. Moderate right atrial enlargement was noted.

PHYSIOLOGIC TRACINGS

Findings

Before Device Implantation

The patient was given a 24-hour Holter monitor 1. The patient's minimum heart rate was 62 bpm, maximum heart rate was 177 bpm, and average heart rate was 103 bpm. The basic rhythm was atrial fibrillation, with the rate varying between 62 and 177 bpm. Very frequent premature ventricular contractions or aberrant beats occurred singly at times and bigeminy in pairs and in runs of ventricular tachycardia or aberrancy 3 to 13 beats in duration. The maximum ventricular tachycardia or aberrant conduction rate was 193 bpm. Also seen were frequent episodes of an accelerated idioventricular rhythm 3 to 4 beats in duration. No symptoms were recorded in the patient's diary.

After Atrioventricular Node Ablation and Device Implantation

The patient was given a 24-hour Holter monitor 2. The basic mechanism was a ventricular pacemaker with fusion beats. The underlying rhythm was atrial fibrillation, with a ventricular rate of 58 to 94 bpm and an average heart rate of 64 bpm. Very frequent premature ventricular or aberrantly conducted beats (31.2% of total ventricular beats) occurred singly and in bigeminy

and in 3- to 4-beat runs of accelerated idioventricular rhythm (AIVR) and in 3- to 11-beat runs of ventricular tachycardia (vs. aberrant beats in a series). The minimum AIVR rate was 75 bpm. The maximum ventricular tachycardia rate was 182 bpm.

COMPUTED TOMOGRAPHY

Findings

Computed tomography (CT) of the heart shows no intracardiac thrombus. Two left and three right pulmonary veins with no pulmonary vein stenosis were noted. All coronary arteries in the right dominant coronary system were patent. Biatrial enlargement and moderately severe left ventricular dilation were observed.

FOCUSED CLINICAL QUESTIONS AND DISCUSSION POINTS

Question

Should a biventricular device or standard dual-chamber implantable cardioverter-defibrillator (ICD) pacemaker be implanted?

Discussion

It is well recognized that the left bundle branch block pattern that ensues with obligate right ventricular pacing after atrioventricular nodal ablation provides electrical dyssynchrony for the contracting myocardium. In light of the patient's symptomatic status and depressed left ventricular function, consideration of cardiac resynchronization therapy CRT is warranted. However, assuming that the basis for his ventricular dysfunction is indeed a tachycardia-mediated cardiomyopathy,[3,6] it is

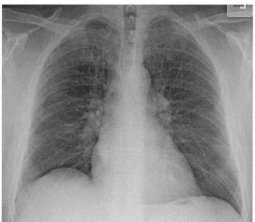 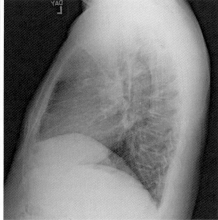

FIGURE 25-3

possible that with effective rate control alone (after atrioventricular node ablation) his ejection fraction may improve. In contrast, obligate right ventricular pacing in the context of depressed left ventricular function does hold the potential for further systolic decline and worsening symptoms of heart failure. The physician caring for him elected to recommend biventricular pacing in favor of right ventricular apical pacing.

Question

Should all patients undergoing CRT with atrial fibrillation and rapid ventricular rates undergo simultaneous atrioventricular node ablation?

Discussion

Atrioventricular node ablation provides the most reliable method for rate control in patients with atrioventricular fibrillation. Randomized controlled trials are still needed to confirm the impact of this procedure on symptom status and survival in patients with atrial fibrillation, heart failure, and biventricular pacing. Several studies, though, have suggested improvements in these fundamental outcomes, and a recent meta-analysis alludes to substantial reductions in all-cause mortality and cardiovascular mortality in those patients who underwent atrioventricular node ablation. In addition, improvements were also seen in the NYHA functional class in the atrioventricular node–ablated groups in contrast to that with medical therapy.[2]

Question

Does evidence suggest that a high premature ventricular contraction burden is a potential cause of CRT nonresponse?

Discussion

It is clear from large studies and registries that a higher percentage of biventricular pacing is associated with improved symptoms and a reduction in mortality.[4] Of interest, it appears that there is potential benefit in improving biventricular percentage pacing above 95%. The Latitude registry has demonstrated that patients with biventricular pacing percentage above 99.6% experienced a 24% reduction in mortality in contrast to the other groups, including patients receiving biventricular pacing more than 95% of the time.[4] Conceptually then, it is not necessary for the patient to sustain 20% or 30% ectopy for the salutary effects of biventricular pacing to be diluted.

Although atrial fibrillation with native conduction appears to be the most frequent offender in reducing biventricular percentage pacing, frequent ventricular ectopy is also recognized.[5] Frequent ventricular ectopy also has been identified as a cause of reversible left

ventricular dysfunction remedial to ablation.[1,6] Moreover, ablation of the premature ventricular contraction focus has been shown to be associated with improvement in left ventricular function and functional class in CRT nonresponders.[5,7] The largest benefit was seen in patients with a preablation premature ventricular contraction burden greater than 22% of their total beats.

FINAL DIAGNOSIS

The final diagnosis is nonischemic cardiomyopathy with persistent atrial fibrillation to which tachycardia or ectopy has likely contributed.

PLAN OF ACTION

The plan for this patient was atrioventricular node ablation and implantation of a biventricular pacemaker, along with subsequent catheter-based premature ventricular contraction ablation.

INTERVENTION

The patient underwent implantation of a biventricular ICD. This was performed without complications using a standard device and delivery system. The coronary sinus lead was placed in a lateral branch of the venous system, and no phrenic stimulation was noted.

At the patient's 3-month follow-up visit, it was noted that he was receiving biventricular pacing only 67% of the time. His device interrogation and 24-hour Holter monitoring showed evidence of frequent ventricular ectopy of two different morphologies. The amiodarone had been discontinued, and his symptomatic status was still NYHA class II to class III. A 24-hour Holter monitor showed that approximately one third of his beats were premature ventricular contractions. A discussion around additional antiarrhythmic therapy (i.e., flecainide or mexiletine) versus ablation was undertaken, and the patient ultimately elected to go ahead with an ablation procedure. Two predominant premature ventricular contractions were mapped and ablated. The first was ablated from an epicardial aspect on the left ventricular summit a safe distance from the left circumflex artery. The second originated from the aortomitral continuity and was ablated from an endocardial approach. The patient was seen 3 months after the procedure. Device interrogation showed biventricular pacing to be occurring 98% of the time.

Findings

The patient's transthoracic echocardiogram at 1 year after atrioventricular node ablation and 9 months after premature ventricular contraction ablation showed a marked improvement in ventricular function with the ejection fraction improving to 45%. In addition, his symptom status was improved to NYHA class II and he continues to actively work on his farm.

Selected References

1. Bogun F, Crawford T, Reich S, et al: Radiofrequency ablation of frequent, idiopathic premature ventricular complexes: comparison with a control group without intervention, *Heart Rhythm* 4:863-867, 2007.
2. Ganesan AN, Brooks AG, Roberts-Thomson KC, et al: Role of AV nodal ablation in cardiac resynchronization: in patients with coexistent atrial fibrillation and heart failure a systematic review, *J Am Coll Cardiol* 59:719-726, 2012.
3. Grogan M, Smith HC, Gersh BJ, et al: Left ventricular dysfunction due to atrial fibrillation in patients initially believed to have idiopathic dilated cardiomyopathy, *Am J Cardiol* 69:1570-1573, 1992.
4. Hayes DL, Boehmer JP, Day JD, et al: Cardiac resynchronization therapy and the relationship of percent biventricular pacing to symptoms and survival, *Heart Rhythm* 8:1469-1475, 2011.
5. Lakkireddy D, Di Biase L, Ryschon K, et al: Radiofrequency ablation of premature ventricular ectopy improves the efficacy of cardiac resynchronization therapy in nonresponders, *J Am Coll Cardiol* 60:1531-1539, 2012.
6. Stulak JM, Dearani JA, Daly RC, et al: Left ventricular dysfunction in atrial fibrillation: restoration of sinus rhythm by the Cox-maze procedure significantly improves systolic function and functional status, *Ann Thorac Surg* 82:494-500, 2006. discussion 500-491.
7. Yarlagadda RK, Iwai S, Stein KM, et al: Reversal of cardiomyopathy in patients with repetitive monomorphic ventricular ectopy originating from the right ventricular outflow tract, *Circulation* 112:1092-1097, 2005.

SECTION 6

Postimplant Follow-Up

Managing Ventricular Tachycardia: Total Atrioventricular Block After Ablation in a Patient with Nonischemic Dilated Cardiomyopathy

Sebastiaan R. D. Piers and Katja Zeppenfeld

Age	Gender	Occupation	Working Diagnosis
42 Years	Female	Beautician	Life-Threatening Electrical Storm from Sustained Monomorphic Ventricular Tachycardia Requiring External Defibrillation

HISTORY

In September 2000 the patient was referred to a cardiologist because of premature ventricular contractions. The 12-lead surface electrocardiogram (ECG) showed sinus rhythm with atypical right bundle branch block (RBBB), a fragmented QRS, and negative T-waves in III, aV_F and V_{1-3}. Echocardiography, a 24-hour Holter ECG, and stress test were reported to be unremarkable. An expectant strategy was adopted.

In December 2009 the patient was hospitalized for sustained monomorphic ventricular tachycardia, with a heart rate of 254 bpm. A coronary angiogram did not show atherosclerosis. Magnetic resonance imaging (MRI) revealed marked thinning and hypokinesia of the basal anterior and anteroseptal wall. The left ventricular end-diastolic volume was 169 mL, left ventricular ejection fraction (LVEF) was 48%. Right ventricular volumes and systolic function were normal. An implantable cardioverter-defibrillator (ICD) was implanted, complicated by pneumothorax.

The patient experienced life-threatening electrical storm as a result of recurrent sustained monomorphic ventricular tachycardia in June 2010. When the emergency service arrived, the twelfth ICD shock was administered for monomorphic ventricular tachycardia resulted in ventricular fibrillation, and the patient lost consciousness. ICD therapy was disabled by a magnet and the patient resuscitated. After successful external defibrillation, acute ventricular tachycardia recurrence

was prevented by intravenous amiodarone. However, despite amiodarone, ventricular tachycardia recurred during admission in her local hospital. The patient was referred for ventricular tachycardia ablation.

The patient's cousin died suddenly at the age of 37. At autopsy a pale and mottled heart was found.

Comments

Although the ECG in 2008 was suspicious and the patient had symptomatic premature ventricular contractions, the echocardiogram, 24-hour Holter ECG, and stress test were reported to be unremarkable. However, contrast-enhanced MRI could have been considered at this time, based on the suspicious ECG.

CURRENT MEDICATIONS

The patient was taking thiamazole 30 mg daily, metoprolol Zoc 100 mg twice daily, calcium carbasalate (Ascal) 100 mg daily, ramipril 2.5 mg daily, oxazepam 10 mg three times daily, and clorazepate 5 mg if needed.

CURRENT SYMPTOMS

The patient received 12 ICD shocks for monomorphic ventricular tachycardia. In the hospital the patient was highly anxious because of the multiple ICD shocks. She did not report chest pain or dyspnea on exertion. The history was otherwise unremarkable.

PHYSICAL EXAMINATION

BP/HR: 115/65 mm Hg/77 bpm
Height/weight: 172 cm, 68 kg
Neck veins: Not distended
Lungs/chest: Unremarkable
Heart: No murmurs
Abdomen: Unremarkable
Extremities: No peripheral edema, peripheral pulses intact in both groins, no murmurs

LABORATORY DATA

Hemoglobin: 8.4 mmol/L
Hematocrit/packed cell volume: 40%
Mean corpuscular volume: 82 fL
Platelet count: $216 \times 10^3/\mu L$
Sodium: 140 mmol/L
Potassium: 4.3 mmol/L
Creatinine: 56 µmol/L
Blood urea nitrogen: 3.3 mmol/L

ELECTROCARDIOGRAM

The ECG recorded sinus rhythm (Figure 26-1) and sustained monomorphic ventricular tachycardia (Figure 26-2) on the first day of admission at the cardiac care unit of the referring hospital.

Findings

The ECG in Figure 26-1 shows sinus rhythm at 72 bpm, pulse rate 140 ms, RBBB QRS 160 ms, QT/QTc 448/469 ms, a fragmented QRS with Q-waves in V_1, I and aV_L, a fragmented S-wave in lead II, V_4 and V_5, a fragmented R-wave in leads V_2 and V_3, and an R' wave in leads I and aV_L.

The ECG in Figure 26-2 recorded monomorphic ventricular tachycardia at 216 bpm, RBBB-like morphology (defined as dominant R in precordial lead V_1), left superior axis, transition V_3, and QRS width of 280 ms.

ECHOCARDIOGRAM

Findings

An echocardiogram of the left ventricle showed no hypertrophy, akinesia of the basal septum and basal

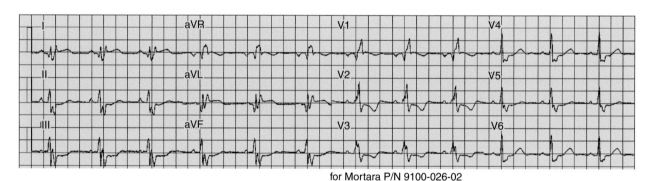

for Mortara P/N 9100-026-02

FIGURE 26-1

FIGURE 26-2

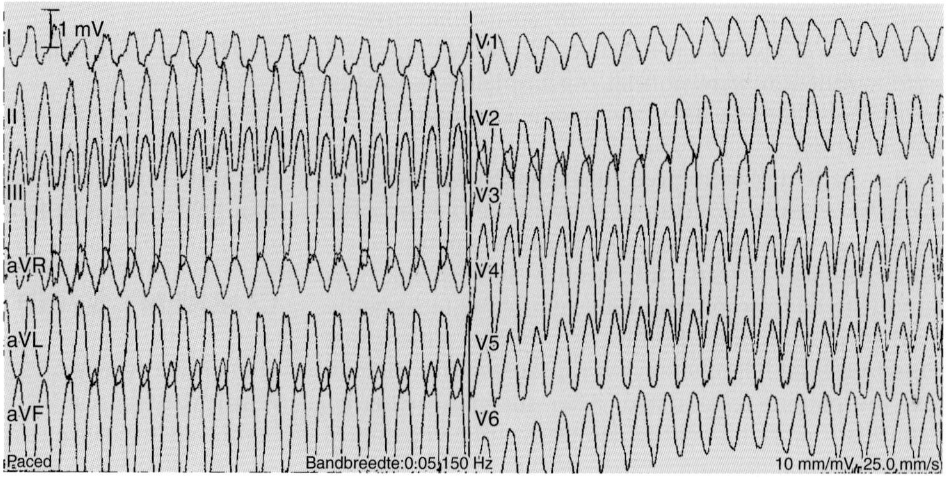

anteroseptal wall, an end-diastolic volume of 170 mL, and LVEF of 35%. The right ventricle was not dilated and tricuspid annular plane systolic excursion was 25 mm.

MAGNETIC RESONANCE IMAGING

Findings

Based on cine magnetic resonance imaging (MRI) images, the LVEF was 40%, with marked hypokinesia of the basal anterior and anteroseptal wall, and the left ventricular end-diastolic volume was 182 mL. The right ventricle showed normal function and dimensions. The short-axis contrast-enhanced MRI slices (Figure 26-3, *A*) demonstrated a transmural scar in the basal anterior and anteroseptal wall. Using custom software, the contours were traced (see Figure 26-3, *B*) to create a three-dimensional scar reconstruction (see Figure 26-3, *C* and *D*).

Comments

The scar distribution is not typical for prior myocardial infarction, because the apical segments are completely spared. However, a scar distribution, involving in particular the basal septum and the adjacent basal anterior wall, has been previously described in patients with nonischemic dilated cardiomyopathy presenting with ventricular tachycardia.

CATHETERIZATION

The decision was made to perform ventricular tachycardia ablation to prevent recurrence of ventricular tachycardia and a potential life-threatening electrical storm. During endocardial ablation, multiple different ventricular tachycardia morphologies could be induced by programmed electrical stimulation (ventricular tachycardic cycle length 200 to 270 ms, most RBBB with inferior axis, one with RBBB and superior axis, and one with LBBB and superior

axis). An electroanatomic map of the left ventricle was created, which revealed a low bipolar voltage area in the basal anteroseptal wall with fragmented electrograms, but no late potentials. For several episodes of ventricular tachycardia, early activation was identified in the basal left ventricle, but only 1 of 11 could be abolished. Although potential ablation target sites could be identified in close proximity to the bundle of His and the proximal left bundle, radiofrequency energy applications were withheld, considering that parts of the reentry circuits may be located deep intramurally or epicardially. The patient was rescheduled for a combined endocardial and epicardial procedure.

During the same admission, the patient underwent combined endocardial and epicardial ventricular tachycardia ablation. Arteriovenous access was obtained, and subxyphoidal puncture was performed. During the procedure, low-voltage areas and fragmented electrograms were identified at the basal and mid-anteroseptal wall, both on the endocardium and the epicardium overlying the septal region and the adjacent basal anterior wall (Figure 26-4, *A* to *D*). Of note, the endocardial low unipolar voltage area was much larger than the endocardial low bipolar voltage area, suggesting a more extensive mid-myocardial or epicardial substrate. Indeed, this area corresponded to the location of an MRI-derived scar (see Figure 26-4, *E*). The epicardial low bipolar and unipolar voltage area could not be explained by epicardial fat, as demonstrated by CT-derived meshes color-coded for epicardial fat thickness (see Figure 26-4, *F*).

During the procedure a total of 17 different ventricular tachycardia morphologies could be induced (the first 9 ventricular tachycardia episodes are shown in Figure 26-5), all related to the scar in the basal septum and basal anterior wall. Several ventricular tachycardia reentry circuit isthmuses were mapped to an area in close proximity to the bundle of His or proximal left bundle. In Figure 26-6, diastolic activity and concealed entrainment are demonstrated at the right ventricular side of the septum for one of these ventricular tachycardic episodes. Despite extensive mapping at the endocardium and epicardium with radiofrequency applications limited to potential entrance or exit sites that were considered to be at safe distance from the bundle of His and left bundle, ventricular tachycardia remained inducible.

FOCUSED CLINICAL QUESTIONS AND DISCUSSION POINTS

Question

Should iatrogenic total atrioventricular block with consecutive pacing be accepted to potentially prevent ventricular tachycardia recurrence in a patient with nonischemic cardiomyopathy who has experienced a life-threatening electrical storm requiring resuscitation despite ICD therapy?

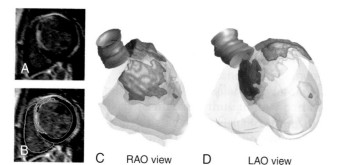

FIGURE 26-3 Based on short axis contrast-enhanced MRI slice (panel **A**) and semi-automatic detection of late enhancement (panel **B**), a 3-dimensional scar reconstruction was created (panels **C** and **D**). The core scar is displayed in red, borderzone in yellow. **LAO** denotes left anterior oblique; **RAO**, right anterior oblique.

Discussion

During right ventricular pacing the ventricles are activated relatively slowly through the myocardium, instead of fast activation through the His-Purkinje conduction system in physiologic conditions. As a result, early activated regions "prestretch" late activated regions, whereas late activated regions "poststretch" early activated regions that are already in the relaxation phase. The resulting dyssynchronous contraction pattern is less effective and may reduce ventricular function. Other potential deleterious effects of right ventricular apical pacing include left ventricular remodeling, functional mitral regurgitation, and left atrial remodeling.[8] In the Mode Selection (MOST) trial, which compared dual-chamber "physiologic" right ventricular apical to pure right ventricular apical pacing in patients with sinus node dysfunction,[6] a strong association was found between high percentages of ventricular pacing and increased rates of heart failure hospitalization. In patients with bradycardia and a normal LVEF, Yu and associates[9] demonstrated that right ventricular–apical pacing results in adverse left ventricular remodeling and a substantial reduction in the LVEF of 7.4%.

Although the adverse effects of right ventricular pacing are well-documented in patients with bradycardia and normal LVEF, only scant data exist on the effect of right ventricular pacing in patients with total atrioventricular block and moderately impaired left ventricular function in the setting of a nonischemic dilated cardiomyopathy without symptoms and signs of heart failure. In the Dual Chamber and VVI Implantable Defibrillator (DAVID) trial, patients with an implantable cardioverter-defibrillator (ICD) with LVEF 40% or less and no indication for ventricular pacing were randomized to ventricular backup pacing at 40/min or dual-chamber rate-responsive pacing at 70/min.[10] The composite end point (death or heart failure hospitalization) occurred more frequently in dual chamber–paced patients than backup-paced patients (84% vs. 73%), suggesting that deleterious effects of right ventricular pacing also may apply to patients with reduced LVEF.

Question

Should right ventricular pacing or biventricular pacing be initiated in case of total atrioventricular block after ablation of the bundle of His and left bundle with preexisting RBBB?

Discussion

In patients who are not in heart failure, without the need for ventricular pacing, insufficient data exist to support a role of biventricular pacing to improve ventricular function. In patients who require frequent ventricular pacing, however, adverse effects of right ventricular pacing may be expected, as outlined earlier. In the study by Yu and colleagues,[9] these deleterious effects could be prevented by biventricular pacing in patients with a normal LVEF who required a pacemaker because of bradycardia. In patients with an LVEF 40% or less, and an indication for ventricular pacing, the small Homburg Biventricular Pacing Evaluation (HOBIPACE) trial demonstrated biventricular pacing to be superior to right ventricular pacing in terms of left ventricular function, quality of life, and exercise capacity.[4]

This patient was considered to potentially benefit from cardiac resynchronization therapy (CRT) because female gender, nonischemic cardiomyopathy, and QRS duration greater than 150 msec consistently have been found to predict greater benefit from CRT. A positive response to CRT has been associated with a reduced risk for ventricular arrhythmia.[7] Thus biventricular instead of right ventricular apical pacing may reduce the risk for recurrent ventricular tachycardia and perhaps electrical storm.

Based on the expected negative effects of right ventricular pacing and the potential higher risk for recurrent ventricular tachycardia or electrical storm, it was decided to implant a biventricular ICD in case of total atrioventricular block.

FINAL DIAGNOSIS

Electrical storm resulted from sustained monomorphic ventricular tachycardia in this patient with nonischemic dilated cardiomyopathy, with ventricular tachycardia reentry circuit sites located in close proximity to the bundle of His and left bundle.

PLAN OF ACTION

The plan for this patient was to perform ablation at the location of the bundle of His and left bundle to abolish all ventricular tachycardia episodes and implant a biventricular ICD in case of total atrioventricular block.

INTERVENTION

All episodes of ventricular tachycardia were abolished and, as expected, complete atrioventricular block occurred. A biventricular ICD was implanted, and biventricular pacing was initiated.

OUTCOME

During 2 years of follow-up, the patient did not develop heart failure and had no recurrence of ventricular tachycardia.

Findings

After 6 months, echocardiography was repeated. The LVEF had increased from 35% to 50%, and the left ventricular end-systolic volume had decreased from 111 mL to 61 mL. Left ventricular function and dimensions were stable during 2 additional years of follow-up, and the patient remained in New York Heart Association class I. The biventricular ICD was interrogated at 6-month intervals, with no ventricular arrhythmia recorded.

Comments

The decision to perform ablation at the location of the bundle of His and left bundle to abolish all ventricular tachycardias has resulted in arrhythmia-free survival, which would have been unlikely in the case of persistent inducibility of the ventricular tachycardia. The impressive increase in LVEF and reduction in left ventricular end-systolic volume at 6-month follow-up and the lack of symptomatic heart failure during further follow-up may be the result of biventricular pacing.

Selected References

1. Arya A, Bode K, Piorkowski C, et al: Catheter ablation of electrical storm due to monomorphic ventricular tachycardia in patients with nonischemic cardiomyopathy: acute results and its effect on long-term survival, *Pacing Clin Electrophysiol* 33:1504-1509, 2010.
2. Carbucicchio C, Santamaria M, Trevisi N, et al: Catheter ablation for the treatment of electrical storm in patients with implantable cardioverter-defibrillators: short- and long-term outcomes in a prospective single-center study, *Circulation* 117:462-469, 2008.
3. Haqqani HM, Tschabrunn CM, Tzou WS, et al: Isolated septal substrate for ventricular tachycardia in nonischemic dilated cardiomyopathy: incidence, characterization, and implications, *Heart Rhythm* 8:1169-1176, 2011.
4. Kindermann M, et al: Biventricular versus conventional right ventricular stimulation for patients with standard pacing indication and left ventricular dysfunction: the Homburg Biventricular Pacing Evaluation (HOBIPACE), *J Am Coll Cardiol* 47:1927-1937, 2006.
5. Nakahara S, Tung R, Ramirez RJ, et al: Characterization of the arrhythmogenic substrate in ischemic and nonischemic cardiomyopathy implications for catheter ablation of hemodynamically unstable ventricular tachycardia, *J Am Coll Cardiol* 55:2355-2365, 2010.
6. Sweeney MO, Hellkamp AS, Ellenbogen KA, et al: Adverse effect of ventricular pacing on heart failure and atrial fibrillation among patients with normal baseline QRS duration in a clinical trial of pacemaker therapy for sinus node dysfunction, *Circulation* 107:2932-2937, 2003.
7. Thijssen J, Borleffs CJ, Delgado V, et al: Implantable cardioverter-defibrillator patients who are upgraded and respond to cardiac resynchronization therapy have less ventricular arrhythmias compared with nonresponders, *J Am Coll Cardiol* 58:2282-2289, 2011.
8. Tops LF, Schalij MJ, Bax JJ. The effects of right ventricular apical pacing on ventricular function and dyssynchrony implications for therapy, *J Am Coll Cardiol* 25(54):764-776, 2009.
9. Yu CM, Chan JY, Zhang Q, et al: Biventricular pacing in patients with bradycardia and normal ejection fraction, *N Engl J Med* 361:2123-2134, 2009.
10. Wilkoff BL, Cook JR, Epstein AE, et al: Dual-chamber pacing or ventricular backup pacing in patients with an implantable defibrillator: the Dual Chamber and VVI Implantable Defibrillator (DAVID) Trial, *JAMA* 288:3115-3123, 2002.

Prevention of Effective Cardiac Resynchronization Therapy by Frequent Premature Ventricular Contractions in a Patient with Nonischemic Cardiomyopathy

Sebastiaan R. D. Piers and Katja Zeppenfeld

Age	Gender	Occupation	Working Diagnosis
65 Years	Male	Clothing Shop Owner	Frequent Idiopathic Premature Ventricular Contractions from the Posteromedial Papillary Muscle Aggravate Symptoms of Heart Failure and Prevent Resynchronization Therapy

HISTORY

In 2002 the patient was diagnosed with Global Initiative for Chronic Obstructive Lung Disease stage II chronic obstructive pulmonary disease and in 2004 with first-degree atrioventricular block. In June 2011 he was admitted for decompensated heart failure. Echocardiography revealed a mildly dilated left ventricle, left ventricular ejection fraction (LVEF) of 20%, and grade III mitral regurgitation. Coronary angiography showed no significant coronary artery disease. Frequent premature ventricular contractions were observed during admission. Medical therapy for heart failure was initiated, and the patient was scheduled for reevaluation.

In October 2011 frequent premature ventricular contractions were reported on a 24-hour Holter monitor (28% of all QRS complexes, with one dominant morphology accounting for 99% of all premature ventricular contractions). Drug therapy with metoprolol 75 mg twice daily was not effective, sotalol was not tolerated, and metoprolol was continued.

In December 2011 the patient was readmitted for intermittent total atrioventricular block reported on a 24-hour Holter monitor. He was in New York Heart Association (NYHA) class III. On an echocardiogram, LVEF was 30%, with grade I to II mitral regurgitation. Despite discontinuation of metoprolol therapy, the total atrioventricular block became permanent. A temporary pacemaker was inserted, followed by cardiac resynchronization therapy defibrillator (CRT-D) implantation.

CURRENT MEDICATIONS

The patient was taking calcium carbasalate (Ascal) 100 mg daily, spironolactone 12.5 mg daily, simvastatin 40 mg daily, perindopril 4 mg daily, furosemide 40 mg daily, and metoprolol 50 mg twice daily.

CURRENT SYMPTOMS

The patient had marked limitation of physical activity (NYHA class III), with no chest pain or collapse.

PHYSICAL EXAMINATION

BP/HR: 125/55 mm Hg/60 bpm
Height/weight: 168 cm/72 kg
Neck veins: Not distended
Lungs/chest: Unremarkable
Heart: Holosystolic murmur, grade 2/6, loudest at the apex
Abdomen: Unremarkable
Extremities: No peripheral edema

LABORATORY DATA

Hemoglobin: 8.8 mmol/L
Hematocrit/packed cell volume: 41.9%
Mean corpuscular volume: 96 fL
Platelet count: NA
Sodium: 138 mmol/L
Potassium: 4.7 mmol/L
Creatinine: 81 μmol/L
Blood urea nitrogen: 7.5 mmol/L

ELECTROCARDIOGRAM

Findings

An electrocardiogram revealed biventricular pacing with frequent premature ventricular contractions and QRS during biventricular pacing at 160 ms (Figure 27-1). Premature ventricular contractions occurred with slightly varying morphology, all right bundle branch block (RBBB) type of morphology (defined as dominant R in precordial lead V_1), left superior axis, transition V_{4-5}.

ECHOCARDIOGRAM

Findings

An echocardiogram showed a dilated left ventricle, no hypertrophy, and an LVEF of 41%, with akinesia of the basal inferolateral wall, no left ventricular thrombus, and grade I to II mitral regurgitation, with eccentric jet along the lateral wall of the left atrium. The mechanism is likely restriction of the posterior mitral leaflet.

PHYSIOLOGIC TRACINGS

Findings

The 24-hour Holter monitor showed sinus rhythm with biventricular pacing, and frequent premature ventricular contractions (33% of all QRS complexes) were seen, 96% of which were monomorphic.

FOCUSED CLINICAL QUESTIONS AND DISCUSSION POINTS

Question

When the patient developed total atrioventricular block in December 2011, did he need biventricular pacing or would right ventricular pacing have been sufficient?

Discussion

In December 2011 the patient had marked limitation of physical activity (NYHA class III), impaired left ventricular function (LVEF 30%), grade I to II mitral valve regurgitation, and an indication for permanent ventricular pacing because of total atrioventricular block. Several studies have demonstrated the deleterious effects of chronic right ventricular pacing, which include intraventricular and interventricular mechanical dyssynchrony, ventricular dilation, and decreased LVEF. Also, right ventricular pacing may further aggravate mitral valve regurgitation,[1] which was already grade I to II at that stage, despite drug therapy. The deleterious effects on left ventricular function may be particularly important in patients who already have left ventricular dysfunction. The Homburg Biventricular Pacing Evaluation (HOBIPACE) trial

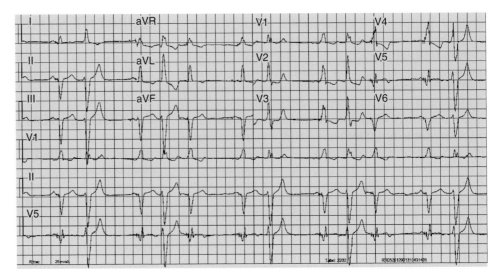

FIGURE 27-1

was the first study to compare biventricular pacing to right ventricular pacing in patients with reduced left ventricular function and a standard indication for permanent ventricular pacing.[5] Using a cross-over design, 30 patients received 3 months of right ventricular pacing and 3 months of biventricular pacing. In contrast to right ventricular pacing, biventricular pacing resulted in smaller left ventricular end-diastolic and end-systolic volumes, a higher LVEF, lower N-terminal prohormone of brain natriuretic peptide concentrations, higher maximum exercise capacity, and better quality of life. According to the current guidelines for cardiac pacing and CRT,[6] CRT may be considered in patients with reduced LVEF who require chronic pacing and in whom frequent ventricular pacing is expected. However, the evidence for this approach is limited, as indicated by the class C recommendation.

Question

Are the premature ventricular contractions likely to affect left ventricular function?

Discussion

The causal relationship between cardiomyopathy and frequent premature ventricular contractions is difficult to define because frequent premature ventricular contractions can induce cardiomyopathy, but nonischemic dilated cardiomyopathy also has been associated with frequent premature ventricular contraction occurrences. Of importance, left ventricular dysfunction induced by premature ventricular contractions may be reversible in patients without an underlying cardiomyopathy. In a study by Bogun and colleagues,[2] for example, 22 patients with frequent idiopathic premature ventricular contractions and LVEF of 50% or less underwent catheter ablation for premature ventricular contractions, after which left ventricular function normalized within 6 months in 82% of patients.[2] However, in patients in whom the underlying cardiomyopathy is causative for the premature ventricular contractions, no data are available on the effect of catheter ablation on left ventricular function. Of note, it may be difficult to differentiate between patients with a premature ventricular contraction–induced cardiomyopathy and those with premature ventricular contractions after impaired left ventricular function. The correct diagnosis may become apparent only if the left ventricular function and dimensions return to normal after successful treatment of the premature ventricular contractions by drug therapy or catheter ablation.

Indeed, in the present case, it is unclear whether the frequent premature ventricular contractions have caused cardiomyopathy or cardiomyopathy causes the ventricular extrasystoles. The lack of frequent premature ventricular contractions during the first admission for decompensated

heart failure does, however, suggest that an underlying cardiomyopathy may be the cause of the frequent premature ventricular contractions. Also, in patients with underlying cardiomyopathy, premature ventricular contractions may further depress left ventricular dysfunction. In the present case, left ventricular function improved after implantation of the CRT-D. However, the patient remained in NYHA class III, which may be due to the frequent premature ventricular contractions and ineffective biventricular pacing.

Question

Based on the 12-lead ECG, what is the most likely site(s) of origin of the premature ventricular contraction(s)? What are the implications?

Discussion

The 12-lead ECG morphology shows an RBBB-like morphology with a superior axis, suggesting an origin in the inferior left ventricle. The precordial transition in V_4 with an RS pattern in V_4 suggests that the origin may be located in the mid-inferior wall, consistent with a site of origin close to the papillary muscle. Indeed, an RBBB-like morphology with superior axis and precordial transition in lead V_{4-6} has been reported to be typical for papillary muscle arrhythmias.[3] This finding has important implications for catheter ablation. Papillary muscle arrhythmias frequently originate from deep within the muscle, which is reflected by large areas of simultaneous activation during electroanatomic mapping. Local activation times typically precede the onset of QRS by only 20 to 30 msec.[7] Origins deep in the muscle may be difficult to abolish by radiofrequency energy applications, because even irrigated tip ablation creates lesions of limited depths if the catheter is stable and in good contact. In addition, a stable position with sufficient contact force can be particularly difficult at the papillary muscle, requiring a transseptal or combined retrograde aortic and transseptal approach. Intracardiac echocardiography may be helpful in such cases.

Question

Is catheter ablation of the premature ventricular contractions indicated?

Discussion

In the European Heart Rhythm Association and Heart Rhythm Society Expert Consensus on Catheter Ablation of Ventricular Arrhythmias, catheter ablation of frequent premature ventricular contractions is recommended if presumed to cause ventricular dysfunction. As outlined earlier, premature ventricular contractions may cause ventricular dysfunction in two ways in the present case: directly, by causing (aggravating) cardiomyopathy, and indirectly, by preventing effective biventricular pacing. The potential benefits of abolishing the frequent premature ventricular contractions are likely to outweigh the potential risks in catheter ablation. Vascular complications include groin hematomas and pseudoaneurysms (~1.4%).[4] The risk for transient ischemic attacks and stroke are considered to be low (<1%) in the introduction of irrigated catheters. Tamponade occurs in approximately 0.7% of cases.

FINAL DIAGNOSIS

Persistent symptoms of heart failure occurred in this patient with CRT-D for total atrioventricular block, likely as a result of frequent premature ventricular contractions that also prevented effective biventricular pacing.

PLAN OF ACTION

The plan for this patient was catheter ablation of premature ventricular contractions.

INTERVENTION

The CRT device was set to DDD mode with right ventricular pacing only, which resulted in stable ventricular bigeminy. The premature ventricular contraction had an RBBB morphology with left superior axis and transition in V_5. The discrepancy between the precordial transition at the outpatient clinic and the laboratory may be caused by small differences in precordial lead placement. The left ventricle was accessed using a retrograde approach via the aorta. The earliest activation was mapped to a wide area around the posteromedial papillary muscle, with the

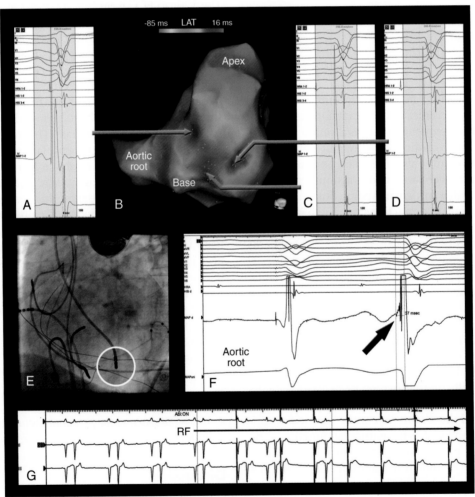

FIGURE 27-2 Electroanatomic activation map of the left ventricle color-coded for local activation time during premature ventricular contractions. The sites with earliest activation are located around the base of the papillary muscle (**B**, *red area*). The local activation times around the papillary muscle were similar (**A, C,** and **D**). Note the subtle differences in the 12-lead electrocardiogram morphology of the premature ventricular contraction, suggestive for slight alterations of the origin itself or the preferential conduction from the origin. The location of the ablation catheter at the successful ablation site on fluoroscopy is displayed in **E**. At this site, the local activation time was 37 msec before the onset of the QRS-complex (**F**). After 8 seconds, the premature ventricular contractions disappeared (**G**).

earliest electrogram occurring at 37 msec before QRS onset (Figure 27-2). Repeated radiofrequency energy applications at the same site temporarily abolished the premature ventricular contraction for only approximately 20 seconds; however, the premature ventricular contraction morphology changed to RBBB, superior axis, and transition in V_3 (with R < S in lead V_6) morphology (Figure 27-3). The earliest activation was mapped to the same area but just remote from the first site, suggesting a shift in the endocardial exit. After a few additional radiofrequency applications, the premature ventricular contractions were abolished and did not recur during a waiting period of 45 minutes. The left ventricular map during right ventricular pacing demonstrated normal bipolar (>1.50 mV) and unipolar (>8.27 mV) voltages and no abnormal electrograms (Figure 27-4). Although these findings make a compact scar in the left ventricle less likely, the presence of a subepicardial scar or diffuse fibrosis cannot be excluded.

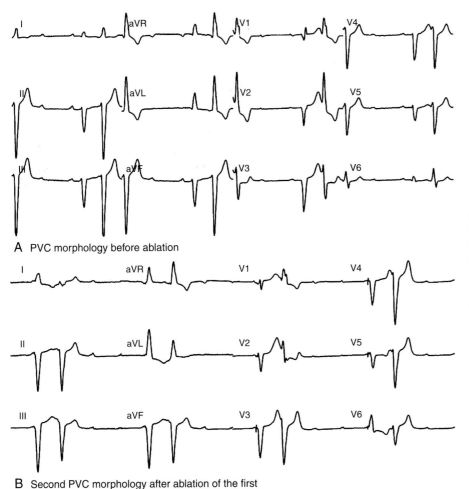

A PVC morphology before ablation

B Second PVC morphology after ablation of the first

FIGURE 27-3 After a radiofrequency application based on activation mapping of the initial premature ventricular contraction *(PCV)* morphology, a change in the 12-lead ECG morphology of the premature ventricular contractions was observed, with a dominant S wave in V_6 suggesting a shift of the PVC exit site.

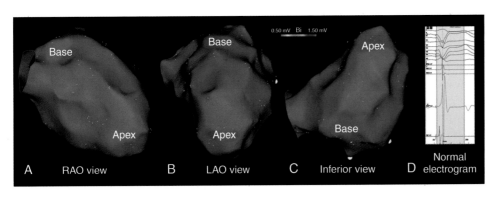

FIGURE 27-4 A to **C,** Electroanatomic map of the left ventricle during right ventricular pacing, color-coded for bipolar voltage (bipolar voltage > 1.50 mV is considered normal and displayed in *purple*). The bipolar voltages and the electrogram morphologies were normal **(D).**

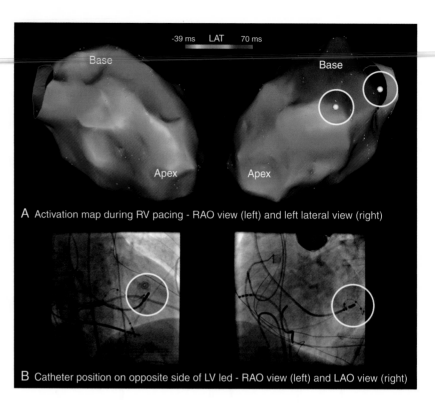

FIGURE 27-5 Electroanatomic map of the left ventricle during right ventricular pacing, now color-coded for local activation time. The sites that were opposite to the left ventricular pacing lead were identified based on fluoroscopy (**B**, *circles*) and subsequently tagged on the map (**A**, *white tags with circles in right upper panel*). The left ventricular pacing lead is located in close proximity to the latest activated site.

A Activation map during RV pacing - RAO view (left) and left lateral view (right)

B Catheter position on opposite side of LV led - RAO view (left) and LAO view (right)

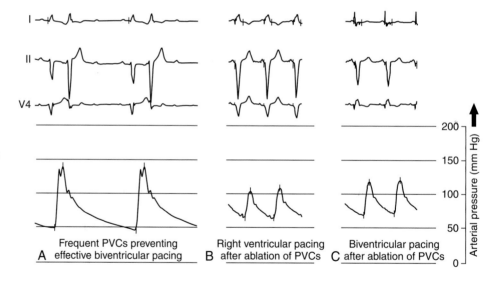

FIGURE 27-6 The frequent premature ventricular contractions (*PVCs*) before ablation did not result in significant cardiac output **(A)**. After ablation of the PVC, right ventricular and biventricular pacing resulted in an almost tripled effective heart rate (**B** and **C**). Of note, the blood pressure was higher during biventricular pacing in contrast to only right ventricular pacing.

A Frequent PVCs preventing effective biventricular pacing

B Right ventricular pacing after ablation of PVCs

C Biventricular pacing after ablation of PVCs

The left ventricular lead was located over the latest activated endocardial area during right ventricular pacing (Figure 27-5). During programmed electrical stimulation, ventricular fibrillation was induced with a basic cycle length (BCL) of 400 and three extras (230, 200, and 200 msec). Successful cardioversion was performed. The device was programmed to biventricular pacing, which was now effective and not limited by premature ventricular contractions. Ventricular pacing resulted in an almost tripled effective heart rate in contrast to that before ablation (Figure 27-6). Biventricular pacing produced higher blood pressures than only right ventricular pacing.

OUTCOME

Three months after ablation the patient had no limitation of physical activity (improvement from NYHA class III before ablation to class I after ablation). A 24-hour Holter monitor revealed that the premature ventricular contractions were reduced from 33% of all QRS complexes before ablation to less than 0.01% after ablation. Echocardiography demonstrated that the left ventricular dimensions had significantly decreased (the left ventricular end-diastolic volume from 151 to 148 mL and the left ventricular end-systolic volume from 89 to 73 mL) and the LVEF increased (from 41% before to 51% after ablation). The mitral regurgitation was still grade I to II. Therefore marked improvement in exercise capacity and significant reverse remodeling of the left ventricle had occurred, which may be the result of abolishment of the premature ventricular contractions and effective biventricular pacing.

Selected References

1. Barold SS, Ovsyshcher IE: Pacemaker-induced mitral regurgitation, *Pacing Clin Electrophysiol* 28:357-360, 2005.
2. Bogun F, Crawford T, Reich S, et al: Radiofrequency ablation of frequent, idiopathic premature ventricular complexes: comparison with a control group without intervention, *Heart Rhythm* 4: 837-863, 2007.
3. Bogun F, Desjardins B, Crawford T, et al: Post-infarction ventricular arrhythmias originating in papillary muscles, *J Am Coll Cardiol* 51:1794-1802, 2008.
4. Bohnen M, Stevenson WG, Tedrow UB, et al: Incidence and predictors of major complications from contemporary catheter ablation to treat cardiac arrhythmias, *Heart Rhythm* 8:1661-1666, 2011.
5. Kindermann M, Hennen B, Jung J, et al: Biventricular versus conventional right ventricular stimulation for patients with standard pacing indication and left ventricular dysfunction: the Homburg Biventricular Pacing Evaluation (HOBIPACE), *J Am Coll Cardiol* 47:1927-1937, 2006.
6. Vardas PE, Auricchio A, Blanc J-J, et al: Guidelines for cardiac pacing and cardiac resynchronization therapy: the Task Force for Cardiac Pacing and Cardiac Resynchronization Therapy of the European Society of Cardiology. Developed in collaboration with the European Heart Rhythm Association, *Eur Heart J* 28:2256-2295, 2007.
7. Yamada T, Doppalapudi H, McElderry HT, et al: Electrocardiographic and electrophysiological characteristics in idiopathic ventricular arrhythmias originating from the papillary muscles in the left ventricle: relevance for catheter ablation, *Circ Arrhythm Electrophysiol* 3:324-331, 2010.

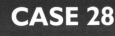

CASE 28

Atrial Fibrillation Therapy in Refractory Heart Failure

Maurizio Gasparini and Edoardo Gandolfi

Age	Gender	Occupation	Working Diagnosis
65 Years	Male	Office Worker	Hypokinetic Dilated Cardio-myopathy with Permanent Atrial Fibrillation and Severe Mitral Valve Regurgitation

HISTORY

A 65-year-old man, affected by permanent atrial fibrillation for more than 10 years experienced worsening mitral valve regurgitation and maladaptive left ventricle remodeling. These conditions led to hypokinetic dilated cardiomyopathy with severe reduction of left ventricular systolic function and repeated hospitalizations for acute heart failure (American College of Cardiology [ACC] and American Heart Association [AHA] stage C heart failure).

The patient was initially treated with drugs for heart failure, associated with a rate control strategy for atrial fibrillation with a combination of beta blockers and digoxin (carvedilol 6.25 mg twice daily; no further titration was possible because of low ventricular rate at rest and low blood pressure). A baseline electrocardiogram (ECG) showed atrial fibrillation with incomplete left bundle branch block (LBBB) and mean heart rate of 78 bpm.

He was subsequently evaluated for surgical treatment of mitral valve incompetence, which was graded as severe (angiographic grade 4+/4+, vena contracta of 0.76 cm, and regurgitant orifice area of 0.44 cm^2). The surgeon did not think surgery was the appropriate first-step therapy in this patient, with an unacceptable level of risk because of severe left ventricular dysfunction and dilation (end-diastolic diameter 70 mm, end-diastolic volume 240 mL, ejection fraction 27%).

Coronary angiography documented the absence of significant coronary stenoses.

Considering left ventricular dysfunction, LBBB, and the persistence of heart failure symptoms, notwithstanding optimized medical therapy (New York Heart Association [NYHA] class III), cardiac resynchronization therapy (CRT) was initiated. On November 2008 a biventricular CRT defibrillator (CRT-D) was implanted and beta blocker dosages were increased.

Six months after discharge the patient reported substantial improvement of symptoms (NYHA II), but experienced two inappropriate implantable cardioverter-defibrillator (ICD) shocks because of a high ventricular rate during atrial fibrillation. ICD control documented suboptimal biventricular pacing percentage during atrial fibrillation (<85%, including fusion and pseudofusion beats). Echocardiography documented a favorable remodeling of the left ventricle (LVEF 27% to 38%, end-diastolic diameter 70 to 64 mm, end-diastolic volume 240 to >200 mL, and severe to mild-moderate mitral regurgitation).

The patient underwent atrioventricular node ablation in March 2009.[1,2] Six months after atrioventricular node ablation (and 1 year after CRT implantation) complete left ventricular reverse remodeling was observed (i.e., LV end diastolic volume 140 mL, LVEF 60%, mild mitral regurgitation); the patient became completely asymptomatic.

However, during subsequent follow-up, the patient showed an extremely difficult control of the international normalized ratio (INR) therapeutic range, with frequent evidence of values above and below the therapeutic range, and had two episodes of corneal hemorrhage. For these reasons, he underwent left atrial appendage occlusion in November 2010.

In March 2011 optimal left atrial appendage occluder positioning was confirmed by cardiac computed tomography and transesophageal echocardiography and oral anticoagulation was safely discontinued.

Comments

Before CRT, titration of beta-blocker therapy was not possible because of a low ventricular rate at rest and low blood pressure. After CRT-D implantation, beta-blocker therapy was optimized, but it was insufficient to warrant complete

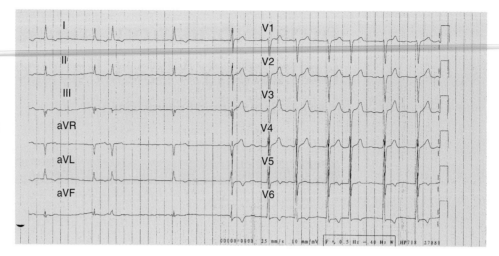

FIGURE 28-1

biventricular pacing (<85%), and two inappropriate ICD shocks on fast atrial fibrillation were observed. Clinical and instrumental benefit was consistent but incomplete.

After successful atrioventricular nodal ablation, 100% effective biventricular pacing was acheived[3] and extremely favorable left ventricular remodeling was then obtained (normal diameters, normal LVEF, and mild mitral valve regurgitation). The patient became asymptomatic.

CURRENT MEDICATIONS

The patient was taking carvedilol 25 mg twice daily, ramipril 5 mg twice daily, furosemide 12.5 mg daily, spironolactone 25 mg daily, warfarin to maintain INR of 2-3 but subsequently discontinued, and aspirin.

Comments

Optimized medical therapy for heart failure was not discontinued even after complete reverse remodeling of the left ventricle. Oral anticoagulant therapy with warfarin was managed with difficulty by the patient and provoked complications such as corneal hemorrhage. The patient then underwent successful left atrial appendage occlusion.

CURRENT SYMPTOMS

The patient was substantially asymptomatic, with dyspnea only with strenuous exertion (NYHA I).

PHYSICAL EXAMINATION

BP/HR: 125/80 mm Hg/55 bpm
Height/weight: 175 cm/73 kg
Neck veins: No jugular venous distention
Lungs/chest: Normal breathing sounds, no congestion signs

Heart: Rhythmic cardiac sounds, 1/6 systolic murmur
Abdomen: Normal
Extremities: Warm

Comments

After extremely favorable reverse remodeling, the patient was asymptomatic with good tolerance to physical activity and dyspnea only after strenuous exertion.

LABORATORY DATA

Hemoglobin: 12.9 mg/dL
Hematocrit/packed cell volume: 38.3%
Mean corpuscular volume: 92.9 fL
Platelet count: 218 × 10³/μL
Sodium: 138 mmol/L
Potassium: 3.6 mmol/L
Creatinine: 0.72 mg/dL
Blood urea nitrogen: 13.5 mg/dL

ELECTROCARDIOGRAM

Findings

The electrocardiogram showed atrial fibrillation, heart rate of 75 bpm, and incomplete LBBB (Figure 28-1). Figure 28-2 shows atrial fibrillation, biventricular pacing, fusion, and pseudofusion beats, and Figure 28-3 shows atrial fibrillation, biventricular pacing, and heart rate of 70 bpm.

Comments

After CRT-D implantation and before atrioventricular node ablation, biventricular pacing was suboptimal (see Figure 28-2). ICD counters always overestimate pacing percentage because of fusion and pseudofusion beats.

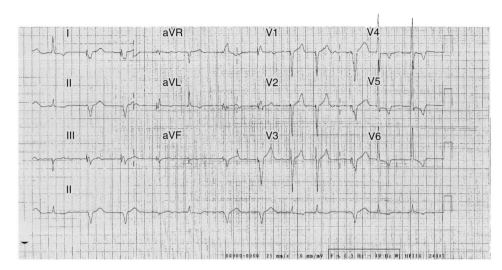

FIGURE 28-2

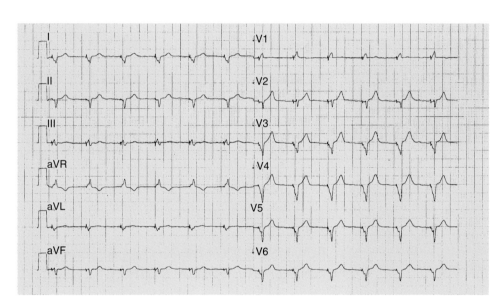

FIGURE 28-3

CHEST RADIOGRAPH

Comments

The chest radiograph before CRT shows an enlarged cardiac silhouette (Figure 28-4). After CRT and left ventricular reverse remodeling (Figure 28-5), the radiographic cardiac silhouette appears normal and was confirmed to be normal at 2 and 3 years from implantation.

ECHOCARDIOGRAM

Comments

Figures 28-6 and 28-7 show the reduction of mitral regurgitation severity after reverse remodeling obtained with combined therapy (medical, CRT, and atrioventricular node ablation).

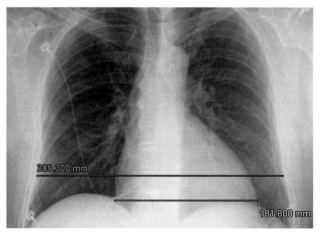

FIGURE 28-4

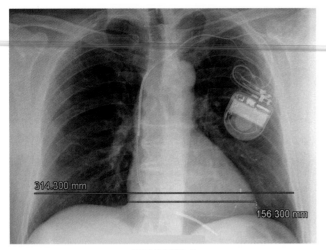

FIGURE 28-5

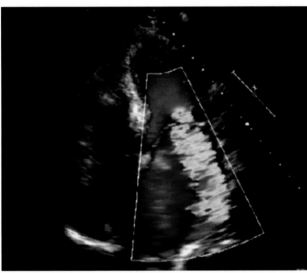

FIGURE 28-6

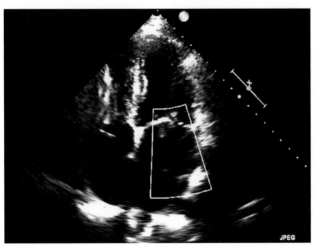

FIGURE 28-7

PHYSIOLOGIC TRACINGS

Findings

The ICD counter highlighted the achievement of near complete biventricular pacing after atrioventricular node ablation, in contrast to unacceptable pacing percentage on medical therapy alone (Figure 28-8).

COMPUTED TOMOGRAPHY

Comments

Postoperative computed tomography revealed optimal left atrial appendage occluder positioning and a complete left atrial appendage (Figure 28-9).

CATHETERIZATION

Findings

Coronary angiography documented the absence of stenotic lesions, excluding a potential ischemic component of the left ventricular dysfunction. Prolonged projections for coronary sinus anatomy visualization were obtained in preparation for left ventricular lead implantation for resynchronization therapy (Figures 28-10 and 28-11).

Comments

FOCUSED CLINICAL QUESTIONS AND DISCUSSION POINTS

Question

How can a patient with permanent atrial fibrillation and severe reduction of left ventricular systolic function associated with severe mitral regurgitation best be treated? Can surgery be considered an effective and safe option?

Discussion

In the presence of severe mitral regurgitation, LVEF usually is overestimated; the actual left ventricular systolic function could be much lower than that measured by echocardiography. In this setting, surgery may be associated with a very high operative risk and the postoperative rise in left ventricular afterload could determine much more severe left ventricular dysfunction.

Question

Can CRT be considered a valid option for this complex condition?

Report of Compass   Pagina 3

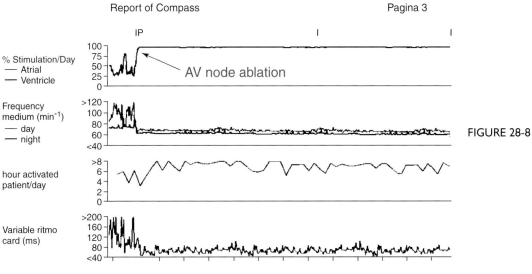

FIGURE 28-8

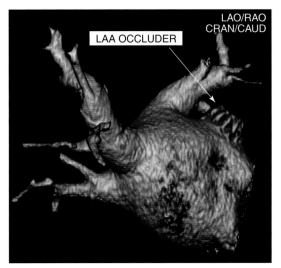

FIGURE 28-9

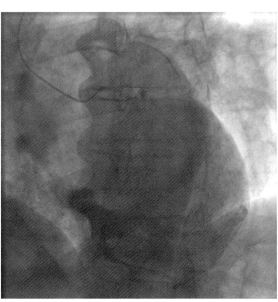

FIGURE 28-11

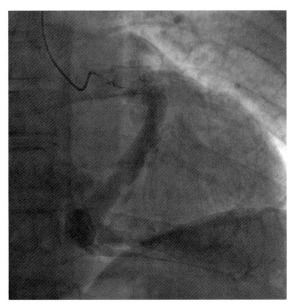

FIGURE 28-10

Discussion

Current guidelines for CRT do not provide a class I recommendation for CRT in patients with heart failure who are in atrial fibrillation, even though evidence exists of benefits similar to those in patients in sinus rhythm,[3,4] particularly if atrioventricular node ablation is performed. In a patient with atrial fibrillation and mitral regurgitation that can be ascribed to left ventricular dyssynchrony resulting from LBBB and adverse left ventricular remodeling, causing a tenting of valve leaflets, CRT is a treatment option that appears to focus on the origin of the problem. Reversal of dyssynchrony and left ventricular reverse remodeling can be associated with a significant reduction of mitral regurgitation.

The extremely favorable outcome in this patient appears to confirm the pathophysiologic explanation of functional mitral regurgitation.

Question

Is atrioventricular node ablation necessary to maximize CRT benefit in patients with atrial fibrillation and heart failure?

Discussion

The evidence of the need for maximization of biventricular pacing percentage to optimize CRT outcome is now confirmed by several studies[5,6] and two meta-analyses.[7] Drug therapy alone is rarely able to cause a dromotropic effect on the atrioventricular node sufficient to permit complete or near complete biventricular pacing, especially during effort. Biventricular pacing percentages derived from ICD counters are always overestimated because of fusion and pseudofusion beats.

Atrioventricular node ablation is the only procedure able to block atrioventricular node conduction in every condition and allow complete biventricular pacing.

FINAL DIAGNOSIS

The patient was diagnosed with ACC and AHA stage B heart failure. He had normal systolic function and normal left ventricle diameters and volumes.

PLAN OF ACTION

The patient was to undergo clinical evaluation, echocardiogram, and ICD interrogation every 6 months. He was provided devices for remote transtelephonic transmission of domestic ICD interrogation.

INTERVENTION

The patient underwent left atrial appendage occluder implantation, warfarin discontinuation, introduction of aspirin and clopidogrel, and subsequent clopidogrel discontinuation. Indetermined ASA assumption.

OUTCOME

The patient experienced maintenance of left ventricular function remodeling through CRT and heart failure medications.

Selected References

1. Gasparini M, Auricchio A, Regoli F, et al: Four-year efficacy of cardiac resynchronization therapy on exercise tolerance and disease progression: the importance of performing atrioventricular junction ablation in patients with atrial fibrillation, *J Am Coll Cardiol* 48:734-743, 2006.
2. Gasparini M, Auricchio A, Metra M, et al: Long-term survival in patients undergoing cardiac resynchronization therapy: the importance of performing atrio-ventricular junction ablation in patients with permanent atrial fibrillation, *Eur Heart J* 29:1644-1652, 2008.
3. Kaszala K, Ellenbogen KA: Role of cardiac resynchronization therapy and atrioventricular junction ablation in patients with permanent atrial fibrillation, *Eur Heart J* 32:2344-2346, 2011.
4. Brignole M, Botto G, Mont L, et al: Cardiac resynchronization therapy in patients undergoing atrioventricular junction ablation for permanent atrial fibrillation: a randomized trial, *Eur Heart J* 32:2420-2429, 2011.
5. Koplan BA, Kaplan AJ, Weiner S, et al: Heart failure decompensation and all-cause mortality in relation to percent biventricular pacing in patients with heart failure: is a goal of 100% biventricular pacing necessary? *J Am Coll Cardiol* 53:355-360, 2009.
6. Hayes DL, Boehmer JP, Day JD, et al: Cardiac resynchronization therapy and the relationship of percent biventricular pacing to symptoms and survival, *Heart Rhythm* 8:1469-1475, 2011.
7. Ganesan AN, Brooks AG, Roberts-Thomson KC, et al: Role of AV nodal ablation in cardiac resynchronization in patients with coexistent atrial fibrillation and heart failure: a systematic review, *J Am Coll Cardiol* 59:719-726, 2012.

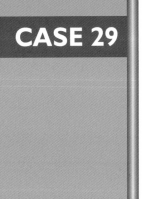

CASE 29

Cardiac Resynchronization Therapy Defibrillator Implantation in Atrial Fibrillation

Erlend G. Singsaas and Kenneth Dickstein

Age	Gender	Occupation	Working Diagnosis
76 Years	Male	Retired Florist	Heart Failure and Atrial Fibrillation with Rapid Ventricular Rate

HISTORY

Since 1980 this patient was treated periodically with venosections as a result of hemochromatosis. He had received medical therapy for hypertension since 1985 and was diagnosed with hypertensive nephropathy in 1994. He had a non-Q anterior myocardial infarction in 1996, with following postinfarction angina pectoris.

The patient was hospitalized in 2004 for unstable angina pectoris. A coronary angiogram demonstrated triple vessel disease, and he successfully underwent coronary artery bypass surgery.

In 2011 he was admitted to hospital because of a paroxysm of atrial fibrillation, which converted spontaneously to sinus rhythm during the stay.

During late winter 2012 the patient experienced increasing exercise intolerance and fatigue. He had no chest pain. He developed pitting edema of the lower extremities, which soon extended above his knees, and he had noticed intermittent palpitation. He had episodes of orthopnea, causing him to sleep sitting in a chair at night.

He was admitted to hospital on April 13, 2012 with signs of congestive heart failure. An electrocardiogram (ECG) showed atrial fibrillation with rapid ventricular response, left bundle branch block (LBBB), and QRS width of approximately 160 ms. An echocardiogram the next day demonstrated a dilated left ventricle with an end-diastolic diameter of 66 mm and obvious dyssynchronous contractility. The left ventricular ejection fraction (LVEF) was reduced, at 20%, because of apical akinesia and inferior and lateral hypokinesia. No significant valvular disease was present. Chest radiography on admission showed cardiac enlargement and signs of pulmonary congestion.

The patient was initially treated with an intravenous diuretic, a beta blocker, an angiotensin receptor blocker, and a mineralocorticoid receptor antagonist, but the uptitration of these drugs was limited by hypotension, renal failure, and a tendency to hyperkalemia. The patient had to be periodically treated with dobutamine and dopamine, and he also received an infusion of levosimendan. Atrial fibrillation and periodic atrial flutter with insufficient rate control was initially treated with amiodarone, and direct current cardioversion was planned. Preparing for cardioversion, transesophageal echocardiography was performed, revealing a thrombus in the left atrial appendage. This finding caused cardioversion to be postponed and amiodarone to be discontinued because rhythm conversion was considered unfavorable in this situation. Instead, digoxin was added. On this treatment the patient showed some improvement clinically and the LVEF increased to approximately 30%, but he was still symptomatic even at minimal physical exertion.

The patient was monitored on telemetry, which revealed short runs of nonsustained ventricular tachycardia. On April 25, 2012, with the patient still hospitalized and on telemetry, a run of ventricular tachycardia degenerated into ventricular fibrillation. He was immediately resuscitated and defibrillated into atrial fibrillation and suffered no neurologic sequelae. Amiodarone was commenced. He had no signs of acute coronary syndrome.

CURRENT MEDICATIONS

The patient was taking bumetanide 4 mg daily, candesartan 16 mg daily, carvedilol 12.5 mg twice daily, hydrochlorothiazide 25 mg daily, spironolactone 12.5 mg daily, atorvastatin 40 mg daily, warfarin 5 mg daily, amiodarone 200 mg twice daily, and digoxin 0.125 mg daily.

Comments

The patient was intolerant to angiotensin-converting enzyme inhibitors because of cough.

CURRENT SYMPTOMS

The patient was experiencing dyspnea and was in New York Heart Association (NYHA) class III. He also had peripheral edema and ventricular tachyarrhythmia.

Comments

The patient had symptomatic heart failure despite optimal pharmacologic therapy.

PHYSICAL EXAMINATION

BP/HR: 134/70 mm Hg/60-110 bpm, irregular
Height/weight: 179 cm/100 kg
Neck veins: Not congested
Lungs/chest: Bilateral basal crepitations
Heart: Systolic murmur grade 2/6; punctum maximum at the right sternal border, radiating to the neck
Abdomen: Modest central obesity
Extremities: Pitting edema just above the ankles

LABORATORY DATA

Hemoglobin: 10 g/dL
Hematocrit/packed cell volume: 35%
Mean corpuscular volume: 94 fL
Platelet count: 187 × 10³/µL

Sodium: 133 mmol/L
Potassium: 4.7 mmol/L
Creatinine: 210 µmol/L
Blood urea nitrogen: 32 mmol/L

Comments

The patient's estimated glomerular filtration rate was 26 mL/min.

ELECTROCARDIOGRAM

Findings

The ECG obtained on admission on April 13, 2012 showed atrial fibrillation with a ventricular rate of 80 to 130 bpm, LBBB, and a QRS width of approximately 160 ms (Figures 29-1 and 29-2). The ECG obtained after cardiac resynchronization therapy defibrillator (CRT-D) implantation on May 10, 2012 demonstrated a high degree of biventricular pacing, despite atrial dysrhythmia. The QRS width was approximately 120 ms (Figures 29-3 and 29-4).

CHEST RADIOGRAPH

Findings

A chest radiograph was obtained on admission. Sternal circlages were noted on the frontal and lateral views. The cardiothoracic ratio was 0.57, which indicated cardiac enlargement. Mild enlargement of the perihilar vessels and Kerley B lines were seen, suggestive of pulmonary congestion (Figures 29-5 and 29-6).

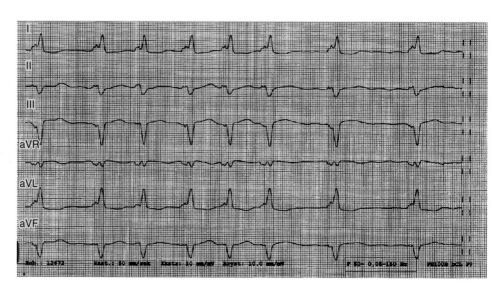

FIGURE 29-1

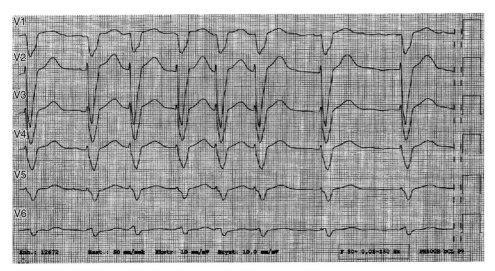

FIGURE 29-2

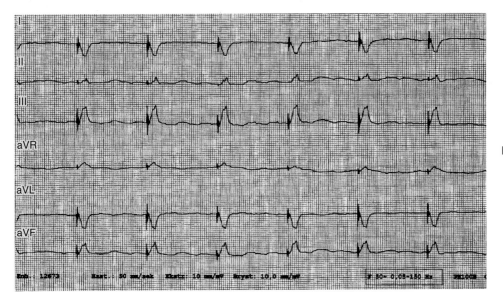

FIGURE 29-3

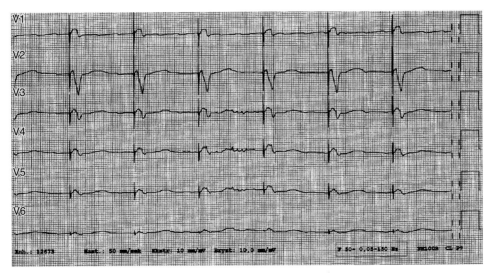

FIGURE 29-4

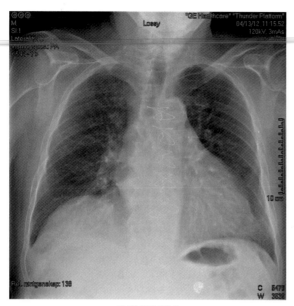

FIGURE 29-5

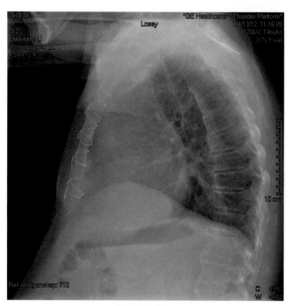

FIGURE 29-6

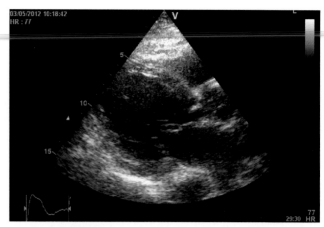

FIGURE 29-7   See *expertconsult.com* for video.

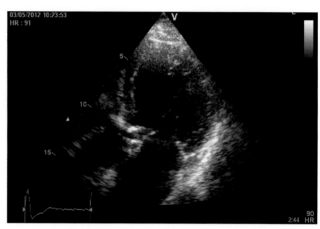

FIGURE 29-8   See *expertconsult.com* for video.

The LVEF was estimated to be 30% (apical two-chamber view not shown). Signs of aortic sclerosis were present, but no stenosis was seen (Figure 29-8).

ECHOCARDIOGRAM

Findings

On the parasternal long-axis echocardiographic view, recorded May 3, 2012, the left ventricle was dilated, with an end-diastolic diameter of 65 mm. The interventricular septum and posterior wall diameters measured 11 mm, and the left atrial anteroposterior diameter was 41 mm (Figure 29-7).

Findings

On the apical view, recorded May 3, 2012, left ventricular contraction was dyssynchronous, with apical hypokinesia.

FOCUSED CLINICAL QUESTIONS AND DISCUSSION POINTS

Question

Does the presence of atrial fibrillation influence the indication for CRT in patients with heart failure?

Discussion

The evidence for the beneficial effects of CRT in patients in heart failure with sinus rhythm is solid. In the current European Society of Cardiology (ESC) guidelines,[9] CRT holds a class IA recommendation in patients remaining symptomatic despite optimal pharmacologic therapy, with an LVEF of 30% to 35% or less and a QRS duration of 130 to 150 ms or greater. Most randomized controlled trials evaluating the effects of CRT in heart failure excluded patients in permanent atrial fibrillation, and data regarding CRT in patients with heart failure and atrial fibrillation are mostly observational. The major challenge for CRT in atrial fibrillation is to obtain a sufficient degree of biventricular pacing, because the positive effect of CRT on outcomes depends on this.

ESC guidelines[9] state that CRT may be considered in patients with permanent atrial fibrillation, NYHA class III, a QRS width of 120 ms or greater, and an LVEF 35% or less. In addition, according to the guidelines, it is mandatory that the patient is pacemaker dependent as a result of an intrinsic slow ventricular rate, the ventricular rate is well controlled (≤60 bpm at rest and ≤90 bpm on exercise) (class IIB, level C), or pacemaker dependency is induced through atrioventricular node ablation (class IIA, level B). The use of CRT in patients with heart failure and atrial fibrillation is well established in clinical practice; the ESC Cardiac Resynchronization Therapy Survey in 140 European centers demonstrated that 23% of all devices were implanted in patients with atrial fibrillation.[1]

Question

Should atrioventricular node ablation be performed routinely following CRT implantation in patients with permanent atrial fibrillation?

Discussion

To ensure maximal efficacy of CRT, it is crucial to obtain a high degree of biventricular pacing. Measures must be taken so the percentage of biventricular pacing is increased to the highest possible level, because a further reduction in mortality has been observed if biventricular pacing is achieved in excess of 98% of all ventricular beats.[5] Even moderately increased ventricular rates during atrial fibrillation pose a substantial challenge for the delivery of efficient CRT, because rapid and irregular intrinsic conduction will compete with pacing.

A subgroup analysis of patients with permanent atrial fibrillation in the Resynchronization/Defibrillation for Ambulatory Heart Failure Trial (RAFT)[6] failed to demonstrate any significant beneficial effect of CRT-D compared to defibrillators without CRT in patients with apparently good rate control. It is important to note that only 34.3% of CRT-treated patients achieved biventricular pacing greater than 95%. Atrioventricular node ablation in patients with atrial fibrillation and CRT theoretically leads to 100% biventricular pacing. Observational data have shown that CRT and atrioventricular node ablation in patients with atrial fibrillation improves left ventricular function and functional capacity to a degree similar to that in patients with CRT with sinus rhythm[4] and significantly reduces cardiovascular and all-cause mortality in

contrast to pharmacologic rate control in patients with atrial fibrillation treated with CRT.[2,3] These observations need to be confirmed in randomized controlled trials. Although a rare event, pacemaker failure is possible after atrioventricular node ablation. Accordingly, it is important to continuously evaluate rate control and efficacy of CRT in patients with atrial fibrillation and consider atrioventricular node ablation if the degree of biventricular pacing is insufficient.

Question

When assessing a patient with CRT and atrial fibrillation, does the device counter accurately quantify the degree of biventricular pacing?

Discussion

Kamath and colleagues[8] examined patients with CRT and permanent atrial fibrillation with a 12-lead Holter monitor and demonstrated that CRT device counters overestimate the degree of biventricular pacing delivered. Although device counters reported greater than 90% biventricular pacing, in some patients substantial proportions of these beats were fusion or pseudofusion beats. Only effectively paced patients with a low degree of incomplete capture responded to CRT. This emphasizes the importance of using Holter evaluation when assessing amount of capture, because device interrogation alone may not reveal the presence of ineffective biventricular pacing.

Question

Does evidence show that chronic right ventricular pacing and atrioventricular node ablation for atrial fibrillation can be prevented by CRT?

Discussion

Atrioventricular node ablation and pacemaker implantation is a treatment option for the subgroup of patients with therapy-resistant atrial fibrillation, allowing efficient control of ventricular rate. On the other hand, the subsequent delayed and dyssynchronous left ventricular contraction during chronic right ventricular pacing may lead to left ventricular dysfunction and adverse remodeling. CRT represents a more appealing, physiologic method of pacing that does not result in adverse left ventricular remodeling. A recent meta-analysis of five randomized controlled trials involving a total of 686 patients examined whether CRT is superior to right ventricular pacing in this setting.[10] CRT resulted in a significant reduction in heart failure hospitalizations, but did not significantly influence mortality, compared to right ventricular pacing. Further studies are necessary to address the effect on clinical outcomes of CRT versus right ventricular pacing in patients with preserved left ventricular function.[7,10]

FINAL DIAGNOSIS

The patient was in NYHA class III, with heart failure resulting from ischemic cardiomyopathy, an LVEF of 20%, atrial fibrillation, and LBBB, with a QRS duration of 160 ms. Ventricular fibrillation was resuscitated.

PLAN OF ACTION

CRT-D implantation was planned for this patient. In addition, when he had undergone adequate anticoagulation, at least 3 weeks after the discovery of left atrial thrombus, a transesophageal echocardiogram was to be performed. If thrombus could be ruled out, he would undergo direct current cardioversion attempting to restore sinus rhythm, with subsequent pharmacologic rhythm control. Later, follow-up would focus on trying to maximize the degree of biventricular pacing achieved. If failure to restore sinus rhythm or recurrence of therapy-resistant atrial arrhythmia causing insufficient CRT delivery should occur, atrioventricular node ablation would be considered.

INTERVENTION

The patient underwent CRT-D implantation on May 4, 2012. Sinus rhythm was restored with amiodarone. When the patient was examined at the outpatient clinic on June 11, 2012, the CRT device counter reported biventricular pacing in 94% of all beats and some brief episodes of atrial fibrillation. To optimize CRT delivery, atrioventricular pace and sense delay were reduced from 200 to 180 ms and 150 to 130 ms, respectively.

At a subsequent outpatient visit on September 11, 2012, acceptable values were found, with 97% biventricular pacing, 0% atrial fibrillation burden, some ventricular ectopic beats, and no runs of ventricular tachycardia.

OUTCOME

In September 2012 the patient was in NYHA class II, had no peripheral edema, and had experienced substantial improvement in clinical status. Echocardiography at this time demonstrated an LVEF of 40% and left-ventricular end-diastolic diameter of 59 mm, which also was an improvement over findings in examinations before the CRT implantation.

Selected References

1. Dickstein K, Bogale N, Priori S, et al: The european cardiac resynchronization therapy survey, *Eur Heart J* 30:2450-2460, 2009.
2. Ganesan AN, Brooks AG, Roberts-Thomson KC, et al: Role of AV nodal ablation in cardiac resynchronization in patients with coexistent atrial fibrillation and heart failure, *J Am Coll Cardiol* 59:719-726, 2012.
3. Gasparini M, Auricchio A, Metra M, et al: Long-term survival in patients undergoing cardiac resynchronization therapy: the importance of performing atrio-ventricular junction ablation in patients with permanent atrial fibrillation, *Eur Heart J* 29: 1644-1652, 2008.
4. Gasparini M, Auricchio A, Regoli F, et al: Four-year efficacy of cardiac resynchronization therapy on exercise tolerance and disease progression, *J Am Coll Cardiol* 48:734-743, 2006.
5. Hayes DL, Boehmer JP, Day JD, et al: Cardiac resynchronization therapy and relationship of percent biventricular pacing to symptoms and survival, *Heart Rhythm* 8:1469-1475, 2011.
6. Healey JS, Hohnloser SH, Exner DV, et al: Cardiac resynchronization therapy in patients with permanent atrial fibrillation: results from the Resynchronization for Ambulatory Heart Failure Trial (RAFT), *Circ Heart Fail* 5:566-570, 2012.
7. Jensen-Urstad M: Should all patients undergoing atrioventricular junction ablation receive cardiac resynchronization therapy? *Europace* 14:1383-1384, 2012.
8. Kamath GS, Cotiga D, Koneru JN, et al: The utility of 12-lead Holter monitoring in patients with permanent atrial fibrillation for the identification of nonresponders after cadiac resynchronization therapy, *J Am Coll Cardiol* 53:1050-1055, 2009.
9. McMurray JJV, Adamopoulos S, Anker SD, et al: ESC guidelines for the diagnosis and treatment of acute and chronic heart failure 2012, *Eur Heart J* 33:1787-1847, 2012.
10. Stavrakis S, Garabelli P, Reynold DW: Cardiac resynchronization therapy after atrioventricular junction ablation for symptomatic atrial fibrillation: a meta-analysis, *Europace* 14:1490-1497, 2012.

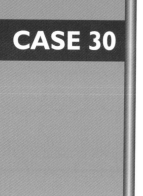

CASE 30

Up and Down in Device Therapy

Beat Andreas Schaer and Christian Sticherling

Age	Gender	Occupation	Working Diagnosis
79 Years	Male	Retired	Right Ventricular Pacing–Induced Impaired Ejection Fraction

HISTORY

The patient underwent bypass surgery (left internal mammary artery to left anterior descending artery and saphenous vein graft to distal right coronary artery) 13 years previously. Three months later, routine Holter electrocardiogram (ECG) monitoring revealed asymptomatic episodes of second-degree and third-degree atrioventricular block. The patient refused pacemaker implantation because of lack of symptoms.

In December 2002 the patient developed dyspnea (New York Heart Association [NYHA] class II). Another 24-hour ECG showed not only high-degree atrioventricular block but also sinus bradycardia. A dual-chamber pacemaker was implanted in February 2003. Follow-up was uneventful, and right ventricular pacing was reported to be almost 100%.

In December 2005 angiography was performed for atypical chest pain and a slight increase in dyspnea. No significant stenosis was present, but his left ventricular ejection fraction (LVEF) had decreased to 25%. Therefore an upgrade to a cardiac resynchronization therapy defibrillator (CRT-D) was carried out in February 2006.

In May 2007 the patient was free from dyspnea and echocardiography showed a normal LVEF of 73%.

The patient remained asymptomatic, and no arrhythmias, apart from paroxysmal atrial fibrillation, were recorded in the implantable cardioverter-defibrillator (ICD) memory. In July 2011 the battery was depleted (elective replacement indicator). Another echocardiogram confirmed a preserved LVEF of 60%. The patient was in NYHA class I. During VVI pacing with 30 bpm, no intrinsic ventricular activity is present.

CURRENT MEDICATIONS

The medications the patient was taking in February 2003 were atorvastatin 10 mg daily and aspirin. In February 2006 he was taking ramipril 7.5 mg daily, metoprolol 50 mg twice daily, torsemide 10 mg daily, atorvastatin 20 mg daily, and aspirin. In July 2011 he was taking ramipril 7.5 mg daily, metoprolol 50 mg twice daily, torsemide 10 mg daily, simvastatin 80 mg daily, and warfarin.

CURRENT SYMPTOMS

The patient had no angina, dyspnea, or peripheral edema.

PHYSICAL EXAMINATION

BP/HR: 115 over 75/72
Height/weight: 181 cm/108 kg, body mass index 33
Neck veins: Normal
Lungs/chest: Normal
Heart: Normal heart sounds
Abdomen: Normal
Extremities: No peripheral edema

LABORATORY DATA

Hemoglobin: 115/75 mg Hg
Hematocrit/packed cell volume: 47%
Mean corpuscular volume: 93 fL
Platelet count: 219 × 10³/μL
Sodium: 143
Potassium: 4.1
Creatinine: 98 μmol/L
Blood urea nitrogen: 8 mmol/L

ELECTROCARDIOGRAM

Findings

The electrocardiogram revealed atrioventricular sequential pacing, paced QRS complex at 168 ms, and positive findings in lead V_1 (Figure 30-1).

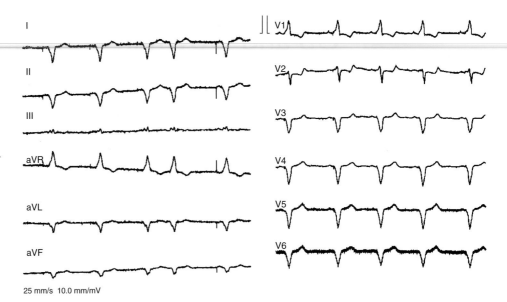

FIGURE 30-1 12-Lead electrocardiogram with cardiac resynchronization therapy "on."

25 mm/s 10.0 mm/mV

ECHOCARDIOGRAM

Findings

The echocardiogram showed the patient's left ventricular end-diastolic volume to be 110 mL, left ventricular end-systolic volume of 43 mL, an LVEF of 60%, left ventricular mass index of 120 g/m^2, and delta P over tidal volume of 15 mm Hg.

FOCUSED CLINICAL QUESTIONS AND DISCUSSION POINTS

Question

Is a downgrade to a CRT pacemaker (CRT-P) an option to consider in this case?

Discussion

No guidelines or randomized trials have addressed this question. Also, no studies evaluated patient preferences in such situations. Cardiologists who hold the opinion "once ICD, always ICD" will perform ICD generator replacement. The reasons downgrading was chosen in this case are as follows:

1. If this patient would present now with a normal LVEF and third-degree atrioventricular block, he would receive a VDD or DDD pacemaker, because no data support "prophylactic" CRT implantation in this situation. In addition, no indication exists for ICD.
2. In a 2011 paper from our group,[3] subgroup analysis of patients with a CRT-D and a primary prevention indication showed that only 1 in 46 patients whose LVEF improved to greater than 35% experienced

ICD therapy beyond the first year (single episode antitachycardia pacing delivered for ventricular tachycardia) during a mean follow-up of 35 months. Device replacement was performed in 22 patients after a mean of 43 months. In none of the 8 patients who had not previously received ICD therapies were ICD therapies observed during an additional follow-up of mean 27 months.
3. Even though the patient most probably will not need ICD therapy, he still has a risk for inappropriate therapy. This risk is approximately 8% in patients with coronary artery disease with a primary prevention indication and a mean follow-up of 30 months.[4] Even if an ICD would be programmed with a cutoff rate of greater than 230 bpm, considerable risk still exists for noise sensing because of lead fracture.

Question

Is downgrading to CRT-P or DDD pacing an option in this patient?

Discussion

Given the fact that the most likely cause for impaired left ventricular function and heart failure in this patient is dyssynchrony induced by right ventricular pacing, downgrading to CRT-P or DDD seems to not be a good idea. In addition, the difference in cost between a DDD device and a CRT-P device is much smaller than between CRT-P and CRT-D.

Question

Is reducing heart failure medication an option to consider in this patient?

Discussion

This patient's condition is obviously much better than before CRT implantation, regarding both LVEF and symptoms. However, the reason for this is unclear (e.g., biventricular stimulation, improved heart failure medication after CRT-D implantation, natural course, teetotalism). Therefore therapy with the angiotensin-converting enzyme inhibitor should be continued. The dosage of the diuretic can be reduced, as long as the patient takes his weight on a regular basis. No evidence shows that beta blockers in patients with normal LVEF improve their prognosis, so the dosage might be reduced or even stopped. On the other hand, if the patient tolerates it, why change a winning strategy?

Question

Should noninvasive stress testing or coronary angiography be done before a treatment decision is made?

Discussion

In nonischemic cardiomyopathy, no stress testing would be indicated. This patient has ischemic heart disease, but is free from angina since the coronary artery bypass graft performed 13 years previously. As long as an ICD is implanted, the patient is potentially protected from deleterious effects of severe ischemia or myocardial infarction, that is, ventricular fibrillation. Apart from treatment of risk factors, no intervention can reduce the risk for infarction, not even percutaneous coronary intervention. However, in patients with stable coronary artery disease, the annual risk[2] for myocardial infarction (~1.5%) or cardiovascular death (~1%) is very low. To exclude severe ischemia as a potential trigger of ventricular fibrillation, myocardial perfusion scintigraphy or stress echocardiography would be the best option (class IIA, level B).[1] In the case of a positive test, coronary angiography should be performed and the stenosis(es) treated. However, this would not change our attitude toward downgrading to CRT-P.

FINAL DIAGNOSIS

The patient was diagnosed with chronic right ventricular pacing–induced impairment of LVEF.

PLAN OF ACTION

The decision was made to upgrade to CRT-D.

INTERVENTION

Downgrade to CRT-P was performed after recovery of LVEF and no arrhythmias during a follow-up of 65 months. Twelve months after downgrading, no ventricular arrhythmias were documented in the CRT-P memory, but he was in atrial fibrillation and cardioversion was suggested.

OUTCOME

The outcome in this patient was favorable.

Selected References

1. Fox K, Garcia MA, Ardissino D, et al: Task Force on the Management of Stable Angina Pectoris of the European Society of Cardiology; ESC Committee for Practice Guidelines (CPG). Guidelines on the management of stable angina pectoris: executive summary: The Task Force on the Management of Stable Angina Pectoris of the European Society of Cardiology, *Eur Heart J* 27:1341-1381, 2006.
2. Fox KM: Efficacy of perindopril in reduction of cardiovascular events among patients with stable coronary artery disease: randomised, double-blind, placebo-controlled, multicentre trial (the EUROPA study), *Lancet* 362:782-788, 2003.
3. Schaer BA, Osswald S, Di Valentino M, et al: Close connection between improvement in left ventricular function by cardiac resynchronization therapy and the incidence of arrhythmias in cardiac resynchronization therapy-defibrillator patients, *Eur J Heart Fail* 12:1325-1332, 2010.
4. Schaer B, Sticherling C, Szili-Torok T, et al: Impact of left ventricular ejection fraction for occurrence of ventricular events in defibrillator patients with coronary artery disease, *Europace* 13:1562-1567, 2011.

Resumption to Sinus Rhythm After Cardiac Resynchronization Therapy in a Patient with Long-Lasting Persistent Atrial Fibrillation

Maurizio Gasparini and Luca Poggio

Age	Gender	Occupation	Working Diagnosis
81 Years	Male	Retired	Ischemic Dilatative Cardiomyopathy with Long-Lasting Persistent Atrial Fibrillation

HISTORY

An 81-year-old patient with type 2 diabetes and hypertension as cardiovascular risk factors sought treatment because of effort-related dyspnea (New York Heart Association [NYHA] class III) and presyncopal episodes. A complete cardiologic assessment was performed. On the baseline electrogram (ECG), atrial fibrillation with incomplete left bundle branch block (LBBB) was found; at transthoracic echocardiography, dilatative cardiomyopathy with reduced left ventricular ejection fraction (LVEF 25%) was the main finding, together with a moderate left atrial dilation (anteroposterior diameter 51 mm) and moderate mitral regurgitation. A 24-hour Holter ECG recording also was performed that evidenced atrial fibrillation with a mean ventricular rate of 90 bpm and no pathologic pauses. Medical therapy was optimized, but in a few months no improvement was observed. The patient therefore received a biventricular implanted cardioverter-defibrillator (ICD) (no atrial lead was implanted because atrial fibrillation was considered permanent).

Six months later, LVEF was slightly improved (30%) and no changes were found in left atrial dimension and mitral regurgitation. Electronic device control also was done, and a suboptimal biventricular pacing percentage was found (82%, Figure 31-1) because of the high rate of atrial fibrillation with spontaneous atrioventricular conduction. No clinical changes were observed. These findings were considered secondary to lack of biventricular full-time pacing, and the patient underwent atrioventricular junction ablation. After 3 months of full-time biventricular stimulation (Figure 31-2), further improvement in LVEF was observed (from 30% to 40%), along with mitral regurgitation and left atrial diameter reduction. The patient reported clinical improvement (no further presyncopal episodes, NYHA class IIB). Surprisingly, at baseline ECG, regular sinus activity was found. The issue was whether to proceed with system upgrade by atrial lead implantation.

Comments

After ICD implantation, only slight instrumental benefit was observed without any clinical improvement. This was due to suboptimal biventricular pacing percentage, because biventricular devices are known to need almost full-time pacing to be effective. We therefore decided to perform atrioventricular node ablation, following which approximately 100% of biventricular pacing was obtained. The positive left ventricular remodeling induced by pacing led to an initial improvement in LVEF and the patient's symptoms. Improving cardiac contractility and ventricular output, thus reducing filling pressure, may have played an important role in reducing atrial stretching, atrial pressure, and, subsequently, left atrial dimensions, removing one of the principal causes of atrial fibrillation. Moreover, mitral regurgitation was reduced as a result of resynchronization therapy. These may be the reasons why sinus rhythm was restored.

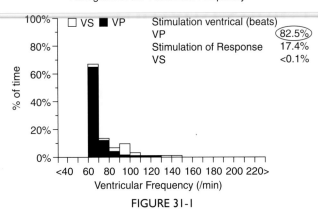

Histogram of the Ventricular Frequency

FIGURE 31-1

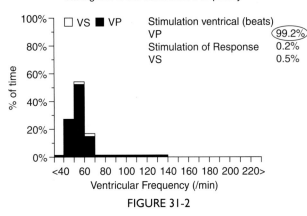

Histogram of the Ventricular Frequency

FIGURE 31-2

CURRENT MEDICATIONS

The patient was taking carvedilol 9.375 mg twice daily, furosemide 25 mg once daily, warfarin 5 mg based on international normalized ratio values, ramipril 5 mg once daily, digoxin 0.125 mg once daily, and amiodarone 200 mg once daily.

Comments

The patient was taking optimal medical therapy for heart failure; an angiotensin-converting enzyme inhibitor and a beta blocker were not fully titrated because of low blood pressure values. Amiodarone was administered even though atrial fibrillation was thought to be permanent as a rate control drug, because carvedilol and digoxin together were not enough. Of course, warfarin also was administered.

CURRENT SYMPTOMS

The patient was in NYHA class IIB, showing improvement after atrioventricular node ablation. Nevertheless, moderate effort-related dyspnea persisted. Despite advanced age, the patient normally engaged in moderate physical activity.

Comments

Improved cardiac contractility, left ventricular reverse remodeling, and reduced filling pressure provided by biventricular pacing, in the presence of optimal medical therapy and after atrioventricular node ablation, led to a better functional class. However, lack of atrial contractility resulting primarily from atrial fibrillation and then desynchronized atrial and ventricular activities once sinus rhythm was restored may have contributed to symptoms patient still reported.

PHYSICAL EXAMINATION

BP/HR: 110/70 mm Hg
HR: 70 bpm
Height/weight: 170 cm/75 kg
Neck veins: Normal jugular veins
Lungs/chest: Normal breath sounds, no signs of congestion
Heart: Rhythmic heart sounds, 1/6 holosystolic murmur
Abdomen: No pathologic findings
Extremities: Warm

Comments

Even in the presence of a desynchronized atrial activity, no signs of congestive heart failure were found, thanks to biventricular pacing–induced improvements. Auscultatory findings related to mitral regurgitation were present.

LABORATORY DATA

Hemoglobin: 14.9 mg/dL
Hematocrit/packed cell volume: 42.9%
Mean corpuscular volume: 96 fL
Platelet count: 155 × 10³/µL
Sodium: 138 mmol/L
Potassium: 4.7 mmol/L
Creatinine: 1.1 mg/dL
Blood urea nitrogen: 18 mg/dL

Comments

Laboratory findings in this patient have always been normal, particularly renal function and electrolytes.

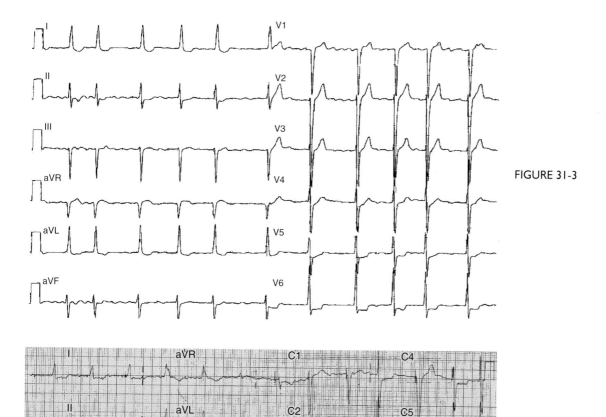

FIGURE 31-3

FIGURE 31-4

ELECTROCARDIOGRAM

Findings

Figure 31-3 shows the baseline ECG, atrial fibrillation with mean ventricular response of 90 bpm, and incomplete left bundle branch block. Figure 31-4 shows the ECG obtained after ICD implantation, showing biventricular pacing with underlying atrial fibrillation; some spontaneously conducted beats are visible. Figure 31-5 shows ECG obtained after atrioventricular junction ablation. Full-time biventricular pacing with underlying atrial fibrillation can be seen. Figure 31-6 is an ECG showing biventricular pacing with underlying desynchronized sinus rhythm, obtained 3 months after atrioventricular junction ablation. Figure 31-7 shows the ECG performed after atrial lead implantation, showing atrial tracked biventricular pacing.

Comments

The figures show electrocardiographic evolution, from the beginning to the three-lead system.

CHEST RADIOGRAPH

Findings

Figure 31-8 presents the chest radiograph obtained after atrial lead implantation.

Comments

No pleural effusion and only a few signs of congestion are present after 3 months of full-time biventricular pacing. The atrial lead had been implanted the previous day.

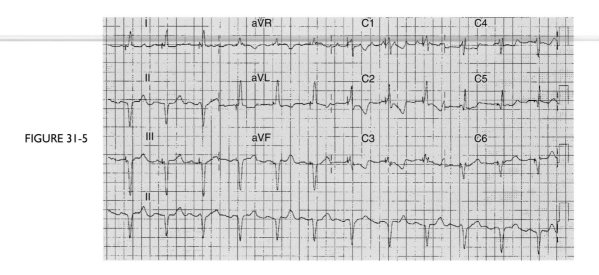

FIGURE 31-5

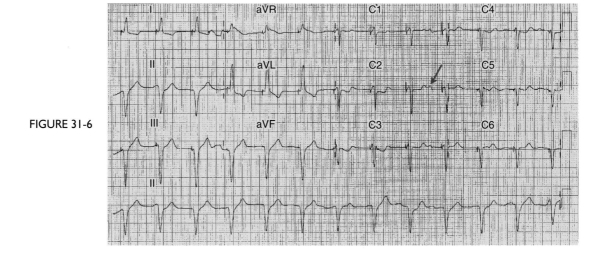

FIGURE 31-6

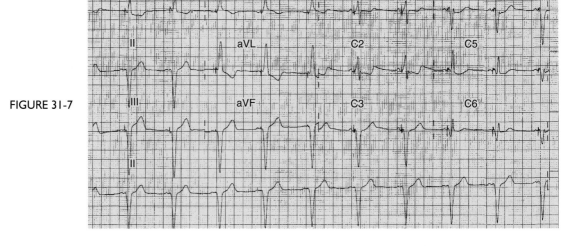

FIGURE 31-7

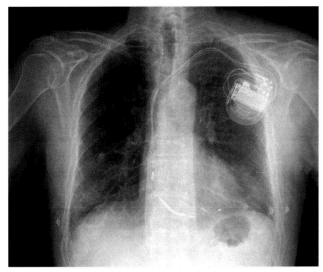

FIGURE 31-8

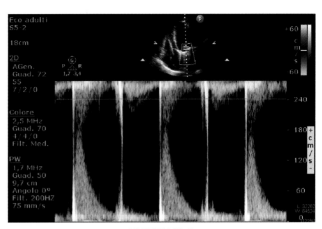

FIGURE 31-9

EXERCISE TESTING

The patient's 6 Minute Walk Test (6MWT) before ICD implantation was 250 m. His 6MWT at the time of atrioventricular node ablation (6 months after implantation) was 270 m. At the time sinus rhythm resumption was discovered (3 months after atrioventricular junction ablation), his 6MWT was 350 m. At 3 months after atrial lead implantation, his 6MWT was 400 m.

Comments

No functional class improvement occurred after biventricular ICD implantation. An improvement was achieved only after atrioventricular node ablation by obtaining 100% biventricular stimulation. Further improvement was obtained after atrial lead implantation.

ECHOCARDIOGRAM

Findings

The echocardiogram obtained before ICD implantation showed a LVEF of 25%, end-diastolic diameter of 65 mm, left atrium diameter of 51 mm, and moderate mitral regurgitation (2+, vena contracta 0.55 cm, and regurgitant orifice area 0.29 cm^2).

Comments

Baseline echocardiography, showing reduced left ventricular systolic function. Left atrial and ventricular dilation were also present, leading to secondary mitral regurgitation.

Findings

The echocardiogram obtained 6 months after ICD implantation revealed a LVEF of 30%, end-diastolic diameter of 62 mm; left atrium diameter of 50 mm; and moderate mitral regurgitation (2+, vena contracta 0.51 cm, and regurgitant orifice area 0.28 cm^2).

Comments

Because of insufficient biventricular pacing, only a small instrumental improvement was observed.

Findings

The echocardiogram obtained 3 months after atrioventricular junction ablation showed a LVEF of 40%, end-diastolic diameter of 58 mm, left atrium diameter of 45 mm, and moderate mitral regurgitation (2+, vena contracta 0.37 cm, and regurgitant orifice area 0.24 cm^2).

Comments

A few months after atrioventricular node ablation, left atrial and ventricular reverse remodeling led to an improvement of systolic function and a reduction in left atrial and ventricular diameters. Secondary mitral regurgitation decreased thereafter.

Findings

The echocardiogram obtained 6 months after atrial lead implantation (Figure 31-9) showed a LVEF of 50%, end-diastolic diameter of 55 mm, left atrium diameter of 43 mm, and mild mitral regurgitation (1+, vena contracta 0.29 cm, and regurgitant orifice area 0.19 cm^2).

Comments

Restoring synchronized atrioventricular activity led to an almost normal LVEF; the left atrium and left ventricle diameters were only slightly higher than normal, and mitral regurgitation also was reduced.

FOCUSED CLINICAL QUESTIONS AND DISCUSSION POINTS

Question

Is biventricular device implantation the right choice in a patient with left ventricular dysfunction and permanent atrial fibrillation (or is it supposed to be)?

Discussion

Most of the studies evaluating the clinical benefits of biventricular pacing have been conducted in patients with sinus rhythm.[3] However, most patients with reduced LVEF may present one or more episodes of paroxysmal or persistent atrial fibrillation, which may become permanent, despite pharmacologic treatment, as a result of concomitant left atrial remodeling. Patients with atrial fibrillation are usually older, carry more comorbidities, and may present lower pacing percentages because of spontaneous conduction. Implanting a biventricular device improves myocardial contractility and ventricular output, reduces filling pressures, and reduces possible associated secondary mitral regurgitation, all of which may lead to the stopping of both atrial and ventricular remodeling (and sometimes also reversing it),[2] thus reducing the likelihood of developing atrial arrhythmias or increasing their number of atrial arrhythmias. Atrioventricular node ablation should be considered in the presence of suboptimal biventricular pacing percentages. Sinus rhythm resumption is not meant to be the goal; however, it is clear that most patients experience clinical benefits and left atrial and ventricular reverse remodeling by biventricular pacing, thus making it a good choice in this patient population.

Question

Is sinus rhythm resumption predictable in this type of patient?

Discussion

A 2010 study conducted on patients with permanent atrial fibrillation and cardiac resynchronization therapy (CRT) found clinical predictors to be left ventricular end-diastolic diameter less than 65 mm, narrow CRT paced QRS (<150 ms), left atrial diameter less than 50 mm, and atrioventricular junction node ablation.[1] In our patient, all four criteria were satisfied, thus making this event quite likely.

Question

Is atrial lead implantation a good choice? Is an actual improvement expected?

Discussion

Once sinus rhythm resumption was found, the patient was in NYHA class IIB with a moderately reduced LVEF (40%). It is reasonable to think that restoring normal atrioventricular synchrony, thus making atria regularly fill ventricles and avoid retrograde flow (which may raise pulmonary pressures) could lead to a further clinical and instrumental improvement.[1] Despite advanced age, considering the active lifestyle and usual level of physical activity, the clinical benefit expected by adding a new lead would be worth the risks related to a new invasive procedure.

FINAL DIAGNOSIS

The final diagnosis in this patient is ischemic dilatative cardiomyopathy with permanent atrial fibrillation, left ventricular function recovery, clinical improvement, and sinus rhythm restoration after atrioventricular junction ablation and full-time biventricular pacing.

PLAN OF ACTION

The plan for this patient was right atrial lead implantation to further improve the patient's symptoms.

INTERVENTION

The intervention performed was right atrial lead implantation.

OUTCOME

The patient was in NYHA class I. Six months after system upgrade, an almost normalized LVEF 50% was found, together with mild left atrial and ventricular dilation and mild mitral regurgitation.

Findings

The procedure resulted in improvement in both clinical and instrumental data.

Comments

Restoring atrioventricular synchrony in the presence of atrial tracked biventricular pacing led to an almost normalized heart function.

Selected References

1. Gasparini M, Steinberg JS, Arshad A, et al: Resumption of sinus rhythm in patients with heart failure and permanent atrial fibrillation undergoing cardiac resynchronization therapy: a longitudinal observational study, *Eur Heart J* 31:976-983, 2010.
2. Kies P, Leclercq C, Bleeker GB, et al: Cardiac resynchronisation therapy in chronic atrial fibrillation: impact on left atrial size and reversal to sinus rhythm, *Heart* 92:490-494, 2006.
3. Vardas PE, Auricchio A, Blanc JJ, et al: European Society of Cardiology. Guidelines for cardiac pacing and cardiac resynchronization therapy: The Task Force for Cardiac Pacing and Cardiac Resynchronization Therapy of the European Society of Cardiology. Developed in Collaboration with the European Heart Rhythm Association, *Eur Heart J* 28:2256-2295, 2007.

SECTION 7

Management of Complications of Cardiac Resynchronization Therapy

Guide Wire Fracture During Cardiac Resynchronization Therapy Implantation and Subsequent Management

Marta Acena, François Regoli, Matteo Santamaria, and Angelo Auricchio

Age	Gender	Occupation	Working Diagnosis
65 Years	Male	Ex-banker, Retired for 2 Years	Guide Wire Fracture During Implantation of Cardiac Resynchronization Therapy Device

HISTORY

A 65-year-old man with ischemic dilated cardiomyopathy, already treated by stenting of the anterior interventricular coronary artery and then by coronary artery bypass graft surgery, received a dual-chamber implantable cardioverter-defibrillator (ICD) 4 years previously for primary prevention of sudden cardiac death. At that moment the electrocardiogram (ECG) showed an incomplete left bundle branch block (LBBB) with a QRS duration of less than 120 ms. The patient was later admitted to the hospital because of acute heart failure decompensation. During the last 6 months his functional capacity progressively declined (currently New York Heart Association [NYHA] class III) despite medical therapy optimization.

Comments

This patient showed progressive worsening of his clinical condition likely atributable to the underlying heart disease (coronary artery disease) and progression of ventricular conduction delay (LBBB on surface ECG).

CURRENT MEDICATIONS

The patient was taking torasemide 10 mg daily, bisoprolol 5 mg daily, spironolactone 25 mg daily, enalapril 10 mg twice daily, aspirin 100 mg daily, and insulin.

CURRENT SYMPTOMS

The patient was experiencing dyspnea at rest, orthopnea, and edema of the inferior extremities.

PHYSICAL EXAMINATION

BP/HR: 107/60 mm Hg/77 bpm
Height/weight: 175 cm/72 kg
Neck veins: Jugular vein distention
Lungs/chest: Pulmonary crepitations
Heart: Regular cardiac tones without murmurs
Abdomen: Soft and painless
Extremities: Edema of the lower extremities

LABORATORY DATA

Hemoglobin: 12.8 g/dL
Hematocrit/packed cell volume: 38%
Platelet count: $320 \times 10^3/\mu L$
Sodium: 136 mmol/L
Potassium: 3.8 mmol/L
Creatinine: 121 mmol/L

ELECTROCARDIOGRAM

Findings

The ECG revealed a heart rate of 76 bpm, a sinus rhythm with a PR interval of 190 ms, and a complete LBBB with a QRS duration of 136 ms (Figure 32-1).

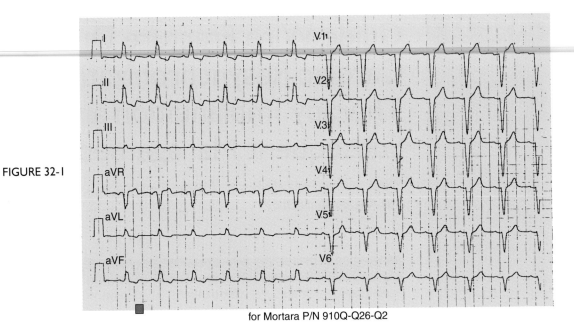

FIGURE 32-1

for Mortara P/N 910Q-Q26-Q2

ECHOCARDIOGRAPHY

Findings

The echocardiogram documented a dilated left ventricle (end-diastolic volume 210 mL) with a severe reduction of the ejection fraction (18%); moderate mitral and tricuspid regurgitation; restrictive mitral flow pattern; left atrium dilation (59 mm); moderate pulmonary arterial hypertension (60 mm Hg); and right ventricle with normal dimensions and function.

CATHETERIZATION

A coronary angiography was performed showing three-vessel disease with patency of all the coronary grafts (left internal mammary artery on anterior interventricular coronary artery, right internal mammary artery on right coronary artery, double venous grafts on circumflex artery).

FOCUSED CLINICAL QUESTIONS AND DISCUSSION POINTS

Question

What would be the next step for the treatment of the heart failure in this patient?

Discussion

An upgrade to a resynchronization device is indicated. The patient already had a dual-chamber ICD for the treatment of ventricular arrhythmias. He had normal chronotropic competence with a preserved day–night variability, and the spontaneous QRS width was 136 ms with a LBBB pattern. The benefit of cardiac resynchronization therapy (CRT) in patients with heart failure with a QRS duration of 120 ms or greater, a LBBB pattern, and an ejection fraction of 35% or less has been demonstrated in many important multicenter trials, such as the Comparison of Medical Therapy, Pacing, and Defibrillation in Chronic Heart Failure (COMPANION)[1] and Cardiac Resynchronization in Heart Failure (CARE-HF) studies.[2] Their consistent results have been summarized in the European Society of Cardiology guidelines of 2013, with an indication of class I and level of evidence B (LBBB pattern, QRS 120-150 ms) for the patient described in this report.[3]

Question

Which position should be considered a target pacing site—a more apical position, a midvein position, or a basal position?

Discussion

A midvein or, better, basal position is the best choice. The impact of the left ventricular lead position on outcome in patients randomized to CRT defibrillator implant in the Multicenter Automatic Defibrillator Implantation Trial–Cardiac Resynchronization Therapy (MADIT-CRT)[4] study has been reported. The study showed that left ventricular leads positioned in the apical region were associated with an unfavorable outcome, suggesting that this lead location should be avoided in CRT.

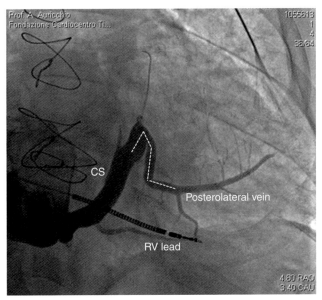

FIGURE 32-2

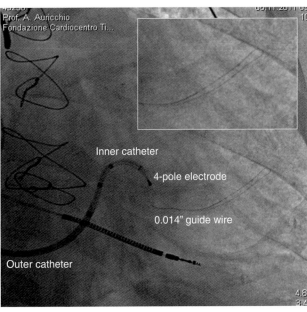

FIGURE 32-3

INTERVENTION

After ICD removal, a 9-French introducer was placed in the left subclavian vein. Then a preshaped 8-French catheter (CPS DirectTM SL II Slittable Outer Guide Catheter with Integrated Valve, St. Jude Medical, St. Paul, Minn.) was used to cannulate the coronary sinus. However, a partial angiography of the coronary sinus was possible because of a prominent valve impeding visualization of the distal section of the coronary sinus. A large and long posterolateral vein presenting a very sharp take-off and a secondary 90-degree curve was visualized (Figure 32-2).

A preshaped inner catheter (CPS Aim SL Slittable Inner Catheter with Integrated Valve, St. Jude Medical) with a 90-degree angle was advanced into the guiding catheter supported by a 0.30-inch Terumo guide wire (Somerset, NJ), and both were gently advanced into the coronary sinus. A successful coronary sinus branch vein subselection was finally achieved. Then a 0.014-inch hydrophilic stiff guide wire (Whisper ES, Abbott, Abbott Park, Ill.) was placed distally into the coronary vein and looped into the same coronary vein (Figure 32-3). The extra-support guide wire was chosen to stretch the tortuous vein and to provide support for a preshaped left ventricular pacing electrode.

A four-pole preshaped electrode (Quartet, St. Jude Medical) was chosen to provide good mechanical stability while allowing significant pacing flexibility by electronic selection of the most appropriate pacing electrodes. The preshaped lead adapted well to the vein tortuosity and diameter; the tip of the lead was placed in the distal section of the vein. Each of the electrodes was tested, and phrenic nerve stimulation was obtained by pacing only the most distal electrode.

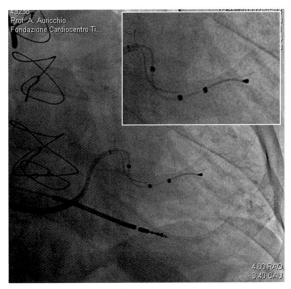

FIGURE 32-4

During the retraction maneuver of the guide wire, the distal part (about 4 cm) was suddenly broken off (Figure 32-4) while the proximal extremity of the fragment protruded into the lumen of the main body of the coronary sinus (Figure 32-5).

Question

What is the next step—leave the wire inside the venous system or try to remove it?

Perforation of the coronary vein may occur, but interference with sensing or pacing might be expected because the guide wire fragment is made of conducting material.

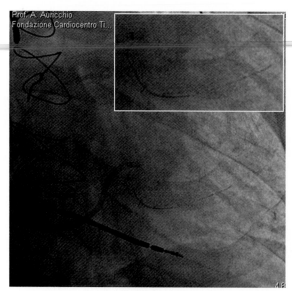

FIGURE 32-5

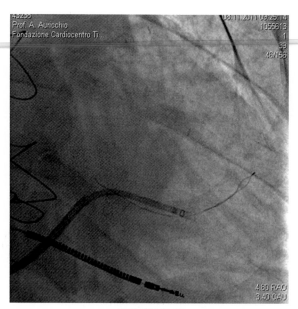

FIGURE 32-7

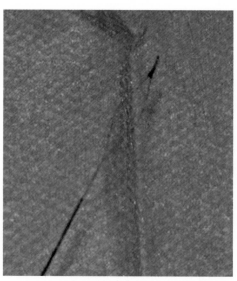

FIGURE 32-6

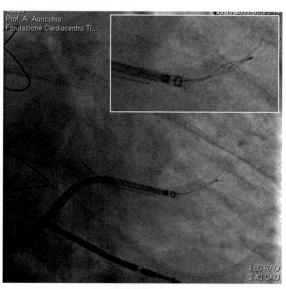

FIGURE 32-8

Several tools are available for removal of foreign material from the circulation system. Retrieval of the guide wire was planned. An endovascular system device (Micro Elite Snare, Radius Medical Technologies, Aston, Mass.) was used that is specifically designed for the retrieval and manipulation of foreign bodies in the cardiovascular system (Figure 32-6). The ultra-small 0.014-inch profile permits delivery through catheters, eliminating the need for exchanges, reducing patient trauma, and saving valuable procedure time. The highly torqueable shaft design allows greater control and maneuverability for better access to distal targets, and the smooth helical loop blends the advantage of a smaller overall distal profile with a longer reach than right-angle loops. Moreover, the radiopaque loop enhances visualization and identification of the device's capture area and sheath location.

The snare was advanced beyond the distal end of the broken wire (Figure 32-7) and pulled back to surround the wire fragment (Figure 32-8). Then, the snare with the captured guide wire fragment was carefully retrieved into the guiding catheter (Figure 32-9). After successful removal, a new guide wire was deployed and the quadripolar permanent pacing lead finally implanted (Figure 32-10). A chest radiograph shows the position of each electrode and the absence of pneumothorax (Figures 32-11 and 32-12).

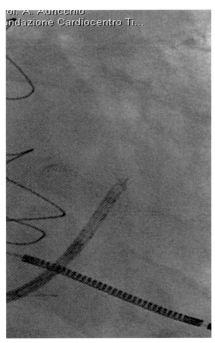

FIGURE 32-9

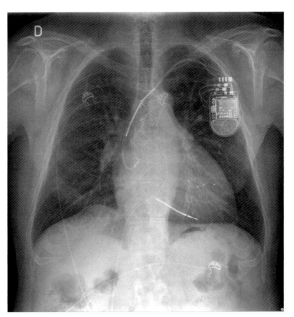

FIGURE 32-11

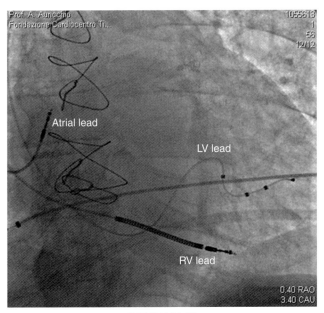

FIGURE 32-10

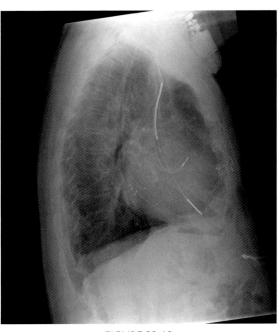

FIGURE 32-12

OUTCOME

The patient was scheduled for a 1-month follow-up after device implantation. The sensed and paced and impedance parameters resulted in within-normal range, and the percentage of biventricular stimulation was 98%. The surgical wound was in a good state of healing and had no signs of infection. From the clinical point of view the patient reported a significant improvement in functional capacity (NYHA class II).

Comments

Do not loop the guide wire within the same vein, to avoid the risk for kinking or fracture.

Selected References

1. Bristow M, Saxon L, Boehmer J, et al: for the Comparison of Medical Therapy, Pacing and Defibrillation in Heart Failure (COMPANION). Cardiac resynchronization therapy with or without an implantable defibrillator in advanced chronic heart failure, *New Engl J Med* 350:2140-2150, 2004.
2. Cleland J, Daubert J, Erdmann E, et al: for the CARE-HF study investigators. Longer-term effects of cardiac resynchronization therapy on mortality in heart failure [the Cardiac REsynchronization-Heart Failure (CARE-HF) trial extension phase], *Eur Heart J* 27:1928-1932, 2006.
3. Brignole M, Auricchio A, Baron-Esquivias G, et al: 2013 ESC guidelines on cardiac pacing and cardiac resynchronization therapy, *Europace* 15(8):1070-1118, 2013.
4. Moss A, Hall W, Cannom D, et al: Cardiac-resynchronization therapy for the prevention of heart-failure events, *N Engl J Med* 361:1329-1338, 2009.

A Difficult Case of Diaphragmatic Stimulation

Bernard Thibault and Paul Khairy

Age	Gender	Occupation	Working Diagnosis
70 Years	Female	Retired	Phrenic Nerve Stimulation After Cardiac Resynchronization Therapy Implant

HISTORY

A 70-year-old woman with nonischemic cardiomyopathy, with New York Heart Association (NYHA) class III symptoms, a left ventricular ejection fraction (LVEF) of 22%, left ventricular end-diastolic dimension of 72 mm, QRS duration of 170 ms, and a left bundle branch block pattern (Figure 33-1) was referred for possible cardiac resynchronization therapy defibrillator (CRT-D) implantation.

Comorbidities included hypertension, type 2 diabetes, dyslipidemia, obesity, and paroxysmal atrial fibrillation well controlled with amiodarone. Workup revealed moderate diffuse coronary artery disease (<40% narrowing), a 6-Minute Walk Test distance of 342 m, and a peak Vo_2 of 13.2 mL/kg/min.

CURRENT MEDICATIONS

Medical therapy was optimized with carvedilol 6.25 mg twice daily, fosinopril 20 mg daily, furosemide 60 mg daily, spironolactone 25 mg daily, amiodarone 200 mg daily, acetylsalicylic acid 80 mg daily, and dose-adjusted warfarin for a target INR 2.0–3.0.

FIRST INTERVENTION

Implantation of the CRT-D device was uneventful. However, the angiogram was of poor quality because of obesity and thus provided little guidance. It was not repeated given the patient's underlying renal dysfunction (i.e., glomerular filtration rate ≤40 mL/min). Three coronary sinus branches were blindly identified. The anterior and posterior branches had septal courses. The bipolar left ventricular lead (1056K, St. Jude Medical, St. Paul, Minn.) was positioned in a long, large-caliber midlateral

branch after confirming the absence of phrenic nerve capture despite high-output (10 V) pacing. Left ventricular pacing thresholds were 3.4 V for the distal electrode and 2.2 V for the proximal ring, both with the right ventricular coil as anode.

Outcome

The following morning, the patient reported symptoms consistent with diaphragmatic stimulation. On interrogation, the best left ventricular capture threshold was 3.75 V (proximal ring to right ventricular coil) and both pacing electrodes elicited phrenic nerve capture at voltages down to 3.25 V. It was impossible to identify a pacing configuration with a left ventricular threshold lower than that of the phrenic nerve capture threshold. The lead appeared to be well positioned on chest radiograph.

SECOND INTERVENTION

A second intervention was therefore performed to rectify the situation. Other potential coronary sinus branches could not be identified. The anterior branch was of small caliber and too far septal and the proximal posterior branch (middle cardiac vein) was deemed unsuitable. A new 1056K left ventricular lead was implanted in the same venous branch. Phrenic nerve capture occurred from both electrodes, but only on deep inspiration. The problem was far less pronounced in a very proximal position. The lead was not wedged into place in the hope that its spiral design would ensure stability.

Outcome

The following day, good functioning of the CRT system was confirmed by interrogation. Nevertheless, the patient presented 1 month later with a dislodged left ventricular lead positioned deeply and anteriorly in the main coronary sinus. Epicardial implantation was considered and discussed, but declined by the patient.

Five years later, she remained with NYHA class III symptoms and had four heart failure–related hospitalizations within 8 months. Her left ventricular systolic function remained stable (LVEF 20%; left ventricular end-diastolic dimension 70 mm). Meanwhile, she developed new-onset complete atrioventricular block and became dependent on right ventricular pacing.

Two months previously, she presented with recurrent presyncope. Intermittent ventricular oversensing (Figure 33-2) resulting from electrical failure of a Riata lead (St. Jude Medical) was documented. The left ventricular lead remained nonfunctional. In addition, a high atrial lead threshold was noted, with a P wave of approximately 1.0 mV.

THIRD INTERVENTION

A backup temporary pacemaker was immediately implanted. Lead extraction was subsequently performed, with all three leads removed by simple traction. Three new leads were implanted, including a quadripolar deeply inserted left ventricular lead (Quartet, St. Jude Medical) in the same lateral branch of the coronary sinus (Figure 33-3). Phrenic nerve capture was present (down to 3.5 V) with the three proximal electrodes but not the distal electrode.

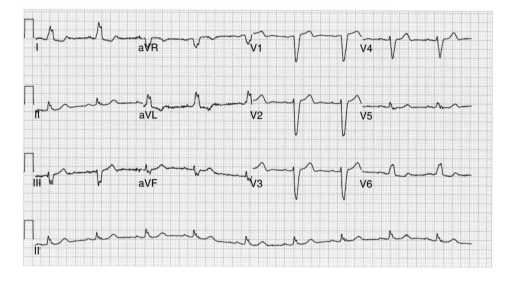

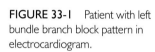

FIGURE 33-1 Patient with left bundle branch block pattern in electrocardiogram.

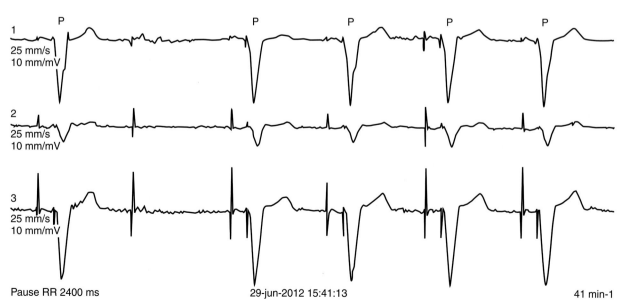

Pause RR 2400 ms — 29-jun-2012 15:41:13 — 41 min-1

FIGURE 33-2 Patient with intermittent ventricular oversensing resulting from electrical failure of a Riata lead (St. Jude Medical).

Outcome

Despite a lack of improvement in LVEF, the patient has not been hospitalized for heart failure during 12 months of follow-up. Effective biventricular pacing is shown in Figure 33-4. On interrogation, a left ventricular pacing threshold of 2.25 V was obtained from the distal electrode in a unipolar configuration (D_1 to right ventricular coil). No phrenic nerve stimulation occurred with up to 7.5 V. For the three other electrodes, the left ventricular pacing threshold was either too high (>4.0 V for the

P_4 ring) or higher than the phrenic nerve capture threshold (M_2 and M_3).

FOCUSED DISCUSSION POINTS

Diaphragmatic contraction resulting from phrenic nerve capture is observed in up to 20% to 30% of CRT implants.[1-3] Unfortunately, it is not always apparent at the time of implantation and may develop in the hours or days that follow. In most instances, the problem may be overcome by reprogramming pacing configurations, pacing output, or both. In a minority of patients, the only options are to reintervene or inactivate left ventricular pacing.[4,6]

Several options are available for reintervention. The new quadripolar left ventricular leads present an attractive solution, offering greater flexibility in programming options.[5,10,11] As this case demonstrates, quadripolar leads also may be considered when standard bipolar left ventricular leads fail to deliver effective CRT.[9] Additional options include implanting a bipolar active fixation lead more proximally within the coronary sinus (e.g., right ventricular lead or Attain Starfix left ventricular lead [Medtronic, Minneapolis, Minn.]). However, such an option may complicate future extraction interventions.[7] Finally, alternative approaches to implanting a left ventricular lead may be considered, either endocardially by a transseptal approach or epicardially by surgical access. In weighing potential options, results from the REPLACE study should be considered, which indicate that the highest risk for device infection occurs in the context of CRT system revision.[8] In this case, a second procedure was initially attempted but failed. The system was entirely revised 6 years later, when reintervention was required for right ventricular lead dysfunction.

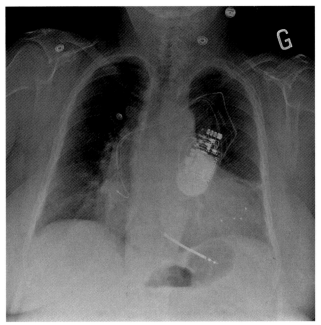

FIGURE 33-3 A posteroanterior chest radiograph is shown depicting the position of the three implanted leads, including a quadripolar left ventricular lead (Quartet, St. Jude Medical) deeply inserted in the lateral branch of the coronary sinus.

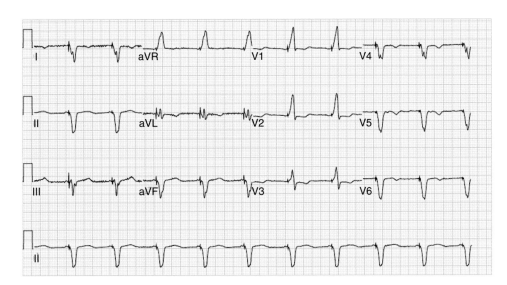

FIGURE 33-4 Patient with effective biventricular pacing shown in electrocardiogram.

Selected References

1. Biffi M, Boriani G: Phrenic stimulation management in CRT patients: are we there yet? *Curr Opin Cardiol* 26:12-16, 2011.
2. Biffi M, Exner DV, Crossley GH, et al: Occurrence of phrenic nerve stimulation in cardiac resynchronization therapy patients: the role of left ventricular lead type and placement site, *Europace* 15:77-82, 2013.
3. Biffi M, Moschini C, Bertini M, et al: Phrenic stimulation: a challenge for cardiac resynchronization therapy, *Circ Arrhythm Electrophysiol* 2:402-410, 2009.
4. Champagne J, Healey JS, Krahn AD, et al: The effect of electronic repositioning on left ventricular pacing and phrenic nerve stimulation, *Europace* 13:409-415, 2011.
5. Forleo GB, Mantica M, Di Biase L, et al: Clinical and procedural outcome of patients implanted with a quadripolar left ventricular lead: early results of a prospective multicenter study, *Heart Rhythm* 11:1822-1828, 2012.
6. Klein N, Klein M, Weglage H, et al: Clinical efficacy of left ventricular pacing vector programmability in cardiac resynchronization therapy defibrillator patients for management of phrenic nerve stimulation and/or elevated left ventricular pacing thresholds: insights from the efface phrenic stim study, *Europace* 14:826-832, 2012.
7. Maytin M, Carrillo RG, Baltodano P, et al: Multicenter experience with transvenous lead extraction of active fixation coronary sinus leads, *Pacing Clin Electrophysiol* 35:641-647, 2012.
8. Poole JE, Gleva MJ, Mela T, et al: Complication rates associated with pacemaker or implantable cardioverter-defibrillator generator replacements and upgrade procedures: results from the replace registry, *Circulation* 122:1553-1561, 2010.
9. Shetty AK, Duckett SG, Bostock J, et al: Use of a quadripolar left ventricular lead to achieve successful implantation in patients with previous failed attempts at cardiac resynchronization therapy, *Europace* 13:992-996, 2011.
10. Sperzel J, Danschel W, Gutleben KJ, et al: First prospective, multi-centre clinical experience with a novel left ventricular quadripolar lead, *Europace* 14:365-372, 2012.
11. Thibault B, Karst E, Ryu K, et al: Pacing electrode selection in a quadripolar left heart lead determines presence or absence of phrenic nerve stimulation, *Europace* 12:751-753, 2010.

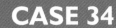
Extraction of a Biventricular Defibrillator with a Starfix 4195 Coronary Venous Lead

John Rickard and Bruce L. Wilkoff

Age	Gender	Occupation	Working Diagnosis
58 Years	Male	Retired	Cardiac Resynchronization Therapy Defibrillator System Infection

HISTORY

A 58-year-old man with ischemic cardiomyopathy with an ejection fraction of 20%, a history of coronary artery bypass graft surgery in 1993, and placement of a biventricular defibrillator (Medtronic Concerto; Guidant 0185 RV ICD lead; Attain Starfix 4195 coronary venous lead) on October 25, 2007 for primary prevention, a history of a left ventricular thrombus, and persistent atrial fibrillation sought treatment at a hospital with fevers, chills, and worsening dyspnea on exertion occurring over the previous 2 months. On admission, blood cultures were drawn that were positive for methicillin-resistant *Staphylococus aureus* (MRSA). A transesophageal echocardiogram suggested a vegetation on the implantable cardioverter-defibrillator (ICD) lead, prompting transfer to a tertiary referral center for complete system extraction.

Comments

Cardiac implantable electronic device (CIED) infection is typically defined as the presence of local warmth, erythema, swelling, edema, pain, or discharge from the device pocket, along with a positive culture from the device, device pocket, blood, or lead. Device-associated endocarditis is defined as the presence of a lead or valvular vegetation on echocardiogram. Prompt removal of the CIED and all leads and administration of a prolonged course of antibiotics is the appropriate management for CIED-related infections. Lead extraction procedures must be performed only at facilities with cardiac surgery programs with experienced cardiac surgeons on site and ready to initiate emergency cardiac

surgery. The facility to which this patient presented lacked such capability, making the transfer to a tertiary referral center with significant experience in lead extraction appropriate.

CURRENT MEDICATIONS

The patient was receiving vancomycin 1 g intravenously twice daily and heparin according to a drip rate nomogram; he was also taking carvedilol 6.25 mg orally twice daily, lisinopril 2.5 mg orally daily, omeprazole 20 mg orally daily, atorvastatin 20 mg orally daily at bedtime, and aspirin 81 mg orally daily.

Comments

Vancomycin is a first-line therapy for MRSA-related bloodstream infections. Staphylococcal species are responsible for 60% to 80% of CIED infections. The optimal duration of antimicrobial therapy for CIED infection is unclear. At least 2 weeks of intravenous antimicrobial therapy is recommended after extraction of an infected device for patients with infected CIED systems, but with positive blood cultures or vegetations the recommendation is usually 4 to 6 weeks. The patient's heparin drip was stopped the night before the planned extraction.

CURRENT SYMPTOMS

The patient was experiencing fatigue, shortness of breath, and nausea.

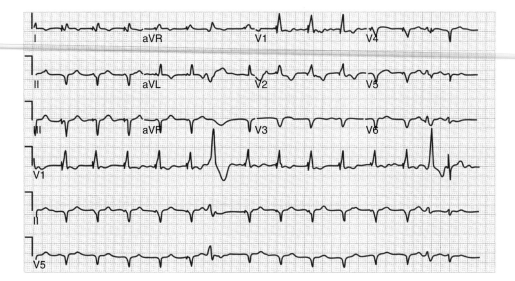

FIGURE 34-1 Preextraction electrocardiogram.

Comments

In patients with a CIED infection, fevers and chills are often absent.

PHYSICAL EXAMINATION

BP/HR: 95/62 mm Hg/87 bpm
Height/weight: 175.25 cm/73 kg
Neck veins: Jugular venous distention at 9 cm at 45 degrees
Lungs/chest: Clear lungs bilaterally with left basilar dullness to percussion; defibrillator site is in the left chest and scar is well healed without erythema or drainage
Heart: Regular rate and rhythm; normal first heart sound (S_1) and second heart sound (S_2); P_2 is not accentuated; no third heart sound (S_3) or fourth heart sound (S_4); no right ventricular heave
Abdomen: Soft, nontender, and nondistended; no appreciable ascites; liver is not pulsatile; a midline surgical incision present in the vicinity of the umbilicus
Extremities: 2+ bilateral pitting edema to the knees

Comments

In all patients thought to have a CIED infection, the device pocket should be inspected carefully for signs of erythema, fluctuance, and drainage. The absence of such signs, however, does not rule out CIED infection.

LABORATORY DATA

Hemoglobin: 10.7 g/dL
Hematocrit/packed cell volume: 33.4%

Mean corpuscular volume: 76.6 fL
Platelet count: 235 × 10^3/μL
Sodium: 133 mmol/L
Potassium: 3.8 mmol/L
Creatinine: 1.0 mmol/L
Blood urea nitrogen: 21 mmol/L

Comments

The patient's white blood cell count was within normal limits. Many patients with CIED infection fail to present with significant leukocytosis.

ELECTROCARDIOGRAM

Findings

The preextraction electrocardiogram shows atrial fibrillation with a biventricular paced rhythm and occasional premature ventricular contractions (Figure 34-1).

CHEST RADIOGRAPH

Findings

Portable chest radiography demonstrated the presence of a Medtronic 4195 Starfix coronary sinus lead in a midmyocardial position (Figure 34-2).

ECHOCARDIOGRAM

Findings

Transesophageal echocardiogram depicts a vegetation on the ICD lead as it crosses the tricuspid valve (Figure 34-3).

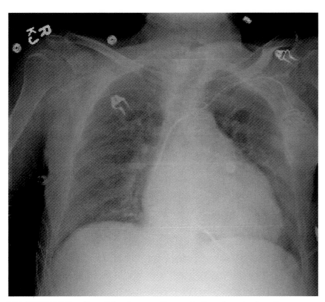

FIGURE 34-2 Portable chest radiograph showing the Starfix coronary venous lead in the midventricular position.

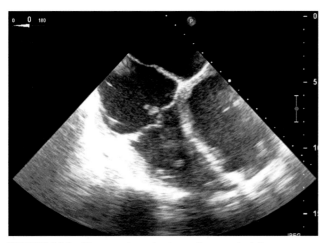

FIGURE 34-3 Transesophageal echocardiogram depicting a vegetation on the implantable cardioverter-defibrillator lead as it crosses the tricuspid valve.

The ejection fraction was 20%. A 1.8- × 0.8-cm mobile echodensity is present attached to the right ventricular lead as it crosses the tricuspid valve.

Comments

The size of the vegetation is important in extraction planning. Some operators will opt for a surgical procedure in patients with large vegetations (>2-3 cm) to limit the risk for septic pulmonary emboli. At our institution, vegetations larger than 3 cm have been extracted. In making the decision on whether to extract leads with large vegetations percutaneously, the comorbidities of the patient need to be thoroughly assessed, the risks of both procedures carefully balanced, and timing and route for reimplantation anticipated in this plan. The

1.8-cm lesion in this case is within reason to undergo percutaneous extraction.

FOCUSED CLINICAL QUESTIONS AND DISCUSSION POINTS

Question

How are CIED infections diagnosed and treated?

Discussion

Patients with CIED infections often present with localized inflammatory changes at the device site, occasionally accompanied by cutaneous erosion. Such a presentation, however, is not uniform, as demonstrated by the current case. Some patients simply initially seek treatment with vague systemic symptoms such as fatigue, anorexia, or decreased functional capacity. On presentation, two sets of blood cultures should be obtained before the initiation of antibiotics. Bacteremia caused by staphylococcal species, in particular, increases the likelihood of CIED involvement. Often, the original imaging study to search for lead or valve infection is a transthoracic echocardiogram. Because of low sensitivity and specificity for picking up vegetations, however, a negative transthoracic echocardiogram cannot rule out the presence of vegetations. A transesophageal echocardiogram is significantly more sensitive than a transthoracic echocardiogram to find lead and valvular vegetations. Even in patients in whom a transthoracic echocardiogram has demonstrated a lead-adherent mass, a transesophageal echocardiogram is still indicated to rule out left-sided valvular involvement. Once a diagnosis of a CIED infection has been made, all components of the CIED system must be removed in a timely fashion followed by a prolonged course of antibiotics.[1,5]

Question

What are the challenges involved with removal of a traditional non–active fixation coronary venous pacing lead?

Discussion

Because of the thin walls of the coronary venous system, coronary venous lead extraction would seem to pose substantial risk for percutaneous extraction.[2] In studies in small animals a high incidence of hemopericardium after coronary venous lead extraction has been noted. In humans, however, an increased complication rate with coronary venous lead extraction has not been borne out. Bongiorni and colleagues[3] reported on a cohort of 37 coronary venous lead extractions.

The age of the coronary venous leads in this study was 19.5 ± 16.5 months. All leads were successfully extracted, with 27 extracted with simple traction alone and the remaining 10 with mechanical dilation. The areas of adhesion for the coronary venous leads were most commonly found in the subclavian vein (60%). In a separate cohort of 173 patients undergoing coronary venous lead extraction from our institution, a total of 76.9% of coronary venous leads were removed using simple traction alone, with the remaining leads requiring the use of a laser-powered sheath. A total of 3.5% of leads required intervention (manual dissection or laser-powered dissection) within the coronary sinus. Major complications were rare, occurring in 1.2% of patients, and minor complications occurred in 7.5% of patients. In a separate cohort of 114 leads from the Mayo Clinic, 91.2% were removed with simple traction alone.[9] Minor complications were reported in 7.2% of patients and major complications in 1.6% of cases. Given the thin-walled nature of the coronary sinus, advancement of dissection sheaths into the coronary sinus itself in difficult cases is discouraged and should be reserved for experienced operators in select patients. Overall, extraction of traditional non–active-fixation coronary venous leads has been shown to be a safe, effective procedure with a low incidence of complications.[4,6-9]

Question

What are the technical challenges involved with removal of the Medtronic Attain Starfix 4195 active fixation coronary venous pacing lead?

Discussion

The Medtronic Attain Starfix 4195 coronary venous lead was approved by the United States Food and Drug Administration in June 2008 as the first active fixation coronary venous lead. The active fixation mechanism consists of three polyurethane lobes that are deployed by advancing tubing around the lead. When deployed, the lobes range from 5 to 24 French in diameter. Acutely, the locking mechanism can be deployed and undeployed. Over time, however, fibrotic tissue ingrowth between the lobes may preclude undeployment. Extraction of Starfix leads can be very challenging. Unlike the case with conventional coronary venous lead extraction, advancement of an extraction sheath into the coronary sinus is often needed with Starfix leads and, in approximately 40% of cases, a sheath must be advanced distally into the coronary sinus tributary itself. Given the high incidence of fibrotic ingrowth and the resultant inability to undeploy the lobes, Starfix lead extraction should be reserved for highly experienced operators at high-volume centers.

Question

What are the challenges associated with reimplantation of a coronary venous lead after extraction of a biventricular pacing system?

Discussion

Successful reimplantation of a coronary venous lead after extraction of a biventricular device is achievable in 80% to 85% of cases, a rate slightly lower than for de novo implants. This slightly lower success rate is likely due to the increased procedural difficulty involved with right-sided procedures (which most reimplants are). In addition, most operators have significantly less experience with right-sided implants. Finally, occlusion of the original coronary venous tributary may be present in up to 50% of cases. Therefore venous tributaries that are difficult to access are occasionally the only available target.

FINAL DIAGNOSIS

The final diagnosis for this patient was CIED-related endocarditis.

PLAN OF ACTION

The plan for this patient was full system extraction.[10]

INTERVENTION

Under general anesthesia, right radial arterial and right femoral venous sheaths were inserted for hemodynamic monitoring and vascular access, respectively. A left infraclavicular incision yielded access for removal of the CIED and leads. The pocket was grossly infected, with purulent material noted. The entire fibrotic capsule and all infected-appearing tissue were debrided. Deep tissue cultures of the pocket were sent for culture. The ICD lead was prepared with an LLD-EZ locking stylet (Spectranetics, Colorado Springs, Colo.). Although the helical screw did not retract, torque was able to be transmitted to the lead tip. The ICD lead was manually unscrewed from the myocardium, and the lead was removed with simple traction. The coronary venous lead was then prepared with an LLD-EZ locking stylet. An attempt was made to undeploy the lobes of the lead locking mechanism. After prolonged efforts, the lobes would not undeploy. Fortunately, after application of gentle traction, the lead was withdrawn into the the brachiocephalic vein, where it became lodged. A 14-French laser sheath was then advanced over the lead, and the lead was

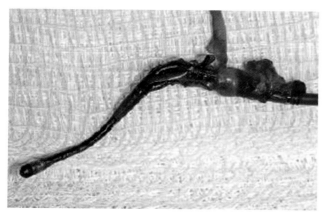

FIGURE 34-4 Tissue ingrowth into the lobes of the Starfix coronary venous lead preventing undeployment.

successfully extracted from the body. On inspection of the lead tip, significant fibrotic growth between the lobes of the lead was noted, with a cast of the cardiac vein trailing from the fibrosis (Figure 34-4). The pocket was irrigated and closed. The patient was treated with a 5-week course of vancomycin.

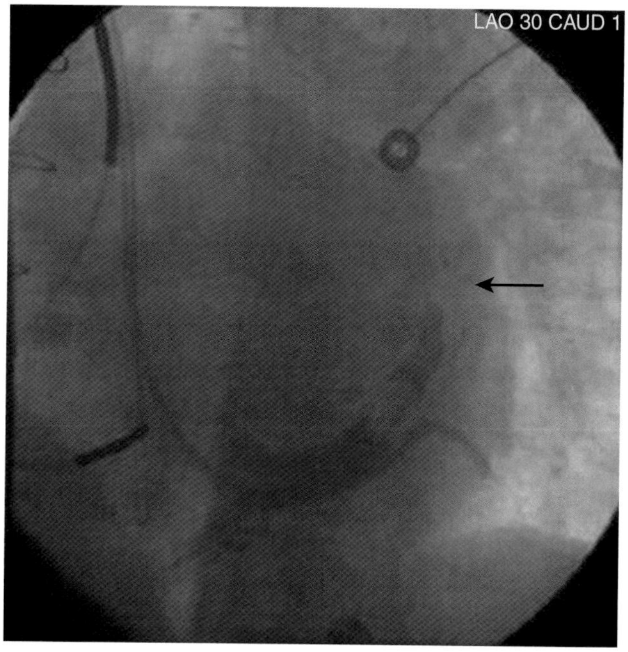

FIGURE 34-5 Occlusion of venous branch from which the Starfix coronary venous lead was extracted.

OUTCOME

After extraction and 10 days of antibiotics with multiple negative blood cultures, the patient was cleared for reimplantation on the right side. A Medtronic 4193 lead was placed in a lateral branch. The patient was discharged to home on 4 weeks of antibiotics.

Findings

A venogram was performed at the time of reimplantation demonstrating a lack of opacification of the high lateral vein from which the Starfix lead was extracted, suggesting complete occlusion of this vein (Figure 34-5).

Comments

Given the significant tissue ingrowth into the locking mechanism, extraction of the Starfix lead is traumatic to the coronary venous system. Although data are lacking, occlusion of the original vessel at time of reimplantation is likely to be significantly higher than that for traditional non–active-fixation coronary venous leads.

Selected References

1. Baddour LM, Epstein AE, Erickson CC, et al: Update on cardiovascular implantable electronic device infections and their management: a scientific statement from the American Heart Association, *Circulation* 3:458-477, 2010.
2. Baranowski B, Yerkey M, Dresing T, et al: Fibrotic tissue growth into the extendable lobes of an active fixation coronary sinus lead can complicate extraction, *Pacing Clin Electrophysiol* 7:e64-e65, 2011.
3. Bongiorni MG, Zucchelli G, Soldati E, et al: Usefulness of mechanical transvenous dilation and location of areas of adherence in patients undergoing coronary sinus lead extraction, *Europace* 1:69-73, 2007.
4. Burke MC, Morton J, Lin AC, et al: Implications and outcome of permanent coronary sinus lead extraction and reimplantation, *J Cardiovasc Electrophysiol* 8:830-837, 2005.
5. Chua JD, Wilkoff BL, Lee I, et al: Dagnosis and management of infections involving implantable electrophysiologic cardiac devices, *Ann Intern Med* 8:604-648, 2000.
6. Maytin M, Carrillo RG, Baltodano P, et al: Multicenter experience with transvenous lead extraction of active fixation coronary sinus leads, *Pacing Clin Electrophysiol* 6:641-647, 2012.
7. Rickard J, Tarakji K, Cronin E, et al: Cardiac venous left ventricular lead removal and reimplantation following device infection: a large single-center experience, *J Cardiovasc Electrophysiol* 23:1213-1216, 2012.
8. Rickard J, Wilkoff BL: Extraction of implantable cardiac electronic devices, *Curr Cardiol Rep* 13:407-414, 2011.
9. Sheldon S, Friedman PA, Hayes DL, et al: Outcomes and predictors of difficulty with coronary sinus lead removal, *J Interv Card Electrophysiol* 35:93-100, 2012.
10. Wilkoff BL, Love CJ, Byrd CL, et al: Transvenous lead extraction: Heart Rhythm Society expert consensus on facilities, training, indications, and patient management, *Heart Rhythm* 7:1085-1104, 2009.

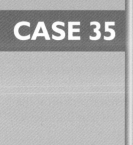

CASE 35

Complications of Cardiac Resynchronization Therapy: Infection

Avish Nagpal and M. Rizwan Sohail

Age	Gender	Occupation	Working Diagnosis
86 Years	Male	Retired Farmer	Infection Related to Cardiac Resynchronization Therapy

HISTORY

An 86-year-old gentleman was seen in the clinic for concerns regarding drainage at the site of his cardiac device on the left chest wall. His history was significant for ischemic heart disease and sinus node dysfunction, for which he had undergone pacemaker placement 2 years previously. At that time, his ejection fraction was estimated to be 38%. More recently, he was found to have New York Heart Association class III symptoms of congestive heart failure despite aggressive medical management. His ejection fraction was found to be 30%, and therefore his device was upgraded to a cardiac resynchronization therapy defibrillator (CRT-D) 6 weeks before presentation. At the time of this procedure, the old right ventricular pacing lead was removed but the chronic atrial lead was left in place. A routine recheck revealed the patient's P wave to be significantly reduced, at 0.2 mV. Device interrogation confirmed that there was no capture on the atrial lead, and therefore he underwent atrial lead revision 3 weeks before presentation. This procedure was complicated by a postoperative hematoma at the surgical site that was managed conservatively. A few days after the procedure, he noticed pain, redness, and drainage from the device pocket in the left chest wall (Figure 35-1) and sought further evaluation at the clinic.

The review of systems in this patient was negative for fever or chills. He did have some fatigue and worsening shortness of breath but did not report chest pain or sputum production.

His other relevant comorbidities included prostate and laryngeal cancer, hypertension, hyperlipidemia, and iron deficiency anemia without an obvious source of bleeding. He had undergone a coronary artery bypass graft in 1994.

CURRENT MEDICATIONS

The patient was taking clopidogrel 75 mg daily, ferrous sulfate 325 mg (65 mg iron) daily, ramipril 5 mg daily, metoprolol 25 mg daily, isosorbide mononitrate 30 mg daily, furosemide 20 mg daily, niacin 1000 mg daily, simvastatin 40 mg daily, and aspirin 81 mg daily.

CURRENT SYMPTOMS

The patient was experiencing erythema, pain, and drainage at the site of device pocket in the left chest wall.

PHYSICAL EXAMINATION

BP/HR: 118/58 mm Hg/68 bpm
Height/weight: 167 cm/85 kg
Neck veins: Jugular vein distention up to the angle of the mandible
Lungs/chest: Bilaterally clear to auscultation
Heart: Normal first heart sound (S_1) and second heart sound (S_2) with grade 3/6 systolic ejection murmur best heard at the base of the heart; skin over the left chest at the device pocket site was erythematous and warm, with purulent discharge from the pocket site; 1 cm dehiscence of surgical incision
Abdomen: Nondistended, soft and nontender, bowel sounds normal
Extremities: No large joint swelling, redness, or tenderness; 2+ pitting edema

Comments

Clinical examination shows dehiscence of surgical incision with purulent drainage and surrounding erythema

221

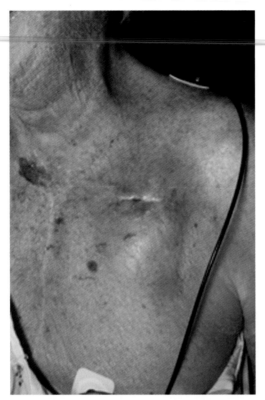

FIGURE 35-1 Pain, redness, and drainage from the device pocket in the left chest wall.

consistent with cardiac device infection. The examination is also concerning for decompensated heart failure, as evidenced by increased jugular vein distention and peripheral edema.

LABORATORY DATA

Hemoglobin: 8.8 g/dL (normal range: 13.5-17.5 g/dL)
Hematocrit/packed cell volume: 38.1% (normal range: 38.8%-50%)
Mean corpuscular volume: 106.8 fL (normal range: 81.2-95.1 fL)
Platelet count: 165 × 10³/μL (normal range: 150-450 × 10⁹/L)
Sodium: 140 mmol/L (normal range: 135-145 mmol/L)
Potassium: 4.5 mmol/L (normal range: 3.6-5.2 mmol/L)
Creatinine: 2.1 mg/dL (normal range: 0.8-1.3 mg/dL)
Blood urea nitrogen: 49 mg/dL (normal range: 8-24 mg/dL)
Leukocytes: 15.8 × 10⁹/L (normal range: 3.5-10.5 × 10⁹/L)

Comments

Routine laboratory tests, including hemoglobin, leukocyte count, platelets, electrolytes, and inflammatory markers such as erythrocye sedimentation rate (ESR) and C-reactive protein (CRP) are neither sensitive nor specific for the diagnosis of cardiac device–related infection. The patient does have anemia and leukocytosis. These findings are not unexpected given the clinical history, which in itself is diagnostic of cardiac device infection.

ELECTROCARDIOGRAM

Findings

Normal sinus rhythm with biventricular pacing.

Comments

Electrocardiogram can provide clues to intracardiac complications of device-related infections such as conduction defects or heart block that may arise secondary to abscess formation.

CHEST RADIOGRAPH

Findings

The chest radiograft revealed a small left pleural effusion with increased pulmonary vascularity and mildly increased perihilar prominence. Lungs were otherwise clear. Sternotomy wires and a left pectoral biventricular implanted cardiac device was seen.

Comments

Chest radiography can sometimes be helpful to detect septic emboli that arise as a result of dislodgement of lead vegetations. Our patient did not have these findings on his chest radiograph. Evidence of decompensated heart failure was present.

ECHOCARDIOGRAM

Findings

Echocardiogram revealed mild left ventricular enlargement with moderate to severely reduced systolic function. The calculated left ventricular ejection fraction was 30%. Moderate to severe generalized left ventricular hypokinesis also was present. Mild right ventricular enlargement was noted, with moderately reduced systolic function. The estimated right ventricular systolic pressure was 50 mm Hg (systolic blood pressure was 131 mm Hg). Calcific aortic valve stenosis (low output, low gradient) with a gradient of 26 mm Hg and calculated valve area of 0.92 cm² was noted.

Comments

The transthoracic echocardiogram did not reveal presence of vegetations. However, because of contiguity between the generator and leads, the patient is at significant risk for developing a more invasive infection if prompt treatment is not initiated. A transesophageal echocardiogram is more sensitive for visualization of valvular or lead vegetations and should be pursued in cases in which a blood culture is reported to be positive.

FOCUSED CLINICAL QUESTIONS AND DISCUSSION POINTS

Question

Based on the available epidemiologic data, what is the most likely pathogen responsible for this infection?

Discussion

The majority of cardiovascular implantable elctronic device (CIED) infections are caused by coagulase-negative staphylococci and *Staphylococcus aureus*. According to an earlier report from our institution, approximately 42% of infections were caused by coagulase-negative staphylococci and 29% of infections were caused by *S. aureus*. Considering that a large proportion of these organisms are resistant to oxacillin, vancomycin typically is used as empiric treatment until susceptibility data are available to guide specific antimicrobial therapy. Other less common organisms implicated as causative agents for CIED infection include other gram-positive cocci (4%), gram-negative cocci (9%), polymicrobial sources (7%), and fungal organisms (2%).[7] Occasionally, the etiologic microorganism cannot be identified, usually because of previous antimicrobial therapy. Therefore every attempt should be made to establish a microbiologic diagnosis before starting empiric antibiotic therapy. Culture-negative cases are often treated with broad-spectrum antibiotics, which places the patient at risk for greater adverse events, including but not limited to renal and hepatic dysfunction, superinfection, and cytopenia. Additionally, increased use of broad-spectrum antibiotics may contribute to the emergence of resistance.

For this patient, swabs of the serous drainage were collected and grew coagulase-negative *Staphylococcus* after 24 hours of incubation.

Question

What is the prevalence of CRT-D infections, and what factors increased the risk for infection?

Discussion

Overall, the rate of CIED infections seems to be rising disproportionately in contrast to the rate of device implantation, despite improvements in surgical techniques such as placement of transvenous leads instead of epicardial electrode patches, more operator experience with a larger volume of implantations, and use of prophylactic antibiotics. This increasing rate of infections has been attributed, in part, to implantation of CIEDs in sicker patients with more comorbidities and more complex procedures.[10] According to a recent study,[5] prevalence of CRT device infection was found to be 4.3% at 2.6 years of follow-up. The annual incidence was calculated to be 1.7% per year.[5] These numbers appear to be higher in contrast to rates of defibrillator or pacemaker infections, which have been reported at 1.2% at a similar time interval in a retrospective study[3] and 1.9 per 1000 device-years in a population-based study.[9] However, the infection rates in the REPLACE registry were reported to be low at 1.3%, similar to the overall incidence of device-related infections, although the follow-up was limited to 6 months and the study was not limited to only CRT devices. It was also observed that the centers that reported more than 5% infection rates used topical antisepsis with povidine-iodine, had lower rates of device implantation, or treated patients with an increased number of comorbidities.[8]

Some studies have evaluated risk factors for CIED infections. However, specific data regarding CRT device infections are limited. In one of the studies previously noted,[5] hemodialysis, increased implantation procedure time, device revision, and CRT-D placement were found to be independent risk factors for device infection on multivariate analysis. Other factors such as placement of epicardial leads and complications at the surgical site, such as hematoma formation, also have been reported to increase the risk for device infection.[6]

Question

What are the clinical manifestations of a cardiac device infection?

Discussion

Clinical presentation of cardiac device infection is variable and depends on timing of onset of infection, causative pathogen, and area of device involvement. The most common manifestation of a cardiac device infection in the early postoperative period includes pain, swelling, redness, and discharge at the surgical site (device generator pocket). Systemic manifestations of infection such as fever, chills, sweating, anorexia, or decompensated heart failure may be absent because of the localized nature of the infection. These systemic manifestations are more prevalent in cases in which the device becomes infected secondary to hematogeneous seeding from a distant source of bloodstream infection, especially with *S. aureus*. Occasionally, patients may present with device or lead erosion without gross inflammatory changes.[7] In these circumstances, the device is assumed to be infected because of contamination from the skin flora. Finally, lead endocarditis may present with either constitutional symptoms or embolic complications such as septic emboli to the lungs.

Question

What diagnostic tests are indicated to confirm CRT infection in this case?

Discussion

Diagnosis of CRT device infection usually is a clinical one. Routine laboratory tests such as leukocyte count, platelet count, ESR, and CRP are frequently obtained but can be normal in cases with localized infection. Blood cultures should be obtained in all cases of suspected CRT device infection, not only to define the extent of infection but also to help establish microbiologic cause and determine the type and duration of antibiotic therapy. A positive blood culture in a patient with suspected infected device should prompt evaluation with a transesophageal echocardiogram to look for vegetations on the device leads or heart valves or complications such as myocardial abscess. Persistently positive blood cultures, in the absence of any other focus of infection, in a patient with a cardiac device suggest device-related endocarditis even in the absence of any echocardiographic evidence of gross vegetation.[2]

All attempts should be made to reach a specific microbiologic diagnosis by obtaining swabs from the generator pocket or device surface for bacterial cultures at the time of explantation. Moreover, pocket tissue and lead tip cultures should be performed to help establish the microbiologic diagnosis. However, positive lead tip cultures should not always be interpreted as evidence of lead endocarditis because lead tips can be contaminated while being pulled percutaneously through an infected device pocket.

The patient described in this case underwent transesophageal echocardiography that did not reveal any vegetations or intracardiac complications such as myocardial abscess formation. Blood cultures were drawn and remained negative after 5 days of incubation.

Question

What would be considered the optimal management of the infected device in this case?

Discussion

Multiple published studies related to cardiac device infections suggest that optimal management of an infected cardiac device includes both the administration of appropriate systemic antibiotics and complete removal of the device, including intracardiac leads. In a large, single-center, retrospective study, conservative treatment with just antibiotics and without device removal was associated with a sevenfold increase in 30-day mortality. Additionally, prompt hardware removal was associated with a threefold decrease in 1-year mortality in contrast to delayed device removal, allowing for initial conservative management with antibiotics alone.[2] These data are consistent with findings from a subsequent study in which relapse rates were observed to be significantly lower with device removal in contrast to hardware retention (2.6% vs. 61.4%).[4]

In contemporary practice, leads are extracted in the majority of cases by percutaneous approach at specialized centers. More invasive procedures, such as sternotomy, are reserved for cases in which the percutaneous procedure cannot be successfully performed or to manage any unintended complication of the percutaneous extraction procedure such as bleeding or vascular perforation. However, the rates of complications associated with percutanous lead removal are very low—less than 1% in experienced medical centers. Treatment algorithms and guidelines have been published by the American Heart Association and support a combined medical and surgical approach involving administration of intravenous antibiotics and complete removal of the infected device, including the generator and all leads, regardless of clinical presentation.[1] Oxacillin, nafcillin, or cefazolin typically is used for treatment of susceptible strains of staphylococci. However, because of high rates of oxacillin resistance seen in species of staphylococci, vancomycin typically is used for empiric treatment until susceptibility data become available. The duration of antibiotic therapy depends on the type of infection. In cases in which infection is limited to the pocket site, 7 to 10 days of antibiotic therapy after device extraction is adequate in most cases. However, cases of device infection associated with bloodstream infection are typically treated with a 14-day course of intravenous antibiotics after device removal. Patients with associated complications in the form of valvular endocarditis, septic thrombophlebitis, or osteomyelitis require a longer course of intravenous antibiotics lasting 28 to 42 days, depending on the particular complication and causative pathogen.

All patients should be assessed for the need for ongoing device therapy before implantation of a new device. Reimplantation, if required, should be done on the contralateral side once the blood culture results are available and pocket infection is under control.

The patient in this case underwent complete percutaneous removal of the device (including generator and leads). He developed transient hypotension during the procedure that responded to intravenous fluid bolus. He was subsequently started on vancomycin intravenously. The susceptibility results revealed the organism to be oxacillin resistant, and he was therefore continued on intravenous vancomycin, which he received for a total of 14 days after device extraction. He underwent replacement of the CRT-D device on the contralateral chest wall 2 days after removal of the infected device. His latest evaluation was performed 2 months after device replacement, and he was found to be symptom free without evidence of relapse or recurrence of the infection.

FINAL DIAGNOSIS

The final diagnosis in this patient was CRT device pocket infection with coagulase-negative *Staphylococcus.*

PLAN OF ACTION

The plan for this patient was combined medical and surgical management.

INTERVENTION

Percutaneous generator and lead extraction was performed in this patient.

OUTCOME

The outcome was complete cure of the infection.

Selected References

1. Baddour LM, Epstein AE, Erickson CC, et al: Update on cardiovascular implantable electronic device infections and their management: a scientific statement from the American Heart Association, *Circulation* 121:458-477, 2010.
2. Le KY, Sohail MR, Friedman PA, et al: Impact of timing of device removal on mortality in patients with cardiovascular implantable electronic device infections, *Heart Rhythm* 8:1678-1685, 2011.
3. Mela T, McGovern BA, Garan H, et al: Long-term infection rates associated with the pectoral versus abdominal approach to cardioverter-defibrillator implants, *Am J Cardiol* 88:750-753, 2001.
4. Pichlmaier M, Knigina L, Kutschka I, et al: Complete removal as a routine treatment for any cardiovascular implantable electronic device-associated infection, *J Thorac Cardiovasc Surg* 142:1482-1490, 2011.
5. Romeyer-Bouchard C, Da Costa A, Dauphinot V, et al: Prevalence and risk factors related to infections of cardiac resynchronization therapy devices, *Eur Heart J* 31:203-210, 2010.
6. Sohail MR, Hussain S, Le KY, et al: Risk factors associated with early- versus late-onset implantable cardioverter-defibrillator infections, *J Interv Card Electrophysiol* 31:171-183, 2011.
7. Sohail MR, Uslan DZ, Khan AH, et al: Management and outcome of permanent pacemaker and implantable cardioverter-defibrillator infections, *J Am Coll Cardiol* 49:1851-1859, 2007.
8. Uslan DZ, Gleva MJ, Warren DK, et al: Cardiovascular implantable electronic device replacement infections and prevention: results from the REPLACE Registry, *Pacing Clin Electrophysiol* 35:81-87, 2012.
9. Uslan DZ, Sohail MR, St Sauver JL, et al: Permanent pacemaker and implantable cardioverter defibrillator infection: a population-based study, *Arch Intern Med* 167:669-675, 2007.
10. Voigt A, Shalaby A, Saba S: Continued rise in rates of cardiovascular implantable electronic device infections in the United States: temporal trends and causative insights, *Pacing Clin Electrophysiol* 33:414-419, 2010.

Nonre-sponders to Cardiac Resynchro-nization Therapy

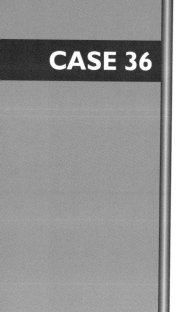

Cardiac Resynchronization Therapy in Non–Left Bundle Branch Block Morphology

John Gorcsan III and Josef J. Marek

Age	Gender	Occupation	Working Diagnosis
62 Years	Female	Retail Sales Agent	Nonischemic Cardiomyopathy

HISTORY

A 62-year-old woman was seen at the cardiology outpatient clinic. Her medical history was significant for the onset of mild heart failure symptoms 2 years previously. She had a past left ventricular ejection fraction (LVEF) of 32% and a diagnosis of nonischemic cardiomyopathy because no significant coronary artery disease was seen on coronary angiography. She was treated medically for heart failure and had undergone implantable cardioverter-defibrillator (ICD) placement. Because she did not have a left bundle branch block (LBBB), she was not considered for cardiac resynchronization therapy (CRT) at the time, with New York Heart Association (NYHA) class II heart failure symptoms. She remained active, working full time, but recently had 6 months of progressive dyspnea on mild exertion, consistent with NYHA class III heart failure symptoms. She was treated with loop diuretics, an angiotensin-converting enzyme inhibitor, and carvidilol. Her medical history is significant for hysterectomy, oophorectomy, appendectomy, tonsillectomy, and mild hypothyroidism. She previously smoked one pack of cigarettes per day but quit smoking 11 years ago.

Comments

This patient has nonischemic cardiomyopathy with an ICD implanted as a primary prevention indication. She experienced 6 months of progressive dyspnea on exertion.

CURRENT MEDICATIONS

The patient was taking furosemide 40 mg daily, enalapril 10 mg twice daily, carvedilol 12.5 mg twice daily, atorvastatin 10 mg daily, levothyroxine 25 mcg daily, and aspirin 325 mg daily.

Comments

This patient was on appropriate pharmacologic therapy for systolic heart failure.

CURRENT SYMPTOMS

The patient was experiencing progressive dyspnea that occurred with everyday activity and occasional ankle swelling. She denied chest pain, paroxysmal nocturnal dyspnea, palpitations, lightheadedness, or syncope.

Comments

These symptoms are consistent with heart failure, in NYHA class III. She was referred for echocardiography and consideration for CRT.

PHYSICAL EXAMINATION

BP/HR: 110/70 mm Hg/65 bpm
Height/weight: 167.6 cm/72.6 kg
Neck veins: Jugular vein distention is estimated to be 10 cm
Lungs/chest: Lungs clear to auscultation, ICD pocket is well healed
Heart: Slightly irregular rhythm with occasional premature beats, grade 1/6 systolic murmur best heard at the left sternal border and increases with inspiration

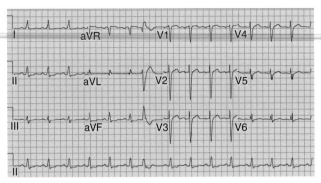

FIGURE 36-1 Electrocardiogram before implant.

Abdomen: No hepatosplenomegaly, aortic enlargement, or bruit

Extremities: Pulses are 2+, mild ankle edema, neurologically intact

Comments

Mild ankle edema supports the diagnosis of heart failure. Systolic murmur at the left sternal border is consistent with known mild tricuspid regurgitation.

LABORATORY DATA

Hemoglobin: 13.3 g/dL
Hematocrit/packed cell volume: 38.6%
Mean corpuscular volume: 89.1 fL
Platelet count: 279 × 10³/μL
Sodium: 140 mmol/L
Potassium: 4.1 mmol/L
Creatinine: 0.6 mg/dL
Blood urea nitrogen: 11 mg/dL

Comments

No laboratory abnormalities were present that would account for worsening heart failure.

ELECTROCARDIOGRAM

Findings

The electrocardiogram (ECG) revealed normal sinus rhythm, occasional premature ventricular complexes, nonspecific intraventricular conduction delay with a QRS width of 140 ms, and nonspecific T-wave changes (Figure 36-1)

Comments

The patient has a widened QRS complex with a duration greater than 120 ms. However, the morphology of the

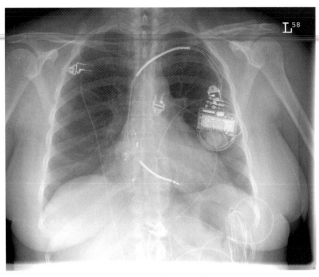

FIGURE 36-2 Chest radiograph.

QRS complex is not a typical LBBB and the QRS duration is intermediately widened (range 120-149 ms).

CHEST RADIOGRAPH

Findings

The chest radiograph showed cardiomegaly with past ICD implantation and evidence of pulmonary vascular congestion (Figure 36-2).

Comments

Evidence of mild congestive heart failure was confirmed on radiography.

ECHOCARDIOGRAM

Findings

The echocardiogram demonstrated global hypokinesia of the left ventricle (Figure 36-3). The LVEF was 28%. Mild mitral regurgitation, mild left atrial enlargement, and evidence of an ICD lead in situ also were seen.

Comments

The echocardiogram is consistent with nonischemic cardiomyopathy and depressed ejection fraction that is slightly less than at the previous visit.

Findings

The six time-strain curves plot the wall thickening toward the center of the left ventricular cavity as

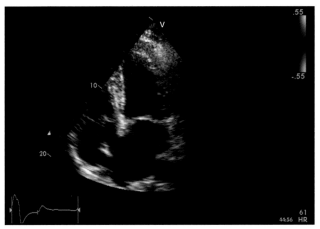

FIGURE 36-3 Apical four-chamber view. See *expertconsult.com* for video.

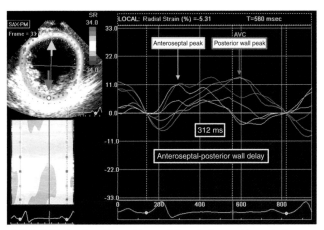

FIGURE 36-4 Speckle tracking radial strain from midventricular short-axis view.

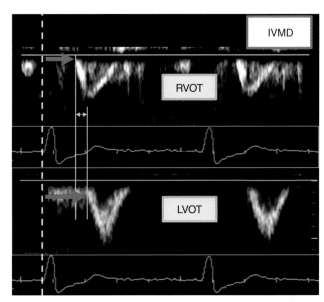

FIGURE 36-5 Pulsed Doppler interventricular mechanical delay *(IVMD). LVOT,* Left ventricular outflow tract; *RVOT,* right ventricular outflow tract.

delay, is 52 ms (left ventricular delay compared with that of the right ventricle) (Figure 36-5). Typically, an IVMD of 40 ms or greater is considered significant interventricular dyssynchrony.[2]

Comments

The IVMD, assessed by this relatively simple pulsed Doppler technique, also demonstrated significant interventricular dyssynchrony.

segmental radial strain. Evidence of significant dyssynchrony with an anteroseptal to posterior wall delay of 312 ms (≥ 130 ms) was present.[2]

Comments

The presence of a typical radial strain pattern of dyssynchrony usually seen in patients with LBBB was noted on echocardiography. Early thickening in the inferoseptal, anteroseptal, and anterior segments was visible (Figure 36-4, *red, yellow,* and *cyan curves*), with later activation in posterior, lateral, and inferior wall (see Figure 36-4, *violet, green,* and *dark blue curves*). This patient has intraventricular mechanical dyssynchrony with a QRS duration of 140 ms and a non-LBBB pattern. Another useful measure of dyssynchrony is 12-site standard deviation by tissue Doppler longitudinal velocities, but this was not performed in this patient.

Findings

The interventricular mechanical delay (IVMD), defined as the difference between left and right ventricle preejection

FOCUSED CLINICAL QUESTIONS AND DISCUSSION POINTS

Question

Does an indication for CRT implantation exist in this patient based on guidelines in the current literature?

Discussion

Although previous CRT guidelines used a QRS width greater than 120 ms regardless of QRS morphology as a criterion, 2012 updated guidelines have changed.[5] CRT is not considered the strongest benefit for patients with an LVEF of 35% or less and NYHA class II, III, or IV symptoms, with a class I indication (strongest level of evidence) only for patients with QRS duration of 150 ms or greater and LBBB morphology. Patients with a QRS of 120 to 149 with LBBB morphology or a QRS of 150 ms or greater and non-LBBB morphology have a class IIA indication, and patients with a QRS of 120 to 149 and non-LBBB morphology have class IIB. These guidelines were based on clinical trial data that did not consider echocardiographic dyssynchrony. This represents a general shift of opinion to focus more on the ECG, with patients with less prolonged QRS durations and atypical QRS morphologies now being viewed as a group with heterogeneous response to CRT. Selection criteria using the ECG result in identifying approximately 30% of patients who are considered nonresponders to CRT. These more limiting guidelines may improve the responder rate, but unfortunately may limit the use of CRT to patients who may benefit. This imposes a significant challenge on clinicians considering implanting CRT devices, because the goal is to help as many patients with heart failure as possible who may benefit from treatment, including device therapy.

Question

What additional information can echocardiographic dyssynchrony provide in the setting of patients with moderately prolonged QRS durations (QRS 120-149 ms)?

Discussion

Evidence from single-center studies[1,3] indicates that echocardiographic dyssynchrony parameters can predict response and long-term prognosis in patients who receive CRT. In particular, patients who lack mechanical dyssynchrony at baseline do not appear to benefit from CRT. In patients with a QRS of 120 to 149 ms, those with significant radial dyssynchrony appeared to have outcomes similar to those of patients with a QRS of 150 ms or greater, whereas patients with a QRS of 120 to 149 ms but without radial dyssynchrony had a significantly lower survival rate (log rank $p = 0.002$). These data support the importance of radial strain dyssynchrony as an adjunct to provide prognostic information in patients with intermediate QRS width (120-149 ms).

Question

What is the role of dyssynchrony in patients with non-LBBB morphology?

Discussion

The greatest level of evidence for CRT response is in patients with LBBB. However, patients with non-LBBB, which includes interventricular conduction delay (IVCD), as in this case, or right bundle branch block (RBBB), have variable response to CRT. Mechanical dyssynchrony has been shown[4] to be less frequently observed in patients with shorter QRS duration and non-LBBB (i.e., radial dyssynchrony 85% in LBBB, 59% in IVCD, and 40% in RBBB). However, in patients with non-LBBB morphology, absence of dyssynchrony

is a strong negative prognostic marker (radial dyssynchrony: hazard ratio [HR] 2.6, 95% confidence interval [CI] 1.47-4.53, $p <0.001$; IVMD: HR 4.9, 95% CI 2.60-9.16, $p <0.001$). Specifically, this study showed that patients with non-LBBB morphology and mechanical dyssynchrony by speckle tracking radial strain or IVMD had significant improvement in LVEF after CRT (23 ± 6 to 31 ± 10, $p = 0.001$), whereas non-LBBB patients who lacked baseline dyssynchrony had no significant improvement in LVEF (25 ± 6 to 27 ± 8, $p =$ not significant) or end systolic volume.

Question

Which dyssynchrony indices should be used in evaluation of patients with a QRS duration less than 150 ms or non-LBBB morphology?

Discussion

Currently, no consensus has been reached as to which dyssynchrony index is best. Although tissue Doppler imaging longitudinal velocity measures, such as 12-site standard deviation or the Yu Index, have been described as useful measures associated with patient outcome,[3] speckle tracking–derived radial strain anteroseptal to posterior wall delay was examined most closely in our study of patients without LBBB. The pulse Doppler–derived IVMD is also important because it reflects a large degree of dyssynchrony and is simple to perform. Dyssynchrony indices associated with patient outcome when examining patients with non-LBBB morphologies and a QRS duration of 120 to 149 ms were speckle tracking radial strain anteroseptal to posterior wall delay and intraventricular mechanical delay.

FINAL DIAGNOSIS

This patient has nonischemic cardiomyopathy and depressed ejection fraction with a history of ICD placement. Because her heart failure symptoms progressed on optimal medical therapy, upgrade to CRT-D was contemplated. The patient has a class IIB indication according to the 2012 guidelines for CRT therapy, which means a less strong indication based purely on the ECG. The speckle tracking and pulsed Doppler dyssynchrony study supports mechanical dyssynchrony being present to a significant degree. This has been associated with improved patient outcomes after CRT.

PLAN OF ACTION

The decision was made to upgrade the patient's ICD device to a CRT-D system.

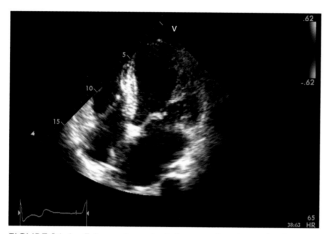

FIGURE 36-6 Echocardiography follow-up after 6 months. See *expertconsult.com* for video.

INTERVENTION

A CRT implantation was performed with successful left ventricular lead positioning in a lateral location. The pulse generator was exchanged for a CRT-D device. No complications occurred during the procedure.

OUTCOME

The postoperative period was uneventful. The symptoms of the patient improved within 2 weeks after CRT to her previous NYHA class II status. At 6 months a follow-up echocardiogram was obtained that showed improvement in overall left ventricular ejection fraction from 28% to 42% (Figure 36-6). No hospitalizations for heart failure occurred in the year of observation after CRT implantation, and the patient enjoyed a more active lifestyle.

Findings

Evidence indicated an increase in ejection fraction to 42%.

Comments

In this setting, upgrade to a CRT device resulted in improvement of symptomatology in left ventricular function. Dyssynchrony echocardiography as an adjunct to the ECG helped the physician select this patient for CRT implantation, and she received significant benefit from this therapy.

Selected References

1. Delgado V, van Bommel RJ, Bertini M, et al: Relative merits of left ventricular dyssynchrony, left ventricular lead position, and myocardial scar to predict long-term survival of ischemic heart failure patients undergoing cardiac resynchronization therapy, *Circulation* 123:70-78, 2011.
2. Gorcsan 3rd J, Abraham T, Agler DA, et al: Echocardiography for cardiac resynchronization therapy: recommendations for performance and reporting—a report from the American Society of Echocardiography Dyssynchrony Writing Group endorsed by the Heart Rhythm Society, *J Am Soc Echocardiogr* 21:191-213, 2008.
3. Gorcsan 3rd J, Oyenuga O, Habib PJ, et al: Relationship of echocardiographic dyssynchrony to long-term survival after cardiac resynchronization therapy, *Circulation* 122:1910-1918, 2010.
4. Hara H, Oyenuga OA, Tanaka H, et al: The relationship of QRS morphology and mechanical dyssynchrony to long-term outcome following cardiac resynchronization therapy, *Eur Heart J* 33:2680-2691, 2012.
5. Tracy CM, Epstein AE, Darbar D, et al: 2012 ACC/AHA/HRS focused update of the 2008 guidelines for device-based therapy of cardiac rhythm abnormalities: a report of the American College of Cardiology Foundation/American Heart Association task force on practice guidelines, *Circulation* 126:1784-1800, 2012.

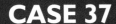

CASE 37

Use of Cardiovascular Magnetic Resonance to Guide Left Ventricular Lead Deployment in Cardiac Resynchronization Therapy

Robin J. Taylor, Fraz Umar, and Francisco Leyva

Age	Gender	Occupation	Working Diagnosis
82 Years	Female	Retired Factory Worker	Heart Failure Caused by Ischemic Cardiomyopathy

HISTORY

An 82-year-old woman who had a myocardial infarction and a coronary artery bypass graft (CABG) in 1997 developed progressive dyspnea and limitation of exercise tolerance to 200 yards (New York Heart Association [NYHA] class III) in 2010. After the diagnosis of systolic heart failure, she was started on medical therapy, but developed bronchoconstriction with beta blockers and a cough on angiotensin-converting enzyme (ACE) inhibitors, and she could tolerate only low doses of an angiotensin receptor blocker. Her medical history included permanent atrial fibrillation and peripheral vascular disease.

Comments

The patient was symptomatic from systolic heart failure and intolerant to medical therapy.

CURRENT MEDICATIONS

The patient was taking clopidogrel 75 mg daily, furosemide 40 mg daily, losartan 50 mg daily, rosuvastatin 10 mg daily, and isosorbide mononitrate XL 60 mg daily.

Comments

The patient experienced bronchoconstriction while on beta blockers, developed a cough on ACE inhibitors, and was intolerant of doses of losartan higher than 50 mg daily.

CURRENT SYMPTOMS

The patient was in NYHA class III. Her exercise capacity was limited at 200 yards by dyspnea, and she had no angina.

Comments

Dyspnea is the main symptom. The patient rarely experienced intermittent claudication.

PHYSICAL EXAMINATION

BP/HR: 98/52 mm Hg/64 bpm (in atrial fibrillation)
Neck veins: Jugular venous pressure not elevated
Lungs/chest: Clear
Heart: First heart sound (S_1) and second heart sound (S_2) of normal intensity, apex beat displaced laterally, soft ejection systolic murmur
Abdomen: Soft, nontender, no organomegaly
Extremities: No pitting edema, weak peripheral pulses

Comments

The patient had cardiomegaly, no evidence of pulmonary edema, and a murmur of mitral regurgitation.

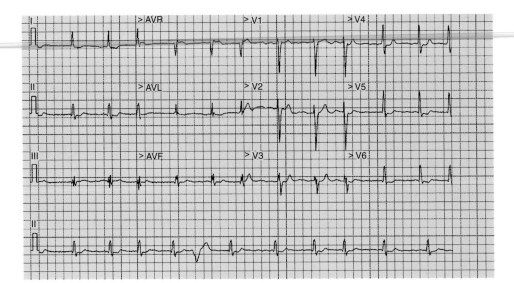

FIGURE 37-1   Pre-implant electrocardiogram.

ELECTROCARDIOGRAM

Findings

The electrocardiogram showed atrial fibrillation with a ventricular response of 97 bpm and a QRS duration of 134 ms (Figure 37-1). There was fragmentation of the QRS complex in leads II, III, aV_F and V_3, with no evidence of a bundle branch block.

Comments

The patient had a high ventricular rate at rest, in the background of intolerance to beta blockers. The QRS duration is in keeping with electrical dyssynchrony. The high ventricular rate raises the possibility of tachyarrhythmia-related left ventricular dysfunction.

CHEST RADIOGRAPH

Findings

The chest radiograph revealed an increased cardiothoracic ratio, no evidence of pulmonary edema, and sternotomy wires (Figure 37-2).

Comments

The findings on chest radiography were in keeping with heart failure without pulmonary edema.

ECHOCARDIOGRAM

Findings

The echocardiogram showed global left ventricular hypokinesia, inferior akinesis, myocardial thinning at

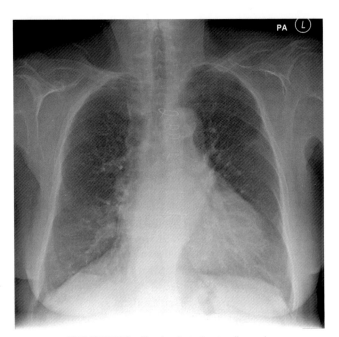

FIGURE 37-2   Pre-implant chest radiograph.

the apex, a pseudospherical left ventricle with severely impaired left ventricular function (LVEF of 29% using Simpson's method), and biatrial dilation (Figure 37-3, *A*).

Comments

The findings on echocardiography were in keeping with ischemic cardiomyopathy.

Findings

The transaortic peak gradient on the echocardiogram was 17 mm Hg, and the mean gradient was 14 mm Hg (see Figure 37-3, *B*).

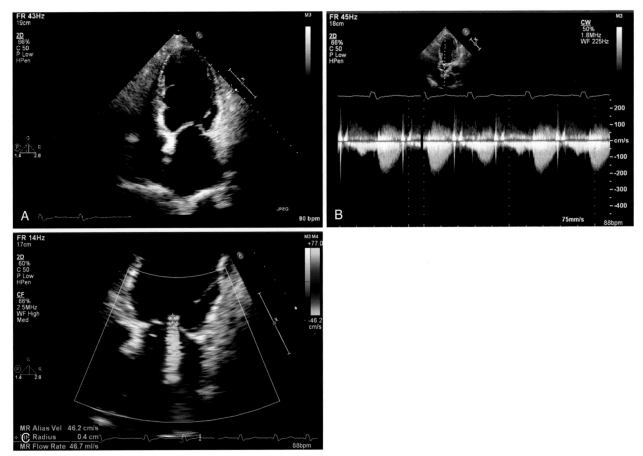

FIGURE 37-3   Pre-implant transthoracic echocardiogram showing an apical. **A,** Apical four-chamber view. **B,** Continuous wave Doppler image through aortic valve. **C,** Color Doppler image through mitral valve.

Comments

The gradient was consistent with mild aortic stenosis (see Figure 37-3, *B*). In the background of severely impaired left ventricular function, the severity of aortic stenosis may be underestimated.

Findings

The mitral regurgitant jet occupied 36% of the left atrial area on the four-chamber view. The proximal isovelocity hemispheric surface area radius was 0.4 cm and the effective regurgitant orifice was 0.2 cm². The valvular leaflets were intact, and dilation of the mitral valve ring and biatrial dilation were present.

Comments

The findings are consistent with moderate mitral regurgitation. The presence of inferior hypokinesis and a previous myocardial infarction raises the possibility of ischemic mitral regurgitation resulting from involvement of the posterior papillary muscle (mitral valve apparatus). Functional dilatation of the mitral valve ring also contributes to the degree of regurgitation.

CORONARY SINUS VENOGRAPHY

Right anterior oblique (RAO) and left anterior oblique (LAO) fluoroscopic coronary sinus venography was performed at the time of cardiac resynchronization therapy (CRT) device implantation, showing veins that might be considered options for left ventricular lead deployment (Figure 37-4, *A*).

Findings

Option 1 in Figure 37-4 is a small-caliber, posterolateral vein draining the mid-lateral segment. This vein has a stenosis in its proximal, tortuous portion (see Figure 37-4, *insert, white arrow*). *Option 2* is a posterolateral vein draining the mid-lateral segment. *Option 3* is a small-caliber, anterolateral vein draining the basal anterior segment.

Comments

Option 1 in Figure 37-4 appears to be a reasonable candidate vein for left ventricular lead deployment. A venoplasty could be performed in the proximal portion and

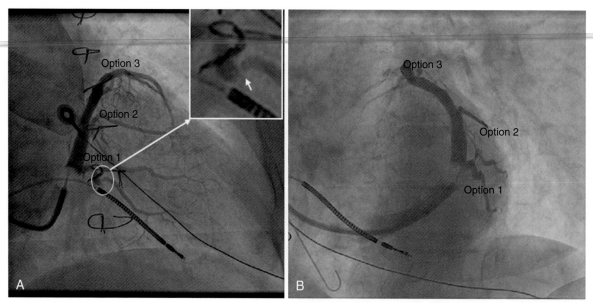

FIGURE 37-4   Coronary sinus venography at implantation. **A,** Right anterior oblique projection. **B,** Left anterior oblique projection.

the vein then straightened using a buddy wire technique. A small-caliber left ventricular lead could then be deployed distally, in the mid-lateral segment.

FEATURE TRACKING CARDIOVASCULAR MAGNETIC RESONANCE IMAGING

Findings

Feature tracking of the basal slice shows that the latest contracting segments in the lateral free left ventricular wall are the basal posterior and the basal inferior segments (Figure 37-5, A, red arrows). Peak circumferential strain in these segments, however, is less than 10%, suggesting myocardial scar. The basal lateral segment appears to not be scarred (peak circumferential strain, −15.81%) and also contracts late (time to peak strain, 414 ms). Note that the earliest contracting segments with a high peak circumferential strain are not scarred (mid-septal and mid-anteroseptal).

Comments

The basal lateral segment appears to be an appropriate target for left ventricular lead deployment.

Findings

Within the mid-cavity the latest contracting segment in the lateral free left ventricular wall is the mid-inferior (see Figure 37-5, B, red arrow). The peak circumferential strain

in this segment, however, is less than 10%, suggesting myocardial scar. The remaining left ventricular free wall segments do not appear scarred, and the latest contracting segments are the mid-anterior and mid-lateral (time to peak circumferential strain of 338 ms for both). The mid-anterior and the mid-lateral segments therefore do not appear to be scarred and are late contracting (see Figure 37-5, B, green arrows). Note that the earliest contracting segments with a high peak circumferential strain are not scarred (mid-septal and mid-anteroseptal).

Comments

The mid-anterior and the mid-lateral segments (Figure 37-5, B, green arrows) appear to be appropriate targets for left ventricular lead deployment

Findings

At the apex the latest contracting segments in the lateral free left ventricular wall are the apical lateral and the apical inferior segments (see Figure 37-5, B, red arrow and green arrow respectively). The apical lateral segment, however, is likely to be scarred (peak circumferential strain <10%). The apical inferior segment appears not to be scarred (peak circumferential strain, −23.05%) and contracts late. Note that the earliest contracting segment with a high peak circumferential strain is the apical septal segment.

Comments

The apical inferior segment appears to be an appropriate target for left ventricular lead deployment.

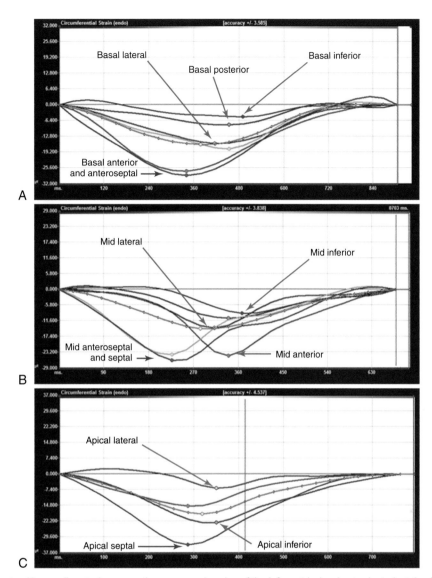

FIGURE 37-5   Feature-tracking cardiovascular magnetic resonance imaging of the left ventricular short axis stack at the **(A)** basal level, **(B)** mid-cavity level, and **C,** apical level.

LATE GADOLINIUM ENHANCEMENT CARDIOVASCULAR MAGNETIC RESONANCE IMAGING

Findings

The left hand panels of Figure 37-6 show basal, mid-cavity, and apical short-axis late gadolinium-enhancement images of the left ventricle. The relevant segments for left ventricular lead deployment, that is, those on the left ventricular free wall, delineated by endocardial, epicardial, and segmental boundaries, are shown in the center panels. In these images, the myocardial scar appears *white* and the viable myocardium appears *black*. The tables on the *right* describe whether scar is present and its pattern. Subendocardial scar is defined as a scar with less than 50% transmurality, whereas a transural scar is defined as that with a transmurality of 51% or greater.

Comments

The only segments that do not appear scarred on late gadolinium-enhanced cardiovascular magnetic resonance (LGE-CMR) are the basal anterior and basal lateral segments. The apical inferior segment, which had a peak circumferential strain of greater than 10% (−23.05%), also appeared scarred on LGE-CMR. This illustrates that the presence of circumferential strain does not necessarily equate to the absence of scar.

FOCUSED CLINICAL QUESTIONS AND DISCUSSION POINTS

Question

Is this patient likely to benefit from CRT?

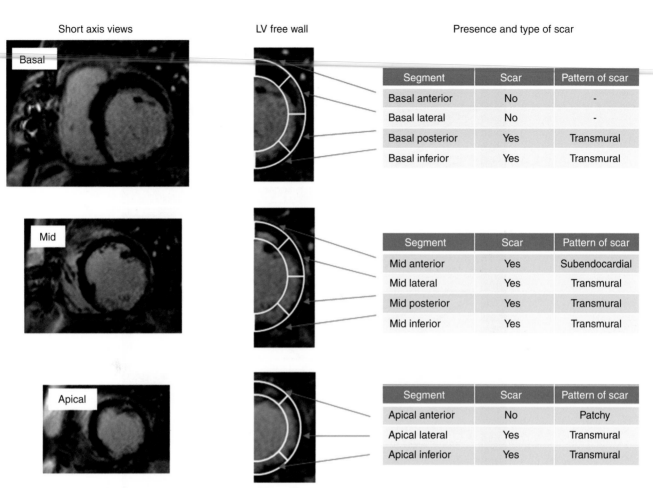

Short axis views	LV free wall	Presence and type of scar

Basal

Segment	Scar	Pattern of scar
Basal anterior	No	-
Basal lateral	No	-
Basal posterior	Yes	Transmural
Basal inferior	Yes	Transmural

Mid

Segment	Scar	Pattern of scar
Mid anterior	Yes	Subendocardial
Mid lateral	Yes	Transmural
Mid posterior	Yes	Transmural
Mid inferior	Yes	Transmural

Apical

Segment	Scar	Pattern of scar
Apical anterior	No	Patchy
Apical lateral	Yes	Transmural
Apical inferior	Yes	Transmural

FIGURE 37-6   Short-axis, late gadolinium enhancement cardiovascular magnetic resonance.

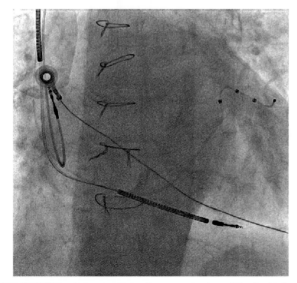

FIGURE 37-7   Anteroposterior fluoroscopic view of the final left ventricular lead position.

Discussion

This patient was in permanent atrial fibrillation. The major outcome trials of CRT, however, have included only patients in sinus rhythm. Notwithstanding, some studies have shown that CRT in the context of atrial fibrillation improves symptoms.[7] Other studies have suggested that CRT in patients in atrial fibrillation is effective only after atrioventricular junction ablation.[2] These findings are encouraging for patients with heart failure and atrial fibrillation, who account for 10% to 25% of patients with heart failure in NYHA class II to III and up to 50% in patients in NYHA class IV. This patient also had a prolonged QRS duration (134 ms) and severely impaired left ventricular function as a result of ischemic cardiomyopathy. It is on this basis that the decision was made to proceed to proceed to implant a CRT defibrillator (CRT-D).

Question

What is the best left ventricular lead position in this patient?

Discussion

Fluoroscopy remains the standard imaging modality for guiding left ventricular lead deployment. As shown at coronary sinus venography (see Figure 37-4), several candidate coronary veins were apparent. As expected after CABG, these veins were generally of small caliber. A posterolateral vein (see Figure 37-4, *option 1*) had a tortuous, proximal segment with a subocclusion that was apparent on the RAO view. This stenosis could be repaired with venoplasty, even in the tortuous segment. After angioplasty, the vein could be straightened using a buddy wire technique. This could allow deployment of a small-caliber (perhaps 4 French) left ventricular lead. A more cranial posterolateral vein (see Figure 37-4, *option 2*) also is an option. This vein drains the mid-lateral segment.

An anterolateral vein (see Figure 37-4, *option 3*) also may be appropriate, on the basis of fluoroscopy. This vein, however, overlies the basal anterior segment, which may be regarded as an inappropriate site for left ventricular lead deployment. In this respect, early CRT studies suggested that the lateral free wall is a better left ventricular pacing site than a more anterior position.[1,3] These findings make mechanical sense, because it is the lateral wall that is typically activated late in the context of a left bundle branch block. Importantly, clinical studies have failed to show superiority of pacing in lateral or posterolateral sites. In a retrospective study of 567 consecutive patients, a posterolateral position (2 to 5 o'clock on the LAO fluoroscopic view) was not associated with a better clinical outcome or echocardiographic response than other positions.[6]

On the basis of the factors discussed previously, most current CRT implanters would be satisfied with *options 1* and *2* (lateral and posterior veins) (see Figure 37-4). Fewer implanters would choose *option 3* (anterolateral vein), particularly because it is a vein of very small caliber.

Question

Should we choose a left ventricular lead position over a late-contracting segment?

Discussion

Single-center echocardiographic studies using tissue Doppler imaging, tissue synchronization imaging, three-dimensional echocardiography, and speckle-tracking echocardiography have shown that a better response to CRT can be achieved if the left ventricular lead is deployed in the area of latest contraction (presumed latest activation).[5]

In this case, we have used feature-tracking cardiovascular magnetic resonance (FT-CMR) for the quantification of myocardial strain. This is a new CMR technique that has been validated against myocardial tagging[4] and uses the same principle as speckle-tracking echocardiography for the quantification of myocardial motion. On the basis of latest contraction segments, we could choose the targets described in the following section.

Basal Segments

As shown in Figure 37-5, *A*, the basal anterior segment contracts earliest (time to peak systolic circumferential

strain, 338 ms), whereas the basal inferior (time to peak systolic circumferential strain, 489 ms) and basal posterior (time to peak systolic circumferential strain, 452 ms) contract the latest. The amplitude of circumferential strain of less than 10% in these segments raises the possibility of myocardial scarring. The only segments that appear not to be scarred are the basal anterior and basal lateral segments, and, of these, the latter contracts latest (time to peak systolic circumferential strain, 414 ms). One of the preferred targets for left ventricular lead deployment using FT-CMR is therefore the basal lateral segment. This site can be reached via the posterolateral vein (see Figure 37-4, *option 2*).

Mid-segments

As shown in Figure 37-5, *B*, the mid-inferior segments contract the latest (time to peak systolic circumferential strain, 367 ms). The low amplitude of strain (−8.85%), however, suggests that this segment is scarred. Of the remaining segments, the mid-anterior segment contracts relatively late (time to peak systolic circumferential strain, 338 ms), as does the mid-lateral segment (time to peak systolic circumferential strain, 310 ms). The latest contracting, nonscarred mid-segments are therefore the mid-anterior and the mid-lateral segments.

Apical Segments

As shown in Figure 37-5, *C*, both the apical lateral and apical inferior segments contract late, in contrast to the apical anterior segment (time to peak systolic circumferential strain of 349 ms and 285, respectively). The apical lateral segment appears scarred (amplitude of peak circumferential strain, −6.67%). Therefore the apical inferior segment is the latest contracting, nonscarred segment on the basis of FT-CMR.

Conclusions from Feature-Tracking Cardiovascular Magnetic Resonance

Candidate targets for left ventricular lead deployment on the basis of FT-CMR are the basal lateral segment, the mid-anterior and the mid-lateral segments, and the apical inferior segment.

Question

Should a left ventricular lead position be chosen over a non-scarred segment, assessed using LGE-CMR?

Discussion

Although myocardial strain can be used as a surrogate for myocardial scarring, the gold standard for detection and quantification of myocardial scarring in vivo is LGE-CMR. Several studies have shown that viability of the paced left ventricular segment also influences the outcome of CRT.

As shown in Figure 37-6, this patient had sustained an extensive myocardial infarction in the territory of the circumflex artery, which extended from the basal to the apical segments, involving the left ventricular free wall but sparing the basal anterior and basal lateral segments. Therefore, on the basis of LGE-CMR alone, the basal anterior and the basal lateral segments are appropriate targets for left ventricular lead deployment. Of these, the basal lateral segment contracts later than the basal anterior segment (see Figure 37-5, *A*). Using the combination of LGE-CMR and FT-CMR, the basal lateral segment is the latest contracting viable segment.

A shown in Figure 37-6, the mid-anterior and the mid-posterior segments were shown to have a peak circumferential strain of –24.78 and –10.71%, respectively, suggesting active contraction. Importantly, LGE-CMR shows that these segments have subendocardial and transmural scars, respectively. All of the apical segments were scarred.

FINAL DIAGNOSIS

The final diagnosis is symptomatic systolic heart failure, with severely impaired left ventricular function despite maximum tolerated medical therapy. In addition, the patient had permanent atrial fibrillation.

PLAN OF ACTION

For this patient the plan was CRT-D implantation, targeting the basal lateral segment for left ventricular lead deployment. A future option is atrioventricular junction ablation.

INTERVENTION

On the basis of the fluoroscopic images alone, an implanter might have been tempted to deploy the left ventricular lead in a posterolateral vein (see Figure 37-4, *option 1*). Although the vein was tortuous and stenosed in its proximal portion, this could have been surmounted by venoplasty and buddy wire technique. However, the segments subtended by this vein were the site of a transmural myocardial infarction. This was clear from the LGE-CMR images and FT-CMR strain analyses, which showed that the latest contracting, viable segment was the basal lateral segment.

To reach the basal lateral segment, the left ventricular lead was deployed in the posterolateral vein (see Figure 37-4, *option 2*). Anticipating some overlap of the pacing electrode with adjacent scar, a quadripolar lead (Quartet, St Jude Medical, St. Paul, Minn.) was selected. Figure 37-7 shows that the distal electrode of the quadripolar left ventricular lead overlies the mid-lateral segment which harbors a transmural scar on LGE-CMR. However, the mid-electrodes overlie the targeted basal lateral segment. At implantation, bipolar pacing thresholds in the distal poles were high (2.75-4.0 V, at a pulse duration of 0.5 ms). Bipolar pacing vectors incorporating the more proximal electrodes were associated with lower thresholds (1.5 to 3.0 V, at a pulse duration of 0.5 ms) but were associated with phrenic nerve stimulation. Pacing from the mid-electrodes (to the right ventricular coil) was associated with the lowest threshold (0.75 V at 0.5 ms, with phrenic nerve stimulation occurring at 4.0 V at 0.5 ms).

OUTCOME

At a 2-month follow-up examination, the patient was in NYHA class I.

Findings

The left ventricular pacing threshold was 0.75 (at 0.5 ms), and phrenic nerve stimulation occurred at 4 V (at 0.5 ms).

Comments

In this patient the combination of FT-CMR and LGE-CMR was used to identify the latest contracting viable segment over the left ventricular free wall in a patient undergoing CRT. Using fluoroscopy alone, some implanters might have selected the posterolateral vein, but this subtended a transmural myocardial scar.

Despite compelling evidence from observational studies, the utility of LGE-CMR has not been assessed by randomized controlled studies. Furthermore, FT-CMR is in its infancy as a technology for the assessment of cardiac dyssynchrony. Further studies are needed to determine whether the combination of these techniques, which can be applied to routine CMR scanning without additional acquisitions, can be used to guide CRT left ventricular lead deployment.

Selected References

1. Butter C, Auricchio A, Stellbrink C, et al: Effect of resynchronization therapy stimulation site on the systolic function of heart failure patients, *Circulation* 104:3026-3029, 2001.
2. Gasparini M, Auricchio A, Metra M, et al: Long-term survival in patients undergoing cardiac resynchronization therapy: the importance of performing atrio-ventricular junction ablation in patients with permanent atrial fibrillation, *Eur Heart J* 29:1644-1652, 2008.
3. Gold MR, Auricchio A, Hummel JD, et al: Comparison of stimulation sites within left ventricular veins on the acute hemodynamic effects of cardiac resynchronization therapy, *Heart Rhythm* 2:376-381, 2005.

4. Hor KN, Gottliebson WM, Carson C, et al: Comparison of magnetic resonance feature tracking for strain calculation with harmonic phase imaging analysis, *Cardiovasc Imaging* 3:144-151, 2010.

5. Khan FZ, Virdee MS, Palmer CR, et al: Targeted left ventricular lead placement to guide cardiac resynchronization therapy: the TARGET study: a randomized, controlled trial, *J Am Coll Cardiol* 59:1509-1518, 2012.

6. Kronborg MB, Albertsen AE, Nielsen JC, et al: Long-term clinical outcome and left ventricular lead position in cardiac resynchronization therapy, *Europace* 11:1177-1182, 2009.

7. Linde C, Leclercq C, Rex S, et al: Long-term benefits of biventricular pacing in congestive heart failure: results from the MUltisite STimulation In Cardiomyopathy (MUSTIC) study, *J Am Coll Cardiol* 40:111-118, 2002.

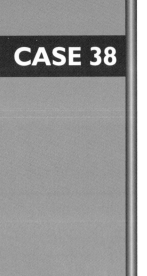

CASE 38

Role of Scar Burden Versus Distribution Assessment by Cardiovascular Magnetic Resynchronization in Ischemia

Jagdesh Kandala and Theofanie Mela

CASE 1

Age	Gender	Occupation	Working Diagnosis
63 Years	Male	Businessman	Acute Coronary Syndrome

HISTORY

A 63-year-old man presented to the emergency room with recent-onset episodic chest discomfort described as "muscle ache." The chest discomfort was radiating to the upper neck and both arms, associated with a tingling sensation. It was not reproducible or worsened on deep inspiration. He recently noticed dyspnea with minimal effort without any associated chest discomfort. However, he denied orthopnea, paroxysmal nocturnal dyspnea, pedal edema, and loss of consciousness.

A year previously, he was diagnosed with coronary artery disease, requiring a bare metal stent insertion for revascularization of 95% obstructive stenosis in the proximal left anterior descending coronary artery. His left ventricular ejection fraction (LVEF) was 38% at the time, and his electrocardiogram (ECG) revealed left bundle branch block (LBBB) morphology. His medical history included 9 months of chemotherapy for non-Hodgkin's lymphoma. Approximately 4 years before the current visit, he was diagnosed with right cavernous meningioma, which was successfully treated with stereotactic radiation therapy without mantle radiation. During the same year, he was treated for benign prostatic hypertrophy with transurethral resection of prostate. He was being treated for depression, anxiety disorder, and hypothyroidism. The patient was married for 35 years and had two grown children. He reported stress at work, was a nonsmoker, and consumed alcohol socially. During the period of chemotherapy, he used marijuana. He had two sisters, who had cardiomyopathy of unclear cause. Both of his sisters died young, at 16 and 42 years of age. The patient's niece was diagnosed with cardiomyopathy at the age of 38 and eventually needed cardiac transplantation.

CURRENT MEDICATIONS

The patient was taking levothyroxine 175 mcg daily, metoprolol 25 mg twice daily, bupropion 150 mg twice daily for depression, valsartan 160 mg daily, hydrochlorthiazide 12.5 mg daily, atorvastatin 40 mg daily, lorazepam 0.5 mg three times daily as needed for anxiety, zolpidem 5 mg daily at bedtime as needed for insomnia, and aspirin 325 mg daily.

CURRENT SYMPTOMS

The patient's current symptoms were chest discomfort of 2 weeks, exertional dyspnea, and reduced exercise tolerance. On examination, he was overweight and not in any apparent distress and had a temperature of 36.8° C (98.2° F) and oxygen saturation of 99% on room air. The neurologic examination was nonfocal.

PHYSICAL EXAMINATION

BP/HR: 147/80 mm Hg/54 bpm
Neck veins: No jugular venous distention
Lungs/chest: Exertional dyspnea, reduced exercise tolerance, respiratory rate of 18 breaths per minute, no crackles, rhonchi, or wheezes
Heart: Regular rate, normal heart sounds, 1/6 holosystolic murmur at the left sternal border, no pericardial rub or gallop
Abdomen: Soft, nontender, no evidence of pedal edema

LABORATORY DATA

Hemoglobin: 13.7 g/dL
Hematocrit: 38.4%
Total leukocyte count: 6200 cells/mm³
Platelet count: 164 × 10³/μL
Sodium: 135 mmol/L
Potassium: 3.9 mmol/L
Chloride: 104 mmol/L
Creatinine: 1.2 mg/dL
Creatine kinase: 88 units/mL
Bicarbonate: 24 mmol/L
N-Terminal brain natriuretic peptide: 258 ng/mL
Blood urea nitrogen: 30 mmol/L
Creatine kinase–myocardial bound: 2.9%
Troponin I and T: Negative

ELECTROCARDIOGRAM

The ECG showed sinus bradycardia at a rate of 55 bpm, first-degree atrioventricular block (PR interval of 210 ms), LBBB unchanged in contrast to ECG obtained 1 month earlier. The QRS duration was 164 ms. No ST-T changes suggestive of ischemia were noted (Figure 38-1).

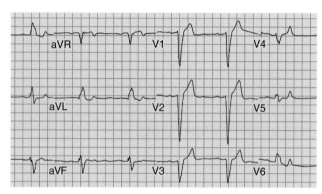

FIGURE 38-1 **Case 1.** Baseline electrocardiogram showing sinus bradycardia, left bundle branch block, and first-degree atrioventricular block.

CHEST RADIOGRAPH

The posteroanterior and lateral radiographic views demonstrated poor inspiration, mild cardiomegaly, and no evidence of infiltrate or effusion (Figure 38-2).

Comments

The patient's chest discomfort and exertional dyspnea in the setting of prior coronary artery disease were concerning for acute coronary syndrome. It was reassuring that the initial myocardial markers were negative. Most important, the patient was not in acute heart failure.

ECHOCARDIOGRAM

The transthoracic echocardiogram showed normally functioning valves in mitral, aortic, tricuspid, and pulmonary positions. The left ventricle was diffusely hypokinetic with some regional variation, which was especially worse in the septum and apex. The LVEF diminished further to 32% in contrast to 38% 8 months previously.

Comments

The patient was admitted to the cardiac care unit. The serial cardiac enzyme examinations and ECGs showed no evidence of acute myocardial infarction.

EXERCISE TESTING

The patient was able to complete a technetium-99m single-photon emission computed tomography (SPECT) myocardial perfusion scan. The exercise test was terminated because of the development of 2:1 atrioventricular block with hypotension. The SPECT perfusion imaging showed fixed perfusion defects in the anterior and septal segments. The left ventricle was dilated, demonstrating global systolic dysfunction.

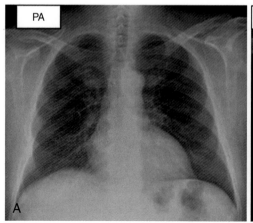
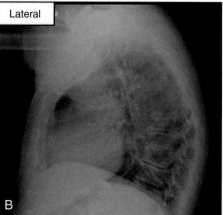

FIGURE 38-2 **Case 1.**
Posteroanterior and lateral views of chest radiograph showing no congestive changes, infiltrate, or effusion.

CARDIAC CATHETERIZATION

Subsequently, coronary angiography was performed that showed no evidence of obstructive coronary artery disease. The proximal left anterior descending artery with a prior bare metal stent was patent. The right coronary artery, the left main coronary artery, and the left circumflex artery showed minor luminal irregularities. No obstructive lesions were present.

CARDIAC MAGNETIC RESONANCE IMAGING

Cardiac magnetic resonance (CMR) with and without gadopentetate dimeglumine showed no evidence of myocardial edema. Delayed enhancement was seen in the subendocardial region of mid-anterior, anterolateral, and lateral apical segment consistent with scar. Scar extent was about 2% of left ventricular mass (Figure 38-3).

FINAL DIAGNOSIS

The patient's final diagnosis was mixed ischemia and non-ischemic cardiomyopathy.

FOCUSED CLINICAL QUESTIONS AND DISCUSSION POINTS

Question

What is the best management strategy to minimize the risk for sudden cardiac death in this patient?

Discussion

The patient had cardiomyopathy with an LVEF of 32% associated with LBBB in the setting of coronary artery disease, as well as New York Heart Association (NYHA) class II heart failure. Further, an added burden of conduction system disease manifested as first-degree atrioventricular block and LBBB on baseline ECG and development of Mobitz type 2 atrioventricular block with exercise, were suggestive of atrioventricular nodal or infranodal disease. In addition, the patient had a family history of cardiomyopathy and sudden cardiac death. Overall, he was at high risk for sudden cardiac death. He met the class I indication for pacing and the primary prevention criteria for implantable cardioverter-defibrillator (ICD) implantation.[7] Increasing the medical therapy, especially beta blocker dosage, was not a viable option because of the bradycardia and relative hypotension. Pacemaker implantation will allow increasing the dosage of beta blockers but not address the sudden cardiac death risk. Overall, the patient has cardiomyopathy with low LVEF and dyssynchrony, as indicated by LBBB and wide QRS that can be best managed with cardiac resynchronization therapy with backup defibrillator (CRT-D).

Question

What further investigation will help in the decision-making process?

Discussion

The patient's cardiomyopathy was much more advanced than the degree of coronary artery disease would explain, raising the possibility of the coexistence of idiopathic dilated cardiomyopathy or sarcoidosis or chemotherapy-induced cardiomyopathy. CMR will not only assess cardiac substrate with better resolution but also determine the scar burden and the scar location. Delayed-enhancement CMR (DE-CMR) or Late Gadolinium Enhancement (LGE)-CMR has been demonstrated to identify and quantify the scar accurately. CMR myocardial tagging can perform radial strain analysis to identify areas of dyssynchrony. An equilibrium contrast CMR can assess diffuse myocardial scar. It is also able to assess coronary venous anatomy that would help identify a suitable branch in an optimal left ventricular segment for left ventricular lead implantation. In addition, CMR is the gold standard for determining left ventricular function and volumes.

Mixed ischemic and nonischemic cardiomyopathy with atrioventricular nodal and intraventricular conduction system disease.

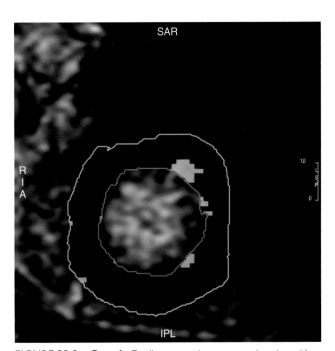

FIGURE 38-3 Case 1. Cardiac magnetic resonance imaging with late gadolinium enhancement suggestive of scar in the anterior and anterolateral segments of left ventricle. Scar burden was estimated to be 2% of the total left ventricular mass.

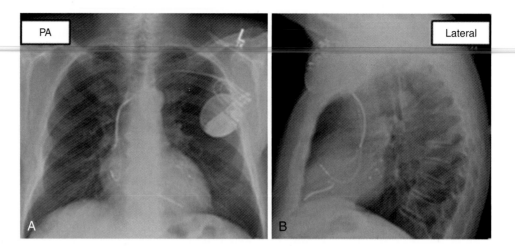

FIGURE 38-4 **Case 1.** Left ventricular lead location in the basal lateral segment on a postimplant chest radiograph.

Question

What factors influenced the beneficial effect of CRT in this patient?

Discussion

The presence of LBBB, wide QRS duration (>150 ms), absence of atrial fibrillation, and optimal left ventricular lead location in a basal lateral segment are predictors of clinical response and left ventricular reverse remodeling.[8] Patients with ischemic cardiomyopathy tend to benefit less from CRT than those with nonischemic cardiomyopathy.[8] This has been attributed to the extent of myocardial viability and the myocardial scar.[8] However, the patient's myocardial scar burden was only 2% of total left ventricular mass, and based on CMR the scar appears to be located away from the region of left ventricular lead pacing site.

PLAN OF ACTION

The plan for this patient is CRT-D implantation. Further optimization of medical therapy was done after pacing had been established.

INTERVENTION

A primary biventricular chamber ICD system was implanted transvenously with final left ventricular lead position in left ventricular basal lateral segments (Figure 38-4). The right ventricular lead location was apico-septal.

OUTCOME

The patient responded well to CRT, with an improvement in exercise capacity. He was able to walk for 1560 feet on the 6-minute walk test (6MWT), in contrast to 1060 feet before CRT. He scored 43 on the Minnesota Living with Heart Failure questionnaire in contrast to 48 at baseline. Subsequently, a 6-month transthoracic echocardiogram demonstrated an improvement in LVEF to 48% and good left ventricular reverse remodeling, demonstrated by a decrease in left ventricular internal dimensions in diastole at 6 months from 45 to 42 mm and in systole from 37 to 30 mm.

CASE 2

Age	Gender	Occupation	Working Diagnosis
64 Years	Male	Teacher	Acute Coronary Syndrome

HISTORY

A 64 year-old man arrived in the emergency room with a 2-day history of exertional shortness of breath and exertional chest pressure. He reported excessive sweating on exertion. However, he denied having nausea, vomiting, dizziness, and palpitations. He had a history of a five-vessel coronary artery bypass graft (CABG). Approximately 9 years later, he required a revision of CABG in addition to bioprosthetic mitral valve replacement. Four years previously, he experienced gastrointestinal bleeding that was thought to have originated from gastritis. In addition he had stage III chronic kidney disease.

CURRENT MEDICATIONS

The patient was taking hydrocholorothiazide 12.5 mg daily, lisinopril 2.5 mg daily, furosemide 20 mg daily orally, atorvastatin 20 mg daily, amiodarone 200 mg daily, atenolol 50 mg daily, gemfibrozil 600 mg daily, and aspirin 81 mg daily.

PHYSICAL EXAMINATION

BP/HR: 125/76 mm Hg/62 bpm
Respiratory rate: 18 breaths/min
Temperature: 37.3° C (99.2° F)
Oxygen saturation: 99% on room air
Height/weight: 180 cm/105 kg
Neck veins: No jugular vein distention
Lungs/chest: Clear
Heart: Regular heart rate with normal heart sounds, no murmur, no pericardial rub or gallop
Abdomen: Soft, nontender
Extremities: Evidence of pedal edema
Neurologic: Unremarkable

LABORATORY DATA

Hemoglobin: 14.9 g/dL
White blood cell count: 10,700 cells/mm^2
Hematocrit: 43.4%
Mean corpuscular volume: 88 fL
Platelet count: 209 × 10^3/μL
Sodium: 141 mmol/L
Potassium: 5.3 mmol/L
Chloride: 108 mmol/L
Bicarbonate: 24 mmol/L
Creatinine: 2.9 mg/dL
Creatine kinase: 88 units/mL
Blood urea nitrogen: 34 mg/dL
N-Terminal probrain natriuretic peptide: 15,776 pg/mL
Creatine kinase–myocardial bound: 2.9%
Troponin I and T: Negative

ELECTROCARDIOGRAM

The ECG showed atrial fibrillation with a heart rate of 62 bpm and intraventricular conduction delay with a QRS duration of 129 ms (Figure 38-5). A few premature ventricular complexes were noted.

CHEST RADIOGRAPH

A portable chest radiographic view demonstrated moderate cardiomegaly. Moderate-sized left-sided pleural effusion was evident.

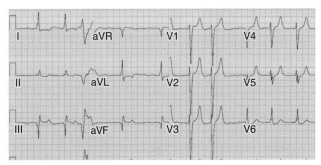

FIGURE 38-5   Case 2. Baseline ECG demonstrating atrial fibrillation and nonspecific interventricular conduction delay.

ECHOCARDIOGRAM

A normally seated bioprosthetic valve was seen in the mitral position with normal leaflet motion. The left ventricle was dilated, with impaired systolic function and an LVEF of 31%. Focal wall thinning and increased reflectivity of the inferior wall were suggestive of scar. The estimated right ventricular systolic pressure was 28 mm Hg.

Comments

The patient was admitted to the intensive care unit to rule out acute coronary syndrome. Subsequent cardiac biomarkers were negative. He underwent myocardial perfusion imaging because of reluctance to perform cardiac catheterization because of compromised renal function.

EXERCISE TESTING

^{99m}Tc sestamibi SPECT imaging at rest and stress revealed fixed perfusion defects at inferior basal, inferior middle, and inferior apical segments. Inferior wall akinesia and hypokinesia without evidence of reversible ischemia were present. The LVEF was 28%.

CARDIAC MAGNETIC RESONANCE IMAGING

CMR with and without gadopentetate dimeglumine demonstrated areas of delayed hyperenhancement in the inferior wall (Figure 38-6). Evidence of transmural infarction in the inferior wall was present, mostly in the apical segment; it was partially transmural in the basal to mid-ventricular segments of the inferior wall. Severe global left ventricular systolic dysfunction was present. The scar extent was estimated to be 12.3% of total left ventricular mass.

Question

How can the difference in response to CRT in the patients in case 1 and case 2 be explained?

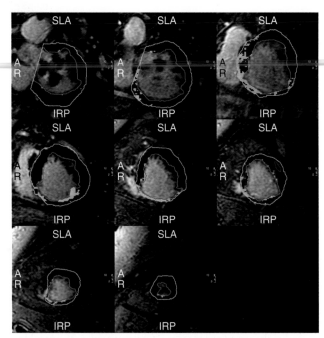

FIGURE 38-6 **Case 2.** Cardiac magnetic resonance imaging demonstrating extensive inferior wall scar. Extent of myocardial scar is 12.3% of the total left ventricular mass.

Discussion

The patient in case 2 responded suboptimally to CRT. Although an improvement in activity level and a modest improvement in LVEF occurred, echocardiographic evidence of left ventricular reverse remodeling was found. Further, his clinical outcome was less than desired. He was hospitalized for congestive heart failure and ventricular arrhythmia. This suboptimal response could be attributed to the ischemic heart disease, higher scar burden, position of the left ventricular lead in the region of scar, relatively narrow QRS (129 ms), and nonspecific intraventricular conduction delay on baseline ECG. In addition, his scar burden level was 12.3% of total left ventricular mass. In a study of 137 patients referred for ICD, DE-CMR was performed to assess scar burden. The study reported fivefold increase in adverse events in patients with myocardial scar of more than 5% of the left ventricular mass.[5] Figures 38-3 and 38-6 show the contrast in the scar burden in the patients in the two cases. In addition, the left ventricular lead in the patient in case 2 was located in the mid-posterolateral wall where partially transmural scar tissue was present, whereas in the patient in case 1 the left ventricular lead was located in a mid-lateral ventricular segment that was away from the scar segment. Left ventricular pacing on an area of scar may result in ineffectual pacing and inadequate resynchronization. A randomized controlled trial, the TARGET study, showed improved clinical outcome when the left ventricular lead was located away from the scar.[10] All of these factors may have played a role in the suboptimal response to CRT seen in the patient in case 2.

Question

Which is more important—myocardial scar location or myocardial scar burden?

Discussion

Scar burden and scar location are increasingly recognized as important determinants of CRT response. Theoretically, higher scar burden implies lesser availability of viable and recruitable myocardium to improve ventricular contraction. Ypenburg and colleagues[15] studied 34 patients and reported an inverse relationship between total scar burden, spatial extent, and transmurality of scar as measured by a 5-point hyperenhancement scale on CMR and change in left ventricular end-systolic volume at 6 months. In a study of 190 patients with ischemic cardiomyopathy,[2] low scar burden (Summed Rest Score <27) as determined by thallium-201 myocardial perfusion imaging had a favorable rate and LVEF improvement in contrast to higher scar burden (SRS ≥27). The scar burden adversely affects CRT response in ischemic and nonischemic cardiomyopathy and hypertrophic cardiomyopathy. In a study of 213 patients with ischemic and nonischemic cardiomyopathy, the authors reported lower LVEF improvement with higher scar burden (>22% as assessed by CMR) in contrast to lower scar burden (<22%). In that study, left ventricular lead location on scar was not a significant predictor of CRT response.[14] However, only 11% of left ventricular leads were located in the region of scar. Conversely, anatomic segmental location of scar tissue was found to have an adverse impact on CRT response in other studies. Bleeker and associates[3] reported worse clinical outcome with transmural scar in a posterolateral segment of the left ventricle independent of scar burden, LVEF, left ventricular end-systolic volume, and QRS duration, although the sample size was much smaller, with only 40 patients. In a similar study, higher heart failure hospitalization rates and death were noted if the left ventricular lead was located in a segment of scar or in the presence of posterolateral scar.[5]

Current evidence, derived mostly from small cohort studies (Table 38-1), underscores the importance of scar burden, segmental scar location, and the relationship between scar tissue and left ventricular lead location. Scar burden and location have the potential to play a role in better patient selection and improvement of the rate of nonresponsiveness to CRT. Further studies are necessary to determine the most appropriate imaging modality to assess scar location, its burden before CRT-D implantation, and its impact on outcome. Furthermore, left ventricular pacing on a region of scar tissue would be ineffectual; therefore avoiding the region of scar tissue during device implantation is a reasonable approach.

TABLE 38-1   Selected Studies Investigating the Impact of Myocardial Scar on Cardiac Resynchronization Therapy Response

Study	Patient Characteristics	Scar Assessment	Conclusions
Mele et al[12] 2009	71 patients with ICM	Echocardiography	Poor CRT response with a higher number of scar segments and closer location to pacing lead
Adelstein et al[1] 2007	50 patients with ICM	Myocardial perfusion Imaging	Higher nonresponse to CRT with higher SPS score, scar density, and greater scar density near the left ventricular lead
Ypenburg et al[15] 2007	34 patients with ICM	DE-CMR	Total scar burden was inversely related to CRT response
Delgado et al[6] 2011	397 patients with ICM	Speckle-tracking radial strain analysis and DE-CMR	Left ventricular lead location on scar was a predictor of worse outcome
Adelstein et al[2] 2011	190 patients with ICM	Thallium-201 SPECT MPI	Higher scar burden (SRS >27) was associated with poor survival
Chalil et al[5] 2007	62 patients with ICM	DE-CMR	Presence of posterolateral scar and pacing on scar were independent predictor of response
Jansen et al[9] 2008	57 patients with ICM + NICM	CMR	Left ventricular dyssynchrony is more important than scar
Ypenburg et al[15] 2007	51 patients with ICM	Technitium-99m SPECT	Both the extent of scar tissue and its location near the left ventricle lead prohibits CRT response
Birnie et al[4] 2009	49 patients with ICM and NICM	Rubidium and fluorine-18-fluorodeoxyglucose PET	Responders had less lateral wall scar than nonresponders but a similar extent of global and septal scar
Bleeker et al[3] 2006	40 patients with ICM	CMR	Posterolateral wall scar was associated with poor response to CRT
Riedlbauchova et al[13] 2009	66 patients with ICM	PET scan	Response to CRT was observed regardless of the presence of total scar and left ventricular lead location in the region of scar or ischemia or hibernation

CMR, Cardiac magnetic resonance; *CRT,* cardiac resynchronization therapy; *DE-CMR,* delayed-enhancement CMR; *ICM,* ischemic cardiomyopathy; *MPI,* myocardial perfusion imaging; *NICM,* nonischemic cardiomyopathy; *PET,* positron emission tomography; *SPECT,* single-photon emission computed tomography; *SRS,* summed rest score; *SPS,* summed perfusion score.

FINAL DIAGNOSIS

The final diagnosis in this patient was ischemic cardiomyopathy, NYHA class II to III heart failure, and left ventricular systolic dyssynchrony, as suggested by the wide QRS, together with chronic renal insufficiency.

Comments

The patient had worsening dyspnea resulting from progressive ischemic cardiomyopathy. Because of the absence of objective evidence of ischemia, his worsening symptoms might be attributed to progressive left ventricular remodeling and dyssynchrony. CRT may help in correcting dyssynchrony and reversing the left ventricular remodeling.

INTERVENTION

CRT-D implantation was performed, and the postimplant chest radiograph showed final left ventricular lead in a mid-ventricular and posterolateral location.

OUTCOME

Six months after CRT device implantation, the patient demonstrated at best modest improvement. Although his LVEF improved from 21% to 28% and he was able to walk to 1080 feet in the 6MWT in contrast to 720 feet before CRT-D, he was only minimally better subjectively. He scored 24 on the Minnesota Living with Heart Failure quality of life score in contrast to

30 before CRT-D implantation. A follow-up echocardiogram at 6 months demonstrated left ventricular internal diameter–diastole of 74 mm and left ventricular internal diameter–systole of 63 mm, in contrast to 71 mm and 63 mm, respectively, on pre-CRT echocardiogram. He was hospitalized twice—for ventricular tachycardia and for worsening congestive heart failure—within a few months of CRT implantation

Selected References

1. Adelstein EC, Saba S: Scar bruden by myocardial perfusion imaging predicts response to cardiac resynchronization therapy in ischemic cardiomyopathy, *Am Heart J* 153:105-112, 2007.
2. Adelstein EC, Tanaka H, Soman P, et al: Impact of scar burden by single-photon emission computed tomography myocardial perfusion imaging on patient outcomes following cardiac resynchronization therapy, *Eur Heart J* 32:93-103, 2011.
3. Bleeker GB, Kaandorp TA, Lamb HJ, et al: Effect of posterolateral scar tissue on clinical and echocardiographic improvement after cardiac resynchronization therapy, *Circulation* 113:969-976, 2006.
4. Birnie D, DeKemp RA, Ruddy TD, et al: Effect of lateral wall scar on reverse remodeling with cardiac resynchronization therapy, *Heart Rhythm* 6:1721-1726, 2009.
5. Chalil S, Foley PW, Muyhaldeen SA, et al: Late gadolinium enhancement-cardiovascular magnetic resonance as a predictor of response to cardiac resynchronization therapy in patients with ischaemic cardiomyopathy, *Europace* 9:1031-1037, 2007.
6. Delgado V, van Bommel RJ, Bertini M, et al: Relative merits of left ventricular dyssynchrony, left ventricular lead position, and myocardial scar to protect long-term survival of ischemic heart failure patients undergoing cardiac resynchronization therapy, *Circulation* 123:70-78, 2011.
7. Epstein AE, Dimarco JP, Ellenbogen KA, et al: ACC/AHA/HRS 2008 Guidelines for device-based therapy of cardiac rhythm abnormalities, *Heart Rhythm* 5:e1-62, 2008.
8. Goldenberg I, Moss AJ, Hall WJ, et al: Predictors of response to cardiac resynchronization therapy in the Multicenter Automatic Defibrillator Implantation Trial with Cardiac Resynchronization Therapy (MADIT-CRT), *Circulation* 124:1527-1536, 2011.
9. Jansen AH, Bracke F, van Dantzig JM, et al: The influence of myocardial scar and dyssynchrony on reverse remodeling in cardiac resynchronization therapy, *Eur J Echocardiogr* 9:483-488, 2008.
10. Khan FZ, Virdee MS, Palmer CR, et al: Targeted left ventricular lead placement to guide cardiac resynchronization therapy: the TARGET study: a randomized, controlled trial, *J Am Coll Cardiol* 59:1509-1518, 2012.
11. Klem I, Weinsaft JW, Bahnson TD, et al: Assessment of myocardial scarring improves risk stratification in patients evaluated for cardiac defibrillator implantation, *J Am Coll Cardiol* 60:408-420, 2012.
12. Mele D, Agricola E, Galderisi M, et al: Echocardiographic myocardial scar burden predicts response to cardiac resynchronization therapy in ischemic heart failure, *J Am Soc Echocardiogr* 22:702-708, 2009.
13. Riedlbauchova L, Brunken R, Jaber WA, et al: The impact of myocardial viability on the clinical outcome of cardiac resynchronization therapy, *J Cardiovasc Electrophysiol* 20:50-57, 2009.
14. Xu YZ, Cha YM, Feng D, et al: Impact of myocardial scarring on outcomes of cardiac resynchronization therapy: extent or location? *J Nucl Med* 53:47-54, 2012.
15. Ypenburg C, Schalij MJ, Bleeker GB, et al: Impact of viability and scar tissue on response to cardiac resynchronization therapy in ischaemic heart failure patients, *Eur Heart J* 28:33-41, 2007.

Difficulties in Prediction of Response to Cardiac Resynchronization Therapy

Silvia Pica, Claudia Raineri, and Stefano Ghio

Age	Gender	Occupation	Working Diagnosis
46 Years	Male	Engineer	Dilated Cardiomyopathy

HISTORY

The patient was diagnosed with myasthenia gravis at the age of 40 years. He reported no cardiologic symptoms until January 2009, when he started experiencing dyspnea on effort. In May 2009 he patient was hospitalized because of congestive heart failure; the echocardiographic examination revealed severe left ventricular dilation and dysfunction. Diuretics and angiotensin-converting enzyme inhibitor therapy were started during the hospitalization, and the patient's condition improved.

The next month the patient was admitted to our hospital for a complete diagnostic workup and therapeutic optimization.

Comments

An association between myasthenia gravis and giant cell myocarditis has been described in the literature. Giant cell myocarditis is a severe autoimmune disease, and anticardiac antibodies have been demonstrated in the serum of affected patients; it is frequently associated with other autoimmune conditions, such as systemic lupus erythematosus, thyroiditis, polymyositis, and myasthenia gravis. Although the pathogenesis is poorly understood, the overall mechanisms for the generation of autoantibodies in giant cell myocarditis include self-sensitization to cardiac antigens in the thymus, production of self-reactive T cells, stimulation of B cells, production of cardiac autoantibodies, and myonecrosis. These antibodies include anti-titin, anti-ryanodine, anti–alpha actinin, anti-actin, and anti-myosin.

CURRENT MEDICATIONS

The patient was taking captopril 25 mg three times daily, furosemide 50 mg once daily, digoxin 0.125 mg once daily, potassium canrenoate 25 mg once daily, warfarin 2.5 mg once daily, pantoprazol 40 mg once daily, pyridostigmine bromide 60 mg once daily, prednisone 12.5 mg every other day.

Comments

Beta blocker therapy was contraindicated because of the myasthenia gravis.

CURRENT SYMPTOMS

The patient was experiencing dyspnea on minimal exertion (New York Heart Association [NYHA] class III).

PHYSICAL EXAMINATION

BP/HR: 85/55 mm Hg/70 bpm
Height/weight: 182 cm/51 kg
Neck veins: No jugular vein distention
Lungs/chest: Clear murmur, no signs of congestion
Heart: Rhythmic first heart sound (S_1) and second heart sound (S_2), no adjunctive murmurs
Abdomen: Treatable abdominal symptoms, peristalsis present
Extremities: Warm, pulses present
Body surface area: 1.7 m²

Comments

The patient had no clinical signs of pulmonary or systemic congestion.

LABORATORY DATA

Hemoglobin: 15.9 g/dL
Hematocrit/packed cell volume: 46.98%
Mean corpuscular volume: 86.9 fL

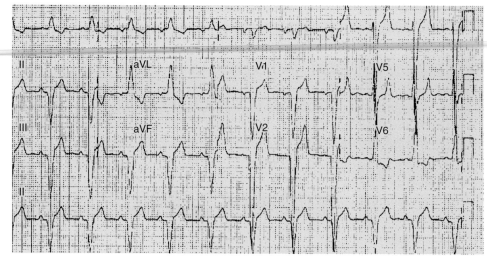

FIGURE 39-1   Preimplant electrocardiogram.

Platelet count: $193 \times 10^3/\mu L$
Sodium: 134 mEq/L
Potassium: 3.8 mEq/L
Creatinine: 1.07 mg/dL
Blood urea nitrogen: 46 mg/dL

ELECTROCARDIOGRAM

Findings

The electrocardiogram (ECG) showed sinus rhythm and complete left bundle branch block (Figure 39-1).

Comments

The ECG clearly suggested the possibility for performing cardiac resynchronization therapy (CRT).

ECHOCARDIOGRAM

Findings

The echocardiogram revealed a left ventricular end-diastolic diameter of 70 mm, end-systolic diameter of 68 mm, mitral annulus diameter of 36 mm, tenting length of 14 mm, and tethering area of 4 cm² (Figure 39-2).

Comments

The patient had severe left ventricular dilation and dysfunction, with tethering of the mitral papillary muscles and dilation of the mitral annulus (see Figure 39-2).

Findings

The echocardiogram showed a left ventricular end-diastolic volume index of 178 mL/m², left ventricular end-systolic volume index of 149 mL/m², left ventricular

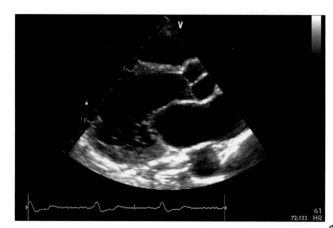

FIGURE 39-2   Parasternal long axis view. See *expertconsult.com* for video.

ejection fraction (LVEF) of 16%, and functional mitral regurgitation of ++/++++.

Comments

Figure 39-3 shows severe left ventricular dilation and dysfunction.

Comments

Figures 39-3 and 39-4 shows severe left ventricular dilation and dysfunction.

Findings

The time delay between anteroseptal and posterior segments at speckle-tracking radial strain analysis is 300 ms (Figure 39-5).[3]

Comments

No clear evidence of septal flash is present. The measurements of aortic and pulmonary preejection periods (not shown in figures) allowed calculation of an interventricular time delay of greater than 40 msec. Tissue

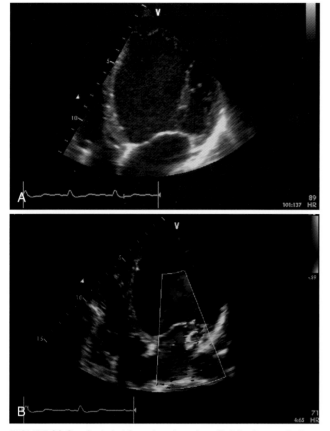

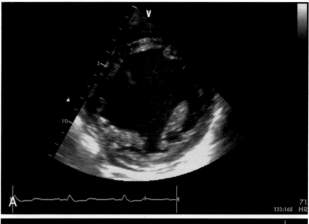

FIGURE 39-3 **A,** Apical four-chamber view. **B,** Mitral regurgitation. See *expertconsult.com* for video.

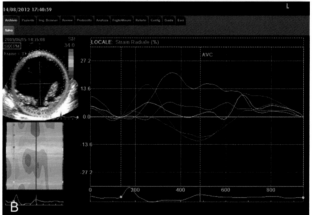

FIGURE 39-5 **A,** Short-axis view at the level of papillary muscles. **B,** Speckle-tracking radial strain analysis. See *expertconsult.com* for video.

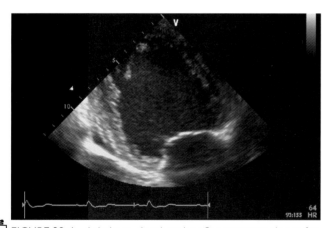

FIGURE 39-4 Apical two-chamber view. See *expertconsult.com* for video.

Doppler analysis (not shown in figures) indicated a time delay between the basal lateral wall and basal septum of greater than 65 msec.

MAGNETIC RESONANCE IMAGING

Findings

Magnetic resonance imaging (MRI) revealed a left ventricular end-diastolic volume of 435 mL, left ventricular end-diastolic volume index of 242 mL/m², left ventricular end-systolic volume of 374 mL, left ventricular end-systolic volume index of 208 mL/m², LVEF of 14%, left ventricular mass of 165 mL, right ventricular end-diastolic volume of 206 mL, right ventricular end-diastolic volume index of 114 mL/m², right ventricular end-systolic volume of 157 mL, right ventricular end-systolic volume index of 87 mL/m², right ventricular ejection fraction of 24%, and left ventricular mass-to-volume ratio of 0.37 (Figure 39-6).

Comments

The patient had severe biventricular dysfunction, with a low left ventricular mass-to-volume ratio (a marker of advanced cardiac remodeling) (see Figure 39-6).

Findings

The delayed enhancement quantification on MRI was 0 mL.

Comments

No fibrosis was seen on MRI (Figures 39-7 and 39-8).

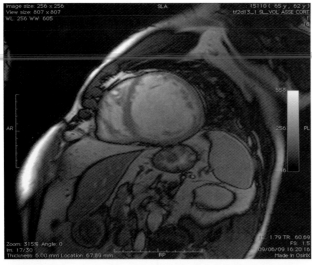

FIGURE 39-6 Cine steady-state free precession sequences. Short-axis stack from the left ventricular base to the apex. See *expertconsult.com* for video.

Findings

The delayed enhancement quantification on MRI was 0 mL.

Comments

No fibrosis was present.[4]

DOBUTAMINE STRESS ECHOCARDIOGRAPHY

Findings

Dobutamine stress echocardiography at 20 mcg/kg/min revealed a left ventricular end-diastolic volume of 295 mL, left ventricular end-diastolic volume index of 173 mL/m^2, left ventricular end-systolic volume of 243 mL, left ventricular end-systolic volume index of 143 mL/m^2, and LVEF of 18% (Figures 39-9 and 39-10).

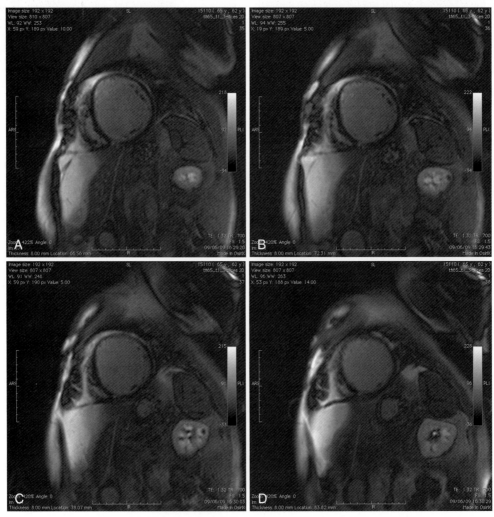

FIGURE 39-7 Late gadolinium (gadopentetate dimeglumine 0.15 mmol/kg) images in short-axis view from the left ventricle base to apex.

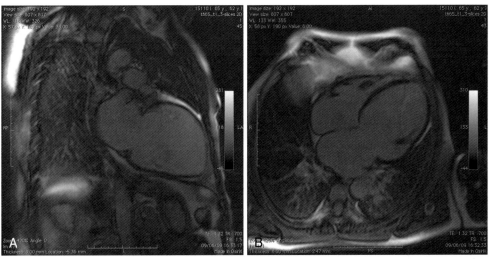

FIGURE 39-8   **A,** Late gadolinium image in two-chamber long-axis view. **B,** Late gadolinium image in four-chamber long-axis view.

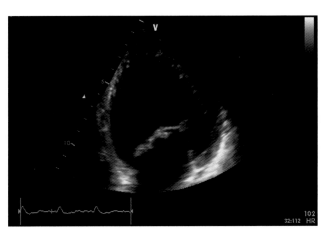

FIGURE 39-9   Apical four-chamber view during dobutamine infusion at 20 mcg/kg/min. See *expertconsult.com* for video.

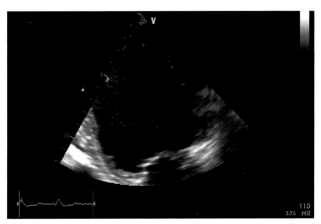

FIGURE 39-10   Apical two-chamber view during dobutamine infusion at 20 mcg/kg/min. See *expertconsult.com* for video.

Comments

In contrast to baseline, during inotropic stimulation a small reduction in left ventricular volumes was noted, but no significant improvement in contractility of the septum occurred and a modest improvement in contractility of the basal lateral wall was seen (Figure 39-9).

Findings

No significant improvement in contractility of the inferior and anterior walls was seen in contrast to baseline.

Comments

During inotropic stimulation no significant improvement was seen in contractility of the inferior and anterior walls (Figure 39-10).[1]

Findings

The calculated time delay between anterior septal and posterior segments at speckle-tracking radial strain analysis was 289 msec, compatible with significant left ventricular dyssynchrony. The appearance of septal flash also was noted. The patient's blood pressure at 20 mcg/kg/min was 100/80 mm Hg.

Comments

During inotropic stimulation a significant worsening of left ventricular dyssynchrony occurred (Figure 39-11).[2,3]

CATHETERIZATION

At right heart catheterization, capillary wedge pressure was 7 mm Hg, pulmonary artery pressure (systolic/mean/diastolic) was 20/10/5 mm Hg, right atrial

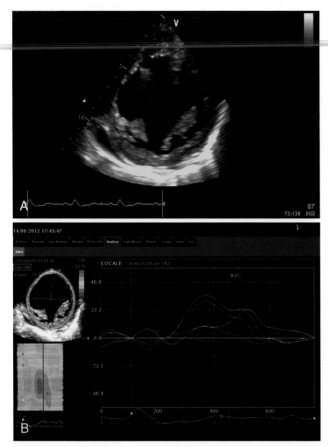

FIGURE 39-11 **A,** Short-axis view at the level of papillary muscles during dobutamine infusion at 20 mcg/kg/min. **B,** Speckle-tracking radial strain analysis during dobutamine infusion. See *expertconsult.com* for video.

pressure was 4 mm Hg, and cardiac index (thermodilution) was 2.29 L/min/m².

Findings

Coronary arteriography was the first examination performed during hospitalization and showed normal coronary arteries.

Comments

Myocardial biopsy was performed and revealed no signs of acute myocarditis, in particular giant cell myocarditis.

FOCUSED CLINICAL QUESTIONS AND DISCUSSION POINTS

Question

Which response to CRT could be predicted in this patient on the basis of left ventricular dyssynchrony analysis?

Discussion

In this patient, significant interventricular and intraventricular dyssynchrony are seen, particularly interventricular (interventricular mechanical delay >40 msec) and intraventricular dyssynchrony (time delay >130 msec between anterior septal and posterior segments on speckle-tracking radial strain analysis and time delay >65 msec between septal and lateral segments on tissue Doppler analysis). Thus, according to extensive literature data, these findings would definitely predict a good response to CRT.

Question

Which response to CRT could be predicted in this patient on the basis of cardiac magnetic resonance (CMR) imaging data?

Discussion

In this case, delayed enhancement is absent, which would support the conclusion that the myocardium is viable; therefore this would predict a positive response to CRT. However, CMR can provide other information. This patient has a low left ventricular mass-to-volume ratio, which might be considered a marker of advanced left ventricular dysfunction (i.e., of a myocardium "too sick to respond to CRT"). CMR information thus is not consistent.

Question

Which response to CRT could be predicted in this patient on the basis of dobutamine stress echo data?

Discussion

Dobutamine infusion elicited only a small increase in left ventricular contractility, which would support the conclusion of the absence of myocardial viability and therefore of a negative response to CRT. However, a clear increase in ventricular dyssynchrony also could be noticed during stress. Therefore even dobutamine stress echo data are difficult to reconcile.

FINAL DIAGNOSIS

The final diagnosis in this patient is primary dilated cardiomyopathy. It was decided to implant a cardiac resynchronization (and antitachycardia) device.

PLAN OF ACTION

The plan for this patient was CRT defibrillator (CRT-D) implantation.

OUTCOME

At 6 months, the patient was in NYHA class II. On echocardiography no improvement in ejection fraction was found (ejection fraction ~15%), but left ventricular end-diastolic and end-systolic volume indices were slightly reduced (respectively, from 178 to 166 mL/m², 7%; and from 148 to 142 mL/m², 4%). According to the reduction in end-systolic volume, the patient was classified as a nonresponder to CRT (the cutoff to define responsiveness is a reduction of at least 15% of end-systolic volume).

INTERVENTION

However, at 6 months the shape of the ventricle clearly changed from a spherical to a more elongate appearance; mitral annulus diameter was reduced to 31 mm, tenting length to 11 mm, and tethering area to 3 cm²; and mitral regurgitation was trivial (in contrast to at least moderate at baseline).

Comments

The first important fact of this case is that no single technique or single parameter allows accurate prediction of response to CRT. The information derived by different techniques often is not consistent, and the best clinical approach is to combine information on dyssynchrony (obtained by several methods) with information on the mechanical substrate amenable to CRT in the failing left ventricle.

The second important point is that not only is predicting the response to CRT difficult but also that defining whether the patient is a positive responder or a negative responder is simplistic. According to the literature, the most commonly accepted definition of a positive response to CRT is a reduction in left ventricular end-systolic volume greater than 15%.

This case also challenges such a definition. The patient did not reach this level of improvement, although he improved subjectively (from NYHA class III to NYHA class II). This can be considered a placebo effect; however, it also could be speculated that the improvement in left ventricular shape and the reduction of mitral regurgitation after CRT may have contributed to the clinical improvement in this patient.

Selected References

1. Muto C, Gasparini M, Peraldo Neja C, et al: Presence of left ventricular contractile reserve predicts midterm response to cardiac resynchronization therapy: results from the LOw dose DObutamine Stress-Echo Test in Cardiac Resynchronization Therapy (LODO-CRT) trial, *Heart Rhythm* 7:1600-1605, 2010.
2. Rocchi G, Bertiniv M, Biffi M, et al: Exercise stress echocardiography is superior to rest echocardiography in predicting left ventricular reverse remodelling and functional improvement after cardiac resynchronization therapy, *Eur Heart J* 30:89-97, 2009.
3. Suffoletto MS, Dohi K, Cannesson M, et al: Novel speckle-tracking radial strain from routine black-and-white echocardiographic images to quantify dyssynchrony and predict response to cardiac resynchronization therapy, *Circulation* 113:960-968, 2006.
4. White JA, Yee R, Yuan X, et al: Delayed enhancement magnetic resonance imaging predicts response to cardiac resynchronization therapy in patients with intraventricular dyssynchrony, *J Am Coll Cardiol* 48:1953-1960, 2006.

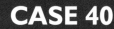

CASE 40

Management of Frequent Ventricular Extrasystoles

David L. Hayes and Samuel J. Asirvatham

Age	Gender	Occupation	Working Diagnosis
83 Years	Male	Retired Veterinarian	Nonresponder to Cardiac Resynchronization Therapy

HISTORY

An 83-year-old man had undergone implantation of a dual-chamber pacemaker 12 years previously for intermittent high-grade atrioventricular block. He did well for several years, but at age 79 experienced symptoms of congestive heart failure. During the initial hospitalization he was found to have significantly reduced left ventricular systolic function, with a left ventricular ejection fraction (LVEF) of 34%. On echocardiography he had global hypokinesis of the left ventricle. An initial pharmacologic stress study revealed equivocal changes in the inferior wall. Because of the equivocal changes a coronary angiogram was performed. No significant coronary artery disease was found, and the patient was classified as having idiopathic dilated cardiomyopathy. The patient was started on an angiotensin-converting enzyme inhibitor, a beta blocker, a diuretic, and low-dose aspirin. He was already taking a lipid-lowering agent. He had resolution of his heart failure symptoms and was discharged after a 5-day hospital stay. Medications were titrated by his local physician over the following 3 months. The patient did well and returned to an active lifestyle and frequent international travel.

At 81 years of age he again began to experience symptoms, with mild dyspnea on exertion and rare episodes of orthopnea. Medications were altered, and the patient improved and managed as an outpatient. His LVEF was minimally changed, at 32%.

The patient returned 11 months later, at age 82, with profound heart failure symptoms. He was hospitalized again, and his LVEF by echocardiography was 26%. An ambulatory monitor reading was obtained, and the patient was noted to have frequent ventricular extrasystoles, representing 25% of ventricular beats during the 24-hour monitoring period.

The physician managing his care thought the opportunity for further optimization of his medical regimen was minimal. The patient was then referred for consideration of upgrade of his dual-chamber pacemaker to a cardiac resynchronization therapy defibrillator (CRT-D).

At the time of the initial referral evaluation, the patient's medical regimen appeared optimal. The recent echocardiogram was reviewed and original measurements and observations confirmed. Pacemaker assessment demonstrated pacemaker dependency. He had frequent ventricular extrasystoles on 12-lead electrocardiogram, and frequent extrasystoles were also noted during auscultation. It was explained to the patient that the frequent ventricular extrasystoles could theoretically improve after a device upgrade, especially if improvement in left ventricular function was realized. If the extrasystoles did not improve, he was told that they might require treatment by pharmacologic suppression and/or an ablation procedure if the foci could be identified.

After a thorough discussion of the potential benefits and risks of CRT-D upgrade, the patient was upgraded to a CRT-D device. The chronic ventricular pacing lead was abandoned and capped. The chronic atrial lead was connected to the new CRT-D pulse generator, and a new right ventricular ICD lead and coronary sinus were placed. The defibrillation threshold was 14 J.

The postimplant chest radiograph is shown in Figure 40-1. Pacing and sensing thresholds checked at the time of discharge were excellent. For the period that the patient was monitored after implant, he continued to have significant ventricular ectopy. He occasionally had pairs and triplets but no longer salvos. The "PVC trigger response" was programmed "on" in an effort to maintain biventricular stimulation. The patient was discharged the day after the CRT-D upgrade and returned a few days later to his home for care to be continued by his cardiologist.

In the months immediately after the procedure the patient thought his peripheral edema was somewhat less noticeable but overall did not feel much improvement. He proceeded with an extended international trip that was intended to last for 5 months at a destination at a considerably higher altitude. Shortly after arrival he

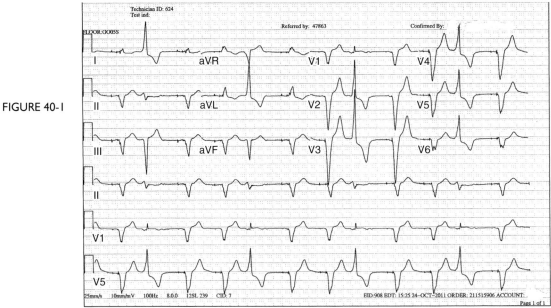

24-OCT-2011 15:13:37

19-AUG-1927 (84 yr)	Vent. rate	76	BPM	Dual chamber electronic pacemaker
Male	PR interval	80	ms	Premature ventricular complexes
	QRS duration	130	ms	Prolonged QT
Room:	QT/QTc	450/506	ms	When compared with ECG of
Loc: 1	P-R-T axes	* −39	166	11-NOV-2010 07:37, no significant change was found

FIGURE 40-1

developed marked dyspnea on exertion to the point that he returned to his home. On return to the lower altitude his symptoms improved minimally.

His local cardiologist added spironolactone to his medical regimen, questioned possible dislodgement of the coronary sinus lead, and referred him for reevaluation of the CRT-D system.

He was reevaluated with chest radiography and echocardiography. On comparison of the postimplant and current radiographs, no significant change in lead positions was appreciated. Pacing and sensing thresholds were excellent. "True" biventricular pacing was noted to be 51%. A 12-lead ambulatory monitor was obtained. Forty percent of his ventricular beats were classified as fusion beats or ventricular extrasystoles. Of the beats classified as premature ventricular contractions, 80% were of the same morphology.

Given the high percentage of ventricular extrasystoles, low percentage of effective biventricular pacing, and, not surprisingly, lack of response to CRT, what options should be considered?

CURRENT MEDICATIONS

The patient was taking carvedilol 25 mg twice daily, furosemide 20 mg twice daily, lisinopril 20 mg daily, naproxen (Aleve) two tablets (250 mg) as needed, and enteric-coated aspirin 81 mg daily.

CURRENT SYMPTOMS

The patient was easily fatigued. He experienced significant dyspnea on exertion at higher altitudes and mild-to-moderate exertional dyspnea at lower altitudes.

PHYSICAL EXAMINATION

BP/HR: 102/64 mm Hg/64 bpm
Height/weight: 183 cm/99.7 kg
Neck veins: Mild distention at 20-degree angle
Lungs/chest: Few bibasilar crackles
Heart: Normal first heart sound (S_1) and second heart sound (S_2), grade 2/6 systolic flow murmur at upper left sternal border, no diastolic murmur, no lift
Abdomen: Overweight, no organomegaly or masses appreciated, bowel sounds normal, unable to distinguish abdominal aorta
Extremities: 1+ pitting pedal edema, pedal pulses difficult to feel, popliteal pulses 2/2, femoral pulses 4/4

LABORATORY DATA

Hemoglobin: 13.6 g/dL
Hematocrit/packed cell volume: 41.8%
Mean corpuscular cell volume: 88.9 fL
Platelet count: $113 \times 10^3/\mu L$

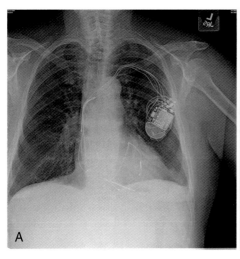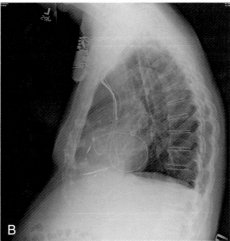

FIGURE 40-2

Sodium: 143 mmol/L
Potassium: 4.3 mmol/L
Creatinine: 1.1 mmol/L
Blood urea nitrogen: 22 mg/dL
N-Terminal probrain natriuretic peptide: 2865 pg/mL

ELECTROCARDIOGRAM

Findings

The electrocardiogram revealed a dual-chamber electronic pacemaker, premature ventricular complexes, and prolonged QT, with no change in contrast to the previous tracing (see Figure 40-1).

CHEST RADIOGRAPH

Findings

The chest radiograph did not reveal significant changes from the previous radiograph. The implantable cardioverter-defibrillator with right atrial, right ventricular, and coronary sinus leads was visualized (Figure 40-2). The heart size was within normal limits. Pulmonary vascularity was at the upper limits of normal. A tiny amount of scarring was noted in the bases. The chest radiograph was otherwise negative.

ECHOCARDIOGRAM

Findings

The echocardiogram revealed mild-to-moderate left ventricular enlargement, moderate-to-severe decrease in left ventricular systolic function, calculated LVEF of 32%, and generalized left ventricular hypokinesis. Some

segmental abnormalities (not depicted graphically) were due to the paced rhythm. Also noted were moderate-to-severe mitral valve regurgitation; moderate tricuspid valve regurgitation resulting, in part, from the device electrode; and moderate-to-severe biatrial enlargement. The findings were consistent with those in moderate pulmonary hypertension. In contrast to the report from November 2010, the rhythm on this echocardiogram was regular, so the quantification of the cardiac magnetic resonance imaging (MRI) is more accurate (see comments in previous report). Visually, however, no significant change was seen in the MRI findings. Tricuspid regurgitation no longer occurred. Side-by-side comparison of images was performed. The right systolic pressure was higher.

FOCUSED CLINICAL QUESTIONS AND DISCUSSION POINTS

Question

Does the premature ventricular contraction morphology matter in terms of CRT nonresponse?

Discussion

The premature ventricular contraction morphology reflects the site of origin for the arrhythmia. For example, in this patient, the left bundle branch block morphology, inferior axis, and positive concordance suggest origin in the basal right ventricular free wall.

Theoretically, premature ventricular contractions that originate in the free wall may be associated with a greater degree of dyssynchrony and thus promote ventricular dysfunction. However, studies suggest that this effect, if present, is minor in contrast to the importance of the overall frequency of the premature ventricular contractions.[2]

If the device senses an event on the right ventricular lead and if premature ventricular contractions occur from the left ventricular free wall, premature ventricular contraction–triggered pacing possibly could occur after ventricular refractoriness has ended and may be proarrhythmic. It appears, however, that this phenomenon is very rare.

Question

At what number of premature ventricular contractions per day should this arrhythmia be considered a cause for CRT nonresponse?

Discussion

Any premature ventricular contraction will result in inhibition of biventricular pacing. In general, if CRT is not being delivered for more than 95% of the beats, consideration to optimize therapy is recommended. Premature ventricular contractions may contribute to or primarily cause cardiomyopathy and heart failure. Typically more than 20,000 beats per day are from the premature ventricular contractions, and treatment with ablation or medication for the premature ventricular contractions may improve ventricular function.[1]

A premature ventricular contraction also may produce continued inhibition of pacing beyond a single beat. For example, if the postventricular atrial refractory period has been extended after a premature ventricular contraction, an ensuing sinus beat will not be tracked. Furthermore, if intrinsic conduction is present through the atrioventricular node, native wide QRS conduction would occur. Now this conducted beat acts as another premature ventricular contraction, in turn resulting in the next sinus beat being in the postventricular atrial refractory period (especially if intrinsic conduction through the atrioventricular node is long), and the phenomenon can be repetitive, significantly decreasing effective CRT.[3]

The device interrogated percentage of biventricular pacing also may be misleading when frequent PVCs occur. Some of the beats may represent the fusion or pseudofusion and be counted as paced beats, but the ventricle is depolarized through the abnormal PVC.

Question

Is it possible to know whether the premature ventricular contractures result from the cardiomyopathy or are causing or contributing to the heart failure process?

Discussion

When cardiomyopathy gives rise to premature ventricular contractions, multiple morphologies could be expected. Monomorphic premature ventricular contractions responsible for the majority of these beats suggest a primary electrical problem that may be giving rise to the cardiomyopathy, and strong consideration should be given to targeting these beats.

At times, considerable doubt may exist as to whether treatment for premature ventricular contraction will improve CRT delivery and the cardiomyopathy itself. Here, when appropriate, a short course of an antiarrhythmic agent, such as amiodarone, can be administered. If the premature ventricular contractions are suppressed and the patient improves significantly, more definitive management such as with radiofrequency ablation for the premature ventricular contraction focus could be considered.

FINAL DIAGNOSIS

The final diagnosis in this patient was nonresponse to CRT because of inadequate biventricular pacing as a result of frequent ventricular ectopy.

PLAN OF ACTION

Options discussed with the patient included an attempt to pharmacologically suppress the ectopy and to attempt ablation of the ectopic foci. The patient wished to avoid another invasive procedure and opted for pharmacologic suppression of the ectopy.

INTERVENTION

The patient was started on amiodarone 200 mg daily and advised to have a repeat ambulatory monitoring examination in 3 to 4 months.

OUTCOME

An ambulatory monitoring examination was completed by the patient's local cardiologist approximately 4 months later. The Holter monitor report noted the heart rate to range from 72 to 116 bpm. Ventricular ectopic beats were said to make up 9% of the total heart beats. This is in contrast to the previous ambulatory monitoring, in which 40% of his total heart beats were ventricular ectopic beats. The biventricular pacing had increased to 90%, and the patient had mild-to-moderate subjective improvement in exercise capability and lessening fatigue.

Selected References

1. Bhushan M, Asirvatham SJ: The conundrum of ventricular arrhythmia and cardiomyopathy: which abnormality came first? *Curr Heart Fail Rep* 6:7-13, 2009.
2. Del Carpio Munoz F, Syed FF, Noheria A, et al: Characteristics of premature ventricular complexes as correlates of reduced left ventricular systolic function: study of the burden, duration, coupling interval, morphology and site of origin of PVCs, *J Cardiovasc Electrophysiol* 22:791-798, 2011.
3. Mullens W, Grimm RA, Verga T, et al: Insights from a cardiac resynchronization optimization clinic as part of a heart failure disease management program, *JACC* 53:765-773, 2009.

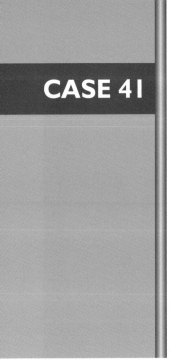

Cardiac Contractility Modulation in a Nonresponder to Cardiac Resynchronization Therapy

Jürgen Kuschyk, Susanne Roeger, and Martin Borggrefe

Age	Gender	Occupation	Working Diagnosis
53 Years	Male	Retired	Dilated and Ischemic Cardiomyopathy with New York Heart Association Heart Failure Class III to IV Symptoms

HISTORY

A 53-year-old man of Greek origin was diagnosed with dilated cardiomyopathy in 1996, at which time his left ventricular ejection fraction (LVEF) was described as moderately to severely reduced and coronary artery disease was initially excluded by angiography. The patient was in New York Heart Association (NYHA) class II and received beta blockers and angiotensin-converting enzyme inhibitors. Cardiac risk factors included arterial hypertension, medically treated type 2 diabetes mellitus, and ongoing smoking. His family history showed no cases of cardiomypathy or sudden cardiac death. His medical history included thalassemia minor (with normal hemoglobin values), hypothyroidism, and chronic gastritis.

In September 2001 the patient was diagnosed with stage III Hodgkin's lymphoma with involvement of mediastinal and cervical lymph nodes and the spleen. In the ensuing months he received chemotherapy according to a modified escalated protocol of bleomycin, etoposide, doxorubicin (Adriamycin), cyclophosphamide, oncovin-vincristine, procarbazine, and prednisone (BEACOPP), followed by radiation therapy. Cardiotoxic anthracyclines were avoided because of the underlying heart condition. Insulin therapy was started for his worsening diabetes.

Over the next few years the patient was followed closely at regular intervals in the oncology outpatient clinic, with imaging studies that excluded relapse of the lymphoma. Echocardiographic and clinical evaluation findings of the heart were stable during this time.

In February 2009 the patient was admitted to the hospital with cardiac decompensation and received intravenous diuretic therapy. Magnetic resonance imaging showed an LVEF of 20% and a left ventricular end-diastolic dimension of 81 mm. An electrocardiogram (ECG) showed normal sinus rhythm with a left bundle branch block (LBBB) and a QRS width of 128 ms. The patient was offered implantation of a biventricular implantable cardioverter-defibrillator (CRT-D), which he refused.

Over the next 2 years the patient's physical condition deteriorated further despite extensive treatment with heart failure medications. In February 2011 he was hospitalized because of progressive dyspnea at rest. Chest progressive radiography revealed pleural effusions. Cardiac catheterization demonstrated two-vessel coronary artery disease with a peripheral occlusion of the left anterior descending artery. A percutaneous coronary intervention was not possible. Magnetic resonance imaging demonstrated a markedly reduced LVEF of 11% (Figure 41-1). ECG findings were unchanged in contrast to those in 2009 with sinus rhythm, borderline LBBB, a QRS width of 130 ms, and a QRS onset to peak R duration of 60 ms in V_5 and V_6 (Figure 41-2). The patient finally consented to the implantation of a CRT-D device, which was performed in February 2011. An atrial electrode (Flextend 2, Boston Scientific, Natick, Mass.) was placed in the right atrial appendage, the right ventricular lead (Endotak Reliance SG, Boston Scientific) was placed in the right ventricular apex, and the left ventricular lead (Acuity Steerable, Boston Scientific) in a posterolateral vein. Good lead impedances and pacing and sensing thresholds were achieved for all three leads. The device parameters were programmed as follows: DDD pacing mode, tracking rate 60 to 130 bpm, paced atrioventricular interval of 130 ms, simultaneous biventricular stimulation with VV delay of 0 ms, and left ventricular electrode configuration of left ventricular tip to left ventricular ring. Despite stable stimulation percentage rates (95%-98%), little change occurred in the patient's physical ability over the following months.

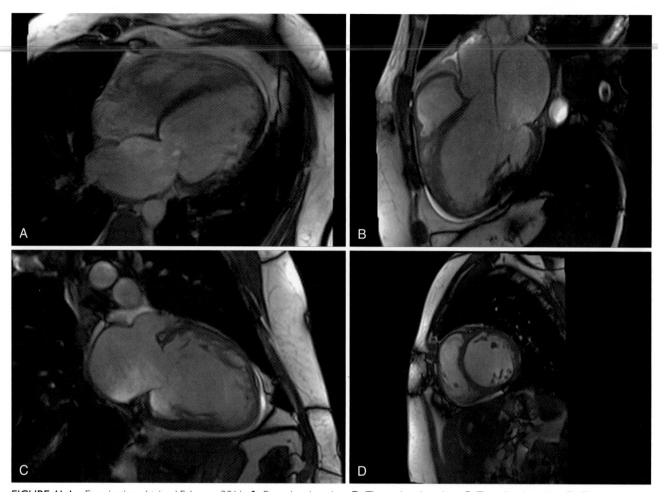

FIGURE 41-1 Examination obtained February 2011. **A,** Four-chamber view. **B,** Three-chamber view. **C,** Two-chamber view. **D,** Short-axis view.

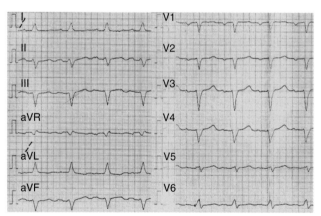

FIGURE 41-2 Electrocardiogram before implantation of the biventricular implantable cardioverter-defibrillator in February 2011.

In August 2011 the patient's fatigue and dyspnea were worsening. Interrogation of the implantable cardioverter-defibrillator (ICD) revealed abnormalities with the atrial lead. Impedance values and pacing and sensing thresholds with the right and left ventricular leads were stable. Chest radiography revealed Twiddler's syndrome (Figure 41-3), with the atrial electrode drawn back into

the left subclavian vein. The patient admitted that he had touched and rotated the device frequently. During the operative revision the device was observed to have been rotated around its axis 18 times. The device was repositioned, and the right atrial electrode was revised successfully.

In February 2012 the patient was hospitalized again because of cardiac decompensation and dyspnea at rest. He had ankle edema and pleural effusions. Device interrogation did not reveal significant ventricular or supraventricular tachyarrhythmias. The patient again required intravenous diuretic therapy.

Although cardiac compensation was achieved, the patient again developed dyspnea after walking only a few meters. His quality of life was measured with a 21-item scale according to the Minnesota Living with Heart Failure Questionnaire, with a score of 79. The N-terminal probrain natriuretic peptide value was elevated to 12.067 ng/L. An exercise test showed highly decreased Vo_2 peak value of 10.7 mL/kg/min with maximum exercise capacity of 40 watts.

The patient's baseline medications, symptoms, physical examination results, laboratory data, and echocardiography

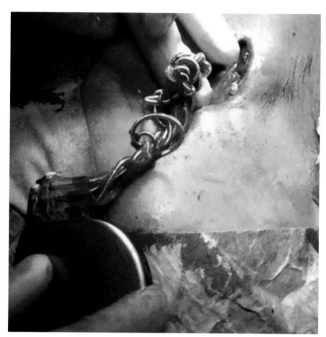

FIGURE 41-3 During the operative revision the device was observed to have been rotated around its axis 18 times.

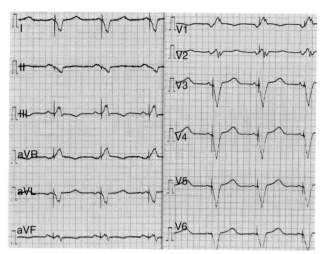

FIGURE 41-4 Electrocardiogram with active biventricular implantable cardioverter-defibrillator stimulation.

are discussed in the following section. The patient ultimately underwent implantation of an Optimizer III device (Impulse Dynamics, Stuttgart, Germany) in March 2012, the results of which will be reviewed in detail.

CURRENT MEDICATIONS

The patient was taking atorvastatin 40 mg daily, carvedilol 37.5 mg daily, torsemide 40 mg daily, spironolactone 12.5 mg daily, enalapril 7.5 mg daily, opipramol 50 mg daily, pantoprazole 20 mg daily, mixed insulin 30 units daily, and aspirin 100 mg daily.

CURRENT SYMPTOMS

The patient was experiencing dyspnea on minimal effort and fatigue.

PHYSICAL EXAMINATION

BP/HR: 120/70 mm Hg/80 bpm
Height/weight: 178 cm/86 kg
Neck veins: Jugular vein distention
Lungs/chest: Percussion dullness
Heart: Regular rate and rhythm without murmur
Abdomen: Soft, flat, and nontender
Extremities: No ankle edema

LABORATORY DATA

Hemoglobin: 12.7 g/dL
Hematocrit/packed cell volume: 41%
Mean corpuscular volume: 82.7 fL
Platelet count: $107 \times 10^3/\mu L$
Sodium: 143 mval/L or 3,289 g/L
Potassium: 3.7 mmol/L
Creatinine: 1.54 mg/dL
Blood urea nitrogen: 77 mg/dL

ELECTROCARDIOGRAM

Findings

The ECG showed normal rate and normal sinus rhythm, LBBB with a QRS width of 128 ms, and QRS onset to peak R time of 60 ms in V_5 and V_6 (see Figure 41-2).

Findings

The ECG showed active biventricular stimulation (Figure 41-4).

Findings

The last three QRS complexes are followed by active high-amplitude Optimizer III stimulation (Figure 41-5).

CHEST RADIOGRAPH

Findings

In Figure 41-6, the *upper arrow* shows the left atrial electrode retracted into the left subclavian vein; the *lower*

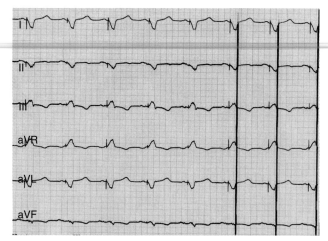

FIGURE 41-5 Electrocardiogram with active stimulation of the Optimizer III system.

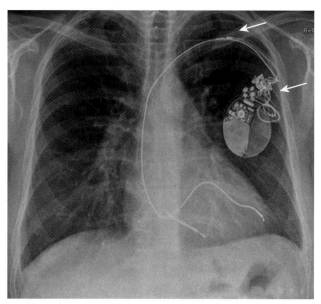

FIGURE 41-6 Chest radiograph from August 2011, 6 months after implantation of the biventricular implantable cardioverter-defibrillator.

arrow shows tightly coiled electrodes that occurred because of rotation of the generator device. The ventricular electrode is still in the proper place in the apex of the right ventricle. The coronary sinus electrode also remains in the proper place in a posterolateral vein.

Findings

A chest radiograph obtained a few hours after implantation of the Optimizer III device (Figure 41-7, *A*) shows the enlarged heart. Follow-up chest radiography shows considerable reduction of cardiac dimensions (see Figure 41-7, *B*).

The following were visualized on chest radiography: the generator of the biventricular ICD (1), Optimizer

III device (2), atrial electrode of the CRT-D (3), ventricular electrode of the CRT-D located in the apex of the right ventricle (4), coronary sinus electrode located in a posterolateral vein (5), atrial sensing electrode of the Optimizer III system (6), upper ventricular stimulation electrode of the Optimizer III (7), and lower ventricular stimulation electrode of the Optimizer III (8).

EXERCISE TESTING

Exercise testing in February 2012, before implantation of the Optimizer III, showed a Vo$_2$ peak of 10.7 mL/kg/min and exercise capacity of 40 W. Exercise testing had to be stopped because of dyspnea and pain in both lower legs.

ECHOCARDIOGRAM

Findings

Echocardiography in February 2012 (Figure 41-8) showed severely decreased ventricular ejection fraction (10%-14%). Figure 41-8, *A*, is a parasternal longitudinal axis view with severe dilation of the left ventricle and left atrium. Figure 41-8, *B*, is a parasternal longitudinal axis view with M-mode Doppler in which septal and posterior wall akinesia are observed.

MAGNETIC RESONANCE IMAGING

Findings

Cardiac magnetic resonance imaging revealed a severely reduced LVEF (11%), left ventricular end-diastolic volume of 375 mL (184 mL/m^2), left ventricular end-systolic volume of 335 mL (164 mL/m^2), ejection volume of 41 mL, septal wall thickness of 7 mm, posterior wall thickness of 7 mm, and left ventricular end-diastolic dimension of 81 mm (see Figure 41-1). The contrast agent revealed transmural late enhancement septal midventricularly to apically.

CATHETERIZATION

Catheterization was performed in February 2011. Cardiac output was 4.4 L/min; cardiac index was 2.1 L/min/m^2; mean right atrial pressure was 14 mm Hg; right ventricular pressure was 61 mm Hg systolic and 21 mm Hg end diastolic; pulmonary artery pressure was 59 mm Hg systolic, 34 mm Hg diastolic, and 44 mm Hg mean; and pulmonary capillary wedge pressure was 30 mm Hg.

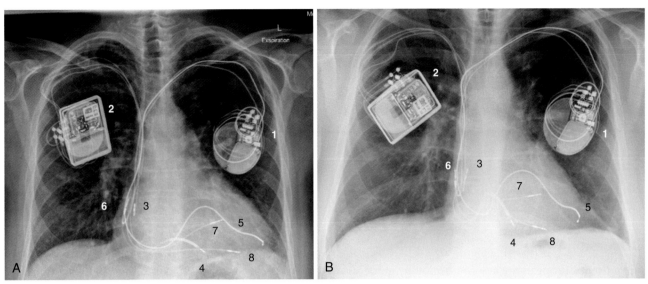

FIGURE 41-7   **A,** Chest radiograph obtained March 2012 after implantation of the Optimizer III device. **B,** Follow-up chest radiograph from July 2012, 4.5 months after implantation of the Optimizer III device. The visualized parts of the two devices are marked with numbers 1-8 to make the identification clearer.

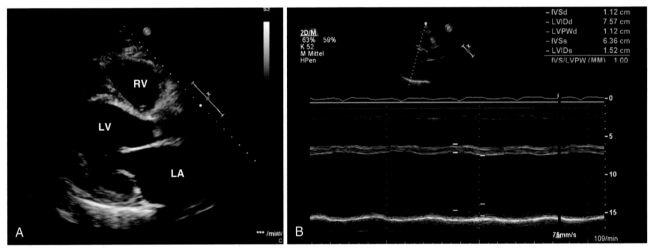

FIGURE 41-8   Echocardiogram.

Findings

The findings on catheterization were two-vessel coronary artery disease with a peripheral occlusion of the left anterior descending artery (100%), outlet stenosis of the first diagonal branch (80%) and small right coronary artery (50%), and left ventriculogram with an LVEF of 10%.

FOCUSED CLINICAL QUESTIONS AND DISCUSSION POINTS

Question

What are indications for CRT? Which patients receive the best clinical results?

Discussion

Cardiac resynchronization therapy has become a standard therapy in patients with heart failure and interventricular and intraventricular conduction disturbances.[5]

CRT with biventricular pacing is an effective adjunctive therapy to pharmacologic management in reducing the rate of hospitalization and death in symptomatic patients with advanced heart failure symptoms (NYHA class III or IV), an ejection fraction of 35% or less, and an intraventricular conduction delay of 120 msec or more.[3,5] Newer data also show favorable outcomes for patients with less advanced heart failure status, for example, patients with NYHA Class II symptoms.[7]

Unfortunately, approximately 40% of the patients are considered nonresponders to CRT. Analyses of prespecified subgroups of patients have demonstrated the best clinical results in patients with a QRS duration of 150 msec or more.[7] Patients with a narrower QRS width are more likely to be nonresponders.

The patient's clinical situation did not improve after CRT implantation. In February 2012, he deteriorated with persistent NYHA class IV symptoms despite successful (95%-97% capture) biventricular pacing. Therefore he was clearly a nonresponder to CRT.

Question

What therapeutic options are available for nonresponders to CRT?

Discussion

The current European Society of Cardiology guidelines for the treatment of patients with persistent severe heart failure symptoms indicate consideration for heart transplantation (if eligible) and left ventricular assist device (LVAD) implantation. The guidelines also suggest that digoxin therapy be considered. However, wait times for heart transplantation are increasingly long and LVAD therapy is not a therapy desired or recommended for all patients. Beyond this, the only other approved (in the European Union) and available therapy for heart failure is cardiac contractility modulation (CCM).

Question

What clinical data exist on the efficacy of treatment with CCM?

Discussion

To date, two multicenter, randomized controlled clinical trials have been conducted.[2,6]

FIX-CHF-4

The FIX-CHF-4 double-blind, double-crossover study was conducted in Europe and included 164 patients with heart failure with ejection fractions of 35% or less and NYHA class II or III.[2] Co-primary end points in the trial were changes in peak oxygen consumption and changes in quality of life assessed by the Minnesota Living with Heart Failure Questionnaire. Secondary efficacy end points consisted of NYHA class and 6-Minute Walk Test. Each of the co-primary end points was significantly improved during the phase with active CCM. The treatment also was shown to be safe.

FIX-CHF-5

The FIX-CHF-5 prospective, randomized, parallel-group, controlled trial was conducted in the United States.[6] It tested the longer term (1 year) safety and efficacy of CCM treatment. A total of 428 patients with NYHA class III to IV, ejection fraction of 35% or less, and narrow QRS were randomized to either CCM or no CCM therapy. This study also showed CCM therapy to be safe in this patient population. In the overall population, CCM therapy significantly improved peak Vo_2, Minnesota Living with Heart Failure Questionnaire results, and NYHA class, but did not improve the ventilatory anaerobic threshold, which was the declared the primary end point. However, in a prespecified subgroup analysis consisting of approximately 50% of the overall population characterized by baseline ejection fraction of 25% or greater and NYHA class III, the primary end point was reached.[1]

Consideration of Both Studies

All patients included in the FIX-CHF-4 and FIX-CHF-5 studies had narrow QRS complexes and were therefore ineligible for CRT. Nevertheless, the patient cohort in the FIX-CHF-4 study had NYHA classes II and III and included a small cohort with QRS duration greater than 130 ms. Our patient was in NYHA class IV, had a wide QRS duration, and already had a CRT-D device in place. Therefore the data of these two studies cannot be used for direct comparison with the situation of the patient in this case.

Question

Are there clinical data on the outcome of CRT nonresponders treated with CCM therapy?

Discussion

To date, little is known about the outcome of CRT nonresponders treated with additional CCM therapy. No randomized clinical data have been published about this very ill group of patients. Case reports and a case series have described first experiences with the technique.[4,8] Näegele and colleagues reported a case series of 16 patients with NYHA class III and IV symptoms in which they showed the feasibility of the method as a useful adjunct in CRT nonresponders when no other options are available. No electrical interference was observed between the CCM therapy and CRT systems, and, in particular, at no time was the CRT-D device found to be delivering inadequate or inappropriate shocks. However, the mortality rate and number of clinical events remained high.

Long-term clinical outcome studies need to be performed to clarify the impact of CCM therapy in nonresponders to CRT. To date, the FIX-CHF-12 study is under way to evaluate clinical follow-up of patients with combined CRT and CCM therapy.

In the patient in this case, the decision was made to add CCM to CRT because of persistent and worsening heart failure symptoms associated with worsening reactive depression caused by immobility and social isolation. When offered the therapy, the patient immediately consented to the operation, although he was informed of the possible risks for infection or mechanical problems with six electrodes in the heart and two implanted generator devices.

FINAL DIAGNOSIS

The final diagnosis in this case was that the patient was a nonresponder to CRT.

PLAN OF ACTION

The plan for this patient was implantation of an additional Opimizer III device.

INTERVENTION

Implantation of the Optimizer III device was performed in March 2012. Ventricular tachycardia detection algorithms of the CRT-D device were turned off during CCM implantation to prevent inappropriate shocks. A submuscular pocket was made in the right subclavian region, and three standard screw-in pacemaker electrodes were introduced into the subclavian vein after venipuncture. One electrode was positioned in the right atrium and used for sensing atrial activity (Tendril ST, 58 cm, St. Jude Medical, St. Paul, Minn.). The other two electrodes (Tendril ST 1888, 65 cm, St. Jude Medical) were positioned on the right ventricular septum. Figure 41-7, A, shows the postoperative chest radiograph with electrode positions, and Figure 41-5 shows the ECG with combined CRT and CCM therapy.

During implantation, left ventricular dP/dt_{max} testing was measured using a 5-French Millar micromanometer catheter placed in the left ventricle. Initially, changes in dP/dt_{max} from baseline with different VV delays (–40 to 40 ms) programmed in the CRT-D device were tested. Changes of VV delay did not induce significant changes from baseline in contrast to a left ventricular VV delay of 0 ms. Subsequently, exclusive left ventricular stimulation was tested (stimulation vector left ventricular ring to right ventricular coil), which showed a mild increase of dP/dt_{max} of 6%. After activation of the Optimizer III device, an increase of dP/dt_{max} from baseline of 18% was achieved.

No cross talk between the devices occurred up to a train delay of 80 ms. The Optimizer III device was programmed to provide therapy for 7 hours per day. Both septal stimulation electrodes were programmed "on." The CCM signal amplitude was programmed to 5.5 V. At the last follow-up examination, device interrogation showed a CCM signal delivery rate of 98%.

OUTCOME

The most recent clinical follow-up examination occurred 4 months after Optimizer III implantation. The patient reported significant improvement of physical ability. He had no dyspnea during activities of daily living, and his formerly constant fatigue has been eliminated. He reported dyspnea only on strong exertion, corresponding to an improvement of overall symptoms from NYHA III to IV to NYHA II. His mental status also was overtly improved. The repeat Minnesota Living with Heart Failure Questionnaire score had decreased to 29 points, a dramatic 50-point reduction. Echocardiography showed increased LVEF to 25% and a reduction in left ventricular end-diastolic and end-systolic dimensions (to 69 and 58 mm, respectively, measured at the level of the mitral leaflet tips in the parasternal long axis).

The patient's N-terminal probrain natriuretic peptide (NT-proBNP) decreased to 3028 ng/L in May 2012. Follow-up exercise testing was also performed at that time, demonstrating an increase in peak Vo_2 to 13 mL/kg/min at 70 W; the patient was without dyspnea, and the test had to be ended early because of orthopedic problems. Figure 41-7, B, shows the follow-up chest radiograph with obvious reduction of the cardiac dimensions.

In the context of a case report, concern always exists that improvements are related to placebo effect. In this case the dramatic clinical improvements observed from CCM therapy were observed after the lack of any clinical effects achieved by CRT implant; had the patient been susceptible to placebo, expectations would have been that these would be observed after the CRT implant. Furthermore, the multiple objective findings (i.e., decreased NT-proBNP, reduced left ventricular dimensions, and improved LVEF) in the face of constant medical therapy also speak against a placebo effect. Although further systematic randomized study needs to be done, the current findings point to the promise of CCM to help at least some patients who are nonresponders to CRT.

Selected References

1. Abraham WT, Nadamanee K, Volosin K, et al: Subgroup analysis of a randomized controlled trial evaluation the safety and efficacy of cardiac contractility modulation in advanced heart failure, *J Card Fail* 17:710-717, 2011.
2. Borggrefe MM, Lawo T, Butter C, et al: Randomized, double blind study of non-excitatory, cardiac contractility modulation electrical impulses for symptomatic heart failure, *Eur Heart J* 29:1019-1028, 2008.
3. Bristow MR, Saxon LA, Boehmer J, et al: Cardiac-resynchronization therapy with or without an implantable defibrillator in advanced chronic heart failure, *N Engl J Med* 350:2140-2150, 2004.
4. Butter C, Meyhofer J, Seifert M, et al: First use of cardiac contractility modulation (CCM) in a patient failing CRT therapy: clinical and technical aspects of combined therapies, *Eur J Heart Fail* 9:955-958, 2007.

5. Cleland JG, Daubert JC, Erdmann E, et al: The effect of cardiac resynchronization on morbidity and mortality in heart failure, *N Engl J Med* 352:1539-1549, 2005.

6. Kadish A, Nademanee K, Volosin K, et al: A randomized controlled trial evaluating the safety and efficacy of cardiac contractility modulation in advanced heart failure, *Am Heart J* 161:329-337, 2011.

7. Moss AJ, Hall WJ, Cannom DS, et al: Cardiac resynchronization therapy for the prevention of heart failure events, *N Engl J Med* 14:1329-1338, 2009.

8. Nägele H, Behrens S, Eisermann C, et al: Cardiac contractility modulation in non-responders to cardiac resynchronization therapy, *Europace* 10:1375-1380, 2008.

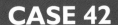

Nonresponders to Cardiac Resynchronization Therapy: Switch-Off If Worsening

Mark H. Schoenfeld

Age	Gender	Occupation	Working Diagnosis
79 Years	Male	Retired Golf Professional	Ischemic Cardiomyopathy, Remote Cardiac Arrest, Congestive Heart Failure, and Left Bundle Branch Block

HISTORY

This 79-year-old man with type II diabetes, hypertension, 2.5 pack per day smoking history for 46 years, and a strong family history of premature coronary disease (father died at 61 years of age of myocardial infarction) suffered a myocardial infarction in 1974 and had cardiac arrest as a result of ventricular fibrillation on the third day of that hospitalization. Coronary revascularization was undertaken with a four-vessel bypass in February, 1999. He developed symptoms of heart failure in 2006, with an echocardiogram showing akinesis of the inferior and posterobasal walls and an ejection fraction of 20% with moderate mitral regurgitation. He was treated with furosemide, carvedilol, candesartan, and statins and continued with New York Health Association (NYHA) class II to III symptoms, with an electrocardiogram demonstrating left bundle branch block (LBBB) with variable QRS durations of 120 to 130 msec. He was thought perhaps to be a candidate for cardiac resynchronization therapy. Outpatient tissue Doppler study confirmed an ejection fraction of 20% but fell short of the usual criteria for left ventricular dyssynchrony. Electrophysiologic study demonstrated easily inducible sustained monomorphic ventricular tachycardia, both at baseline and after procainamide challenge, prompting implantation of a single-chamber Medtronic defibrillator using the left cephalic vein. His ejection fraction was 25% in 2009. With progressive symptoms of heart failure in 2010 despite maximal medical therapy, and with a QRS duration of 140 msec, the decision was made to upgrade his device to a cardiac resynchronization therapy (CRT) system. The left subclavian system was still patent, allowing for passage of an active fixation atrial lead and a coronary sinus lead.

Venography demonstrated that his coronary venous anatomy was limited, with few branches available and most atretic, consistent with his diabetes. One branch served as a reasonable target, with acceptable pacing thresholds without phrenic nerve stimulation. His paced QRS duration narrowed, but symptoms of heart failure have persisted. His level of depression worsened with the death of his wife, and he had occasional dietary indiscretion. Atrioventricular optimization was performed. With ongoing symptoms despite maximal medical therapy and dietary modification, and in an effort to maximize longevity of the implantable cardioverter-defibrillator (ICD), the left ventricular lead was inactivated 1 year later.

CURRENT MEDICATIONS

The patient was taking carvedilol 6.25 mg twice daily, furosemide 100 mg daily, potassium chloride 20 mEq daily, glyburide 2.5 mg daily, simvastatin 20 mg daily, amlodipine 5 mg daily, fish oil 1000 mg daily, and aspirin 81 mg daily.

CURRENT SYMPTOMS

The patient experienced dyspnea at 100 yards and one flight of stairs and had occasional orthopnea.

PHYSICAL EXAMINATION

BP/HR: 100/65 mm Hg/70 bpm
Height/Weight: 172.5 cm/74 kg

Neck veins: 9 cm H_2O
Chest: Bibasilar crackles
Heart: Apex dyskinetic and laterally displaced, second heart sound (S_2) paradoxically split, grade II to VI mitral regurgitation murmur, summation gallop
Abdomen: Soft, nontender, active bowel sounds, liver edge down 2 fingerbreadths, span 10 cm
Extremities: 1+ bipedal edema

LABORATORY DATA

Hemoglobin: 14.2 g/dL
Hematocrit/packed cell volume: 43%
Mean corpuscular volume: 91.7 fL
Platelet count: 180 × 10^3/μL
Sodium: 139 mEq/L
Potassium: 4.4 mEq/L
Creatinine: 1.09 mg/dL
Blood urea nitrogen: 21 mg/dL

ELECTROCARDIOGRAM

Findings

Figure 42-1 shows a biventricular paced sinus rhythm, heart rate of 66 bpm, and paced QRS of 136 msec.

CHEST RADIOGRAPH

Findings

The coronary sinus venogram obtained at the time of implant shows the posteroapical branch selected and final position of the leads (Figures 42-2 and 42-3). Figure 42-4 demonstrates lead position in a different patient in whom the apical position of the coronary sinus lead is even more exemplary of an apical and nonbasal position.

FOCUSED CLINICAL QUESTIONS AND DISCUSSION POINTS

Question

What defines a nonresponder in the CRT population, and at what point would this patient be considered a nonresponder?

Discussion

It is widely recognized that the definition of response and nonresponse to CRT varies considerably, whether by clinical parameters (i.e., changes in NYHA classification

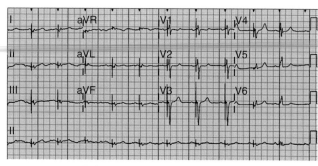

FIGURE 42-1   Electrocardiogram.

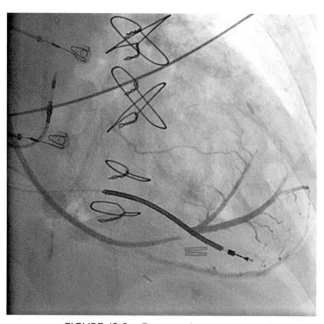

FIGURE 42-2   Coronary sinus venogram.

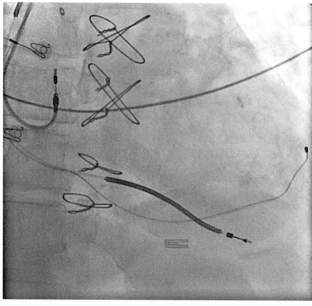

FIGURE 42-3   Chest radiograph of final coronary sinus lead position corresponding to venogram in Figure 42-2.

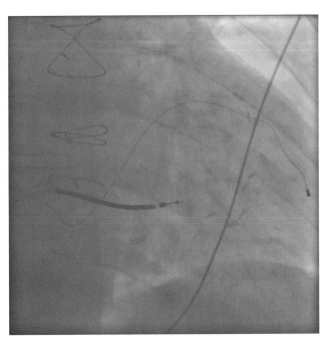

FIGURE 42-4 Chest radiograph in a different patient in whom the apical position of the coronary sinus lead is a better example of an apical coronary sinus lead position.

or hospitalizations for heart failure), imaging criteria (i.e., changes in ejection fraction, dyssynchrony, or stroke volume), or survival.[1-8] Until universal agreement is achieved on this subject, it is difficult to define a predictor of success or, conversely, when to define failure. The patient described is on maximal medical therapy, has ongoing symptoms of heart failure despite CRT with persistent depression of ejection fraction, and would be considered a nonresponder by most clinicians. The length of time to be waited in any individual case before considering CRT a failure is unclear. This is an important issue because prematurely deactivating the coronary sinus lead, although minimizing current drain on the device, may preclude demonstration of a delayed response to CRT.

Question

What may have contributed to this patient's nonresponse to CRT?

Discussion

As noted, predictors of response have been the subject of much investigation and a comprehensive understanding of this issue has yet to be achieved. A longer baseline QRS duration, as suggested by various trials (LBBB >150 msec), more basal position of the left ventricular lead, and lack of demonstration of significant intraventricular dyssynchrony by tissue Doppler imaging may have contributed to a lack of response in this case.

Question

What alternative strategies were available to this patient?

Discussion

Given the observation that the patient had atretic diabetic changes in the coronary venous tree, little else was available in the way of otherwise optimizing lead position because only one branch was sizable enough to engage. Interventional procedures such as venodilation have been employed in highly experienced centers provided the anatomy is reasonable and the approach feasible. Employment of newer quadripolar coronary sinus leads allowing for alternative pacing polarities and locations would not likely have helped in this individual.[9] Epicardial lead placement is an alternative approach, but it is more invasive and there is no guarantee that it would resolve the issue of nonresponse in this case. Atrioventricular optimization was undertaken in this patient without success.

Question

Under what other circumstances might the left ventricular lead be deactivated or left inactive from the time of implant— that is, in addition to being a CRT nonresponder?

Discussion

If the lead dislodges and no other stable position is an option, attempting invasive repositioning of the coronary sinus lead may be deemed a greater risk. If multiple positions have been assessed and the safety margin between effective left ventricular pacing and phrenic nerve stimulation is too narrow, the decision may be made to inactivate the left ventricular lead. The same applies if the left ventricular pacing threshold is unacceptably high. In some situations, a prophylactic coronary sinus lead may have been implanted, such as in a patient with a rapid ventricular response to atrial fibrillation who may require eventual atriventricular node ablation, resulting in cardiac desynchronization. In such cases in which a high incidence of right ventricular pacing may be anticipated in the future, the coronary sinus lead may be left inactive until coronary sinus pacing is required.

FINAL DIAGNOSIS

This patient was nonresponsive to CRT, possibly reflecting more apical or less basal position of coronary sinus lead versus shorter baseline QRS duration or less evidence of baseline mechanical dyssynchrony.

PLAN OF ACTION

The plan for this patient was deactivation of the coronary sinus lead after continued observation of nonresponse and continuation of medical therapy.

INTERVENTION

Deactivation of coronary sinus lead was performed by programming left ventricular lead function to the "off" position.

OUTCOME

At the time of publication, the patient was still alive, albeit with ongoing symptoms of heart failure and profound depression. ICD deactivation also could be considered in the future if comorbid conditions prevail, as suggested by Heart Rhythm Society guidelines on management of patients with cardiac implantable electronic devices.[10]

Selected References

1. Chung ES, Leon AR, Tavzzi L, et al: Results of the predictors of response to CRT (PROSPECT) Trial, *Circulation* 117:2608-2616, 2008.
2. Delgado V, Van Bommel RJ, Bertini M, et al: Relative merits of left ventricular dyssynchrony, left ventricular lead position, and myocardial scar to predict long-term survival of ischemic heart failure patients undergoing cardiac resynchronization therapy, *Circulation* 123:70-78, 2011.
3. Fornwalt BK, Sprague WW, BeDell, et al: Agreement is poor among current criteria used to define response to cardiac resynchronization therapy, *Circulation* 121:1985-1991, 2010.
4. Goldenberg I, Moss AJ, Hall WJ, et al: Predictors of response to cardiac resynchronization therapy in the multicenter automatic defibrillator implantation trial with cardiac resynchronization therapy (MADIT-CRT), *Circulation* 124:1527-1536, 2011.
5. Hsing JM, Selzman KA, Leclercq C, et al: Paced left ventricular QRS width and ECG parameters predict outcomes after cardiac resynchronization therapy: PROSPECT-ECG substudy, *Circ Arrhythm Electrophysiol* 4:851-857, 2011.
6. Khan FZ, Virdee MS, Palmer CR, et al: Targeted left ventricular lead placement to guide cardiac resynchronization therapy: the TARGET study: a randomized, controlled trial, *J Am Coll Cardiol* 59:1509-1518, 2012.
7. Knappe D, Pouleur AC, Shah AM, et al: Dyssynchrony, contractile function, and response to cardiac resynchronization therapy, *Circ Heart Fail* 4:433-440, 2011.
8. Singh JP, Klein HU, Huang DT, et al: Left ventricular lead position and clinical outcome in the Multicenter Automatic Defibrillator Implantation Trial-Cardiac Resynchronization Therapy (MADIT-CRT) Trial, *Circulation* 123:1159-1166, 2011.
9. Burger H, Schwarz T, Ehrlich W, et al: New generation of transvenous left ventricular leads: first experience with implantation of multipolar left ventricular leads, *Exp Clin Cardiol* 16:23-26, 2011.
10. Lampert R, Hayes DL, Annas GJ, et al: HRS expert consensus statement on the management of cardiovascular implantable electronic devices (CIEDs) in patients nearing end of life or requesting withdrawal of therapy, *Heart Rhythm* 7:1008-1026, 2010.

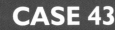
Recognition of Anodal Stimulation

Joseph Y. S. Chan

Age	Gender	Occupation	Working Diagnosis
68 Years	Male	Retired Businessman	Ischemic Cardiomyopathy

HISTORY

This 68-year-old man had a history of non-ST elevation myocardial infarction in 2008 and percutaneous coronary intervention with incomplete revascularization to triple-vessel disease. He developed atrial fibrillation and congestive heart failure in 2010. An echocardiogram showed a left ventricular ejection fraction (LVEF) of 19%, left ventricular end-diastolic volume of 146 mL, and left ventricular end-systolic volume of 119 mL. The QRS width was 144 msec. He remained in New York Heart Association (NYHA) class III while on optimal medical therapy for heart failure. He received a cardiac resynchronization therapy (CRT) pacemaker with bipolar right ventricular lead in the right ventricular apex and bipolar left ventricular lead positioned at the posterior branch of the great cardiac vein together with atrioventricular nodal ablation in 2010. On follow-up, anodal stimulation was detected on device interrogation and testing and the anodal stimulation threshold was 2.0 V at 0.4 msec, which was only slightly higher than the left ventricular lead pacing threshold, at 1.5V at 0.4 msec. The left ventricular lead output was set at 3.0 V at 0.4 msec, which was above the anodal stimulation threshold. No V-V delay was set for the patient. At follow-up examination at 6 months, improvement in symptoms with NYHA class II was noted. An echocardiogram showed an increase in LVEF to 25% and reduced left ventricular end-systolic volume of 91 mL.

CURRENT MEDICATIONS

The patient was taking clopidogrel 75 mg daily, simvastatin 20 mg daily, lisinopril 10 mg daily, carvedilol 12.5 mg twice daily, and aspirin 80 mg daily.

CURRENT SYMPTOMS

The patient's heart failure symptom has improved to NYHA class II. He enjoys light exercise mainly in terms of brisk walking and reports no angina.

PHYSICAL EXAMINATION

BP/HR: 100/70 mm Hg/70 bpm
Height/weight: 160 cm/68 kg
Neck veins: Not engorged
Lungs/chest: Clear
Heart: Apex displaced laterally and downward, no murmur
Abdomen: Soft, no mass
Extremities: Normal

LABORATORY DATA

Hemoglobin: 12.8 g/dL
Mean corpuscular volume: 92.8 fL
Platelet count: 181 × 10³/mm³
Sodium: 138 mmol/L
Potassium: 4.4 mmol/L
Creatinine: 97 mmol/L
Blood urea nitrogen: 8.6 mmol/L

ELECTROCARDIOGRAM

Findings

Figure 43-1, *A*, shows biventricular pacing at maximum output that resulted in anodal stimulation and triple site stimulation (i.e., right ventricular ring, right ventricular tip, and left ventricular tip). Figure 43-1, *B*, shows biventricular pacing below the anodal stimulation threshold, with subtle change in aV$_L$ and aV$_{R'}$ in contrast to triple site stimulation. In Figure 43-1, *C*, further decrement in left ventricular lead output can be seen, which resulted in loss of left ventricular capture, with the electrocardiogram (ECG) morphology basically the same as in right ventricular pacing alone. As shown in Figure 43-1, *D*, on testing by left ventricular pacing alone at maximum output, the ECG is very similar to what would be seen with biventricular pacing because of simultaneous right ventricular ring

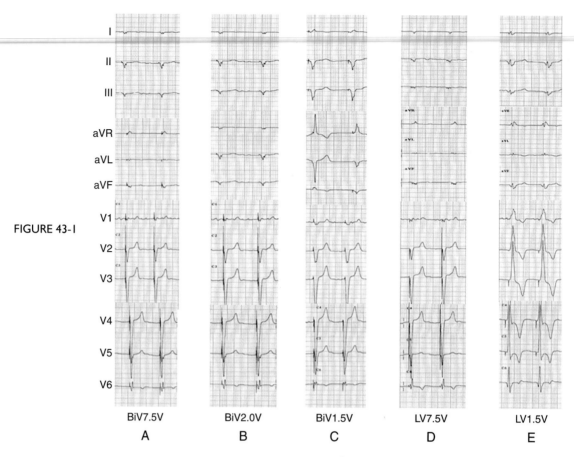

FIGURE 43-1

BiV7.5V	BiV2.0V	BiV1.5V	LV7.5V	LV1.5V
A	**B**	**C**	**D**	**E**

anodal stimulation and left ventricular pacing. Decrement of left ventricular lead output, as seen in Figure 43-1, *E*, led to loss of anodal stimulation and activation starts from the left ventricular pacing lead with marked change in ECG morphology.

FOCUSED CLINICAL QUESTIONS AND DISCUSSION POINTS

Question

How is anodal stimulation recognized in a patient with a CRT?

DISCUSSION

Most CRT devices use a bipolar lead for right ventricular pacing and a unipolar or bipolar lead for left ventricular pacing. Configuration of the left ventricular tip or ring as the cathode and the right ventricular lead ring as the anode is sometimes employed to prevent phrenic nerve stimulation or optimize the threshold for the left ventricular lead. In this configuration, potentially the right ventricular ring electrode can capture the myocardial tissue directly and result in the

phenomenon of anodal stimulation.[1,2,4,5] Anodal stimulation typically occurs with high left ventricular lead output,[1,2,4,5] and it is demonstrated by a change in 12-lead ECG morphology during increment of pacing output above pacing threshold during left ventricular only pacing (with the right ventricle output programmed off). In the presence of anodal stimulation, the ECG morphology is the same as simultaneous left and right ventricular (biventricular) pacing. It is reported that anodal stimulation can be detected in 78.4% of cases.[2] Anodal stimulation can also be seen during biventricular pacing when the QRS morphology becomes narrower at high left ventricular lead pacing output. This can be observed in only 41.4% of cases.[2] In this case report, very subtle change was observed that best could be appreciated in leads aV_L and aV_R, with loss of anodal stimulation when left ventricular lead output was decremented to 2.0 V at 0.4 msec when testing in the biventricular pacing configuration (see Figure 43-1). With further decrease in left ventricular lead output to 1.5 V, loss of left ventricular capture and only right ventricular capture were noted. Loss of anodal stimulation was more obvious when tested in the left ventricular pacing alone configuration. The reason why anodal stimulation may not be apparent when testing with biventricular pacing is because of the close proximity of the right ventricular lead ring and tip so that triple site stimulation may not cause significant change in QRS morphology in contrast to biventricular pacing.

One obvious question is whether anodal stimulation resulted in suboptimal CRT. In a small case study, 3 of 46 patients with left ventricular tip to right ventricular ring configuration were noted to have anodal stimulation and all of them were nonresponders to CRT.[3] Also, in a study of the hemodynamic effect of anodal stimulation by echocardiogram, no statistical difference was found in the hemodynamic effect of anodal stimulation on biventricular pacing. However, in 2 patients, worsening of hemodynamic status was noted with the presence of anodal stimulation.[7] Obviously, these studies are small in sample size and no definitive conclusion can be drawn. Another potential drawback of anodal stimulation is the elimination of the effect of V-V delay because of simultaneous capture of the right ventricular ring (anodal stimulation) and left ventricular tip.[6]

FINAL DIAGNOSIS

This patient had clinically detectable anodal stimulation. As a result the device was to allow triple site stimulation, with favorable response in terms of functional class and left ventricular reverse remodeling after CRT.

PLAN OF ACTION

The plan for this patient was to enable triple site pacing.

Selected References

1. Bulava A, Ansalone G, Ricci R, et al: Triple-site pacing in patients with biventricular device-incidence of the phenomenon and cardiac resynchronization benefit, *J Interv Card Electrophysiol* 10:37-45, 2004.
2. Champagne J, Healey JS, Krahn AD, ELECTION Investigators, et al: The effect of electronic repositioning on left ventricular pacing and phrenic nerve stimulation, *Europace* 13:409-415, 2011.
3. Dendy KF, Powell BD, Cha YM, et al: Anodal stimulation: an underrecognized cause of nonresponders to cardiac resynchronization therapy, *Indian Pacing Electrophysiol J* 11:64-72, 2011.
4. Tamborero D, Mont L, Alanis R, et al: Anodal capture in cardiac resynchronization therapy implications for device programming, *Pacing Clin Electrophysiol* 29:940-945, 2006.
5. Thibault B, Roy D, Guerra PG, et al: Anodal right ventricular capture during left ventricular stimulation in CRT-implantable cardioverter defibrillators, *Pacing Clin Electrophysiol* 28:613-619, 2005.
6. van Gelder BM, Bracke FA, Meijer A: The effect of anodal stimulation on V-V timing at varying V-V intervals, *Pacing Clin Electrophysiol* 28:771-776, 2005.
7. Yoshida K, Seo Y, Yamasaki H, et al: Effect of triangle ventricular pacing on haemodynamics and dyssynchrony in patients with advanced heart failure: a comparison study with conventional bi-ventricular pacing therapy, *Eur Heart J* 28:2610-2619, 2007.

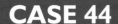

CASE 44

Significant Residual or Worsening Mitral Regurgitation (MitraClip)

François Regoli, Marta Acena, Tiziano Moccetti, and Angelo Auricchio

Age	Gender	Occupation	Working Diagnosis
76 Years	Female	Retired	Cardiac Resynchronization Therapy Nonresponder with Persistent Severe Mitral Regurgitation

HISTORY

This 76-year-old female patient was referred to us for persistent heart failure symptoms in New York Heart Association [NYHA] class III to IV and severe functional mitral regurgitation (FMR) despite optimal therapeutic management combining medication, previous biventricular implantable cardioverter-defibrillator (ICD) (cardiac resynchronization therapy defibrillator [CRT-D]) implant, and atrioventricular node ablation for competing atrial fibrillation rhythm. Four months previously a CRT-D device was implanted based on conventional class I indication—drug-refractory symptomatic heart failure (NYHA class III to IV) because of postactinic cardiomyopathy (the patient had previously received radiotherapy for non-Hodgkin lymphoma) with severe left ventricular systolic dysfunction (left ventricular ejection fraction [LVEF], 29%); the electrocardiogram (ECG) showed significant ventricular conduction delay with complete left bundle branch block and 130-msec QRS complex duration. Atrial fibrillation was the underlying atrial rhythm. Besides severe left ventricular dysfunction, the transthoracic echocardiogram performed before CRT-D device implant showed a mildly dilated left ventricle (end-diastolic voume 186 mL and end-systolic volume 132 mL) and severe functional mitral regurgitation determined by failed coaptation of mitral valve leaflets resulting from symmetric dilation of the mitral anulus. Shortly after CRT-D implant, the patient underwent catheter ablation of the atrioventricular node as a result of recurring high ventricular rate atrial fibrillation.

After 4 months of CRT, both symptoms and mitral regurgitation remained unchanged. The patient was therefore evaluated for percutaneous edge-to-edge mitral valvuloplasty with a MitraClip (Abbott Laboratories, Abbott Park, Ill).[1]

CURRENT MEDICATIONS

The patient was taking acenocoumerol 1 mg adjusted to international normalized ratio value, captopril 10 mg daily, carvedilol 12.5 mg daily, spironolactone 50 mg daily, torsemide 20 mg adjusted according to weight, and metolazone 2.5 mg daily if body weight greater than 50 kg.

Comments

The medication profile of the patient is typical for advanced-phase heart failure, with low dosages of an angiotensin-converting enzyme inhibitor and beta blockers and weight-adjusted dosages of diuretics.

CURRENT SYMPTOMS

The patient was unable to walk up a single flight of 12 steps without stopping because of breathlessness (NYHA class III to IV) and unable to perform the 6-Minute Walk Test.

PHYSICAL EXAMINATION

BP/HR: 90/60 mm Hg/70 bpm
Height/weight: 165 cm/47 kg
Neck veins: Jugular vein congestion
Lungs/chest: Presence of crackles in the midbasal fields
Heart: Mitral valve murmur 3/6
Abdomen: Normal
Extremities: Presence of moderate peripheral edema

LABORATORY DATA

Hemoglobin: 9 g/dL
Mean corpuscular volume: 73 fL
Platelet count: 212 × 10³/μL
Sodium: 138 mmol/L
Potassium: 3.9 mmol/L
Creatinine: 113 mmol/L
Blood urea nitrogen: 18 mmol/L

Comments

Life expectancy considering the patient's demographic, clinical, and laboratory data was calculated using the Seattle Heart Failure Model.[2] Estimated life expectancy for this patient was considered to be very poor, with a median life expectancy of 2.6 years and estimated survival of only 69%, 48%, and 16% at 1, 2, and 5 years, respectively.

ELECTROCARDIOGRAM

Findings

Constant biventricular paced rhythm was seen in VVI modality at 70 bpm (Figure 44-1). The vertical axis in the peripheral leads demonstrated a QRS duration of 120 msec. The underlying atrial rhythm was atrial fibrillation.

ECHOCARDIOGRAM

Findings

Figure 44-2 shows the transthoracic echocardiographic apical four-chamber view with color Doppler before (see Figure 44-2, *A*) MitraClip positioning.

Comments

A preprocedural transthoracic echocardiogram showed a mildly dilated left ventricle (end-diastolic volume 186 mL and end-systolic volume 132 mL) with severe systolic dysfunction (LVEF 26%). Severe functional mitral regurgitation was present, with a marked central regurgitant jet resulting from symmetric dilation of the annulus and consequent lack of leaflet coaptation. Lack of important alterations of leaflet morphology and movement implicate anatomomorphologic integrity of valve leaflets, chordae, and papillary muscles. Increased hemodynamic stress of mitral regurgitation is suggested by biatrial dilation, increased artery pulmonary pressure (45 mm Hg), hypokinesia of the right ventricle, and grade II tricuspid insufficiency.

FIGURE 44-1

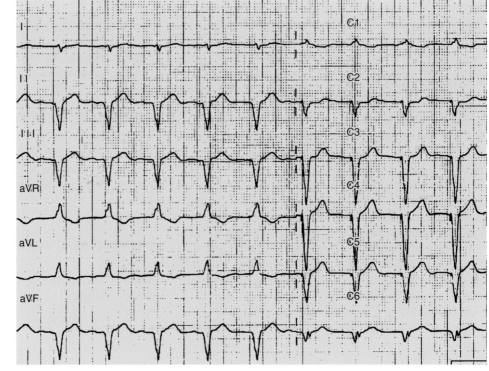

FOCUSED CLINICAL QUESTIONS AND DISCUSSION POINTS

Question

Why is the patient considered a suitable candidate for percutaneous mitral valve repair rather than surgical valve repair?

Discussion

The patient is an extremely compromised CRT nonresponder who continued to be symptomatic because of persistent severe functional mitral regurgitation. Based on EUROSCORE II,[3] the patient's surgical mortality risk was estimated at 17.8%. Furthermore, surgical approach in patients with CRT with indication for valve repair is not supported by prospective, randomized evidence.

As far as percutaneous edge-to-edge mitral valvuloplasty by MitraClip is concerned, one multicenter, prospective, longitudinal study has demonstrated the clinical benefit in this patient subgroup.[4] This study has shown that MitraClip repair of clinically and hemodynamically significant FMR after CRT improves symptoms and produces reversal of maladaptive remodeling in approximately 70% of these patients.

Question

What kind of mitral regurgitation disorder is most amenable to correction by MitraClip?

Discussion

Functional mitral regurgitation is most amenable to repair by MitraClip. Different from primary mitral regurgitation, functional mitral regurgitation (also termed *secondary mitral regurgitation*) is determined by geometric distortion of the subvalvular apparatus, secondary to left ventricular enlargement and remodeling as a result of idiopathic cardiomyopathy or coronary artery disease. The underlying condition in a patient with CRT produces tethering (apical and lateral papillary muscle displacement, and annular dilation) and reduced closing forces because of left ventricular dysfunction (reduced contractility or left ventricular dyssynchrony). It is important to emphasize that in functional mitral regurgitation, valve leaflets and chordae are structurally normal.[5] Besides precise evaluation of the mitral regurgitation grade, echocardiographic examinations (both transthoracic and transesophageal) should assess the following aspects to prepare the patient for mitral valve repair by MitraClip:

1. Presence of annulus dilation resulting from underlying heart disease
2. Anatomomorphologic integrity of the other anatomic constituents of the mitral valve, namely the leaflets and chordae
3. Structural and hemodynamic "repercussions" of mitral regurgitation on other cardiac chambers and on pulmonary arterial pressure

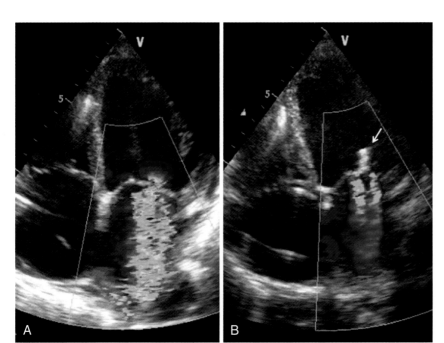

FIGURE 44-2

FIGURE 44-3

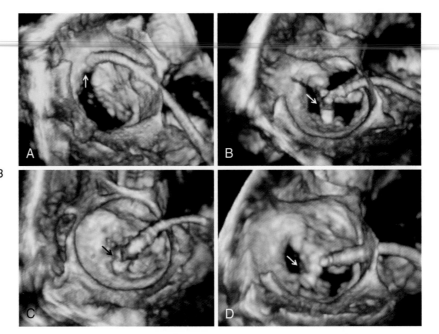

Question

What is the recommended time from CRT implantation to indicate MitraClip in case of persistent moderate-to-severe mitral regurgitation? Why is such a time frame recommended?

Discussion

The patient with CRT should be considered eligible for MitraClip in the case of persisting symptoms associated with unchanged moderate or severe mitral regurgitation after 3 to 6 months of CRT. This preset time frame is recommended based on the established knowledge that CRT-induced reversal of maladaptive left ventricular remodeling, which usually occurs within the first 6 months after device implantation, may reduce mitral regurgitation.[6,7] In the present case, it is important to emphasize that MitraClip intervention was not delayed to 6 months, because the clinical condition of the patient was extremely compromised with little or no therapeutic margin.

FINAL DIAGNOSIS

This patient had persistent severe functional mitral regurgitation and was a symptomatic CRT nonresponder.

PLAN OF ACTION

Mitral regurgitation was addressed by a percutaneous approach based on positioning of the MitraClip.

INTERVENTION

In general anesthesia and under continuous hemodynamic and transesophageal monitoring, the MitraClip delivery system is positioned by the transseptal catheterization approach. This system includes the clip at the tip, a steerable guiding catheter, and a clip delivery system to open, close, and release three-dimensional images.

Figure 44-3 shows intraprocedural transesophageal echocardiographic images during MitraClip positioning *(arrows)*. After transseptal catheterization, the clip, located at the tip of the MitraClip delivery system, is advanced across the mitral valve and into the left ventricle (see Figure 44-3, *A*) with the clip closed. The clip is then opened (see Figure 44-3, *B*), and slight retraction of the system toward the atrium in a central position is performed, thus capturing the valve leaflets. The clip is then closed (see Figure 44-3, *C*) at the desired position. If the position is suboptimal or inadequate, the maneuver may be repeated several times. After a satisfactory position has been achieved with resulting effective mitral regurgitation reduction, the clip is released (see Figure 44-3, *D*) and the delivery system removed. Postprocedural chest radiograph shows the correct position of the MitraClip device *(arrows)* in anteroposterior (Figure 44-4, *A*) and lateral (see Figure 44-4, *B*) projections.

OUTCOME

The outcome in this patient was satisfactory.

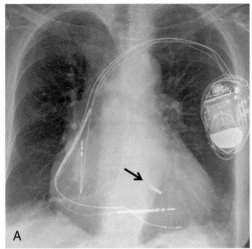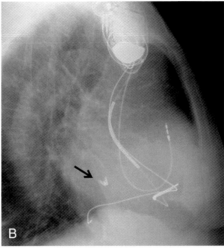

FIGURE 44-4

Findings

Transthoracic echocardiogram showed that MitraClip allowed a remarkable reduction of mitral regurgitation from grade IV to grade II. As a result, artery pulmonary pressure reduced to 35 mm Hg, right ventricular hypokinesia was no longer present, and tricuspid insufficiency reduced to grade I (see Figure 43-2).

After 2 years and 9 months of follow-up, the patient was clinically stable in NYHA class III. The echocardiogram revealed persistence of severe left ventricular (LVEF, 25%) systolic dysfunction, but residual grade II mitral regurgitation and left ventricular diameters (end-diastolic diameter to end-systolic diameter ratio, 66/58 mm) remained stable.

Calculation of Seattle Heart Failure Score based on the patient's demographic, clinical, laboratory, and therapeutic characteristics at last follow-up yielded an estimated mean life expectancy of 5.6 years, suggesting an increase in life expectancy of 2 years, compared to the preprocedural estimate.

Selected References

1. Feldman T, Kar S, Rinaldi M, et al: EVEREST Investigators. Percutaneous mitral repair with the MitraClip system: safety and midterm durability in the initial EVEREST (Endovascular Valve Edge-to-Edge REpair Study) cohort, *J Am Coll Cardiol* 54:686-694, 2009.
2. Levy WC, Mozaffarian D, Linker DT, et al: The Seattle Heart Failure Model: prediction of survival in heart failure, *Circulation* 113:1424-1433, 2006.
3. Roques F, Michel P, Goldstone AR, et al: The logistic EuroSCORE, *Eur Heart J* 24:882-883, 2003.
4. Auricchio A, Schillinger W, Meyer S, et al: PERMIT-CARE Investigators. Correction of mitral regurgitation in nonresponders to cardiac resynchronization therapy by MitraClip improves symptoms and promotes reverse remodeling, *J Am Coll Cardiol* 58:2183-2189, 2011.
5. Vahanian A, Alfieri O, Andreotti F, et al: Guidelines on the management of valvular heart disease (version 2012), *Eur Heart J* 33:2451-2496, 2012.
6. Boriani G, Gasparini M, Landolina M, et al: InSync/InSync ICD Italian Registry Investigators. Impact of mitral regurgitation on the outcome of patients treated with CRT-D: data from the InSync ICD Italian Registry, *Pacing Clin Electrophysiol* 35:146-154, 2012.
7. Di Biase L, Auricchio A, Mohanty P, et al: Impact of cardiac resynchronization therapy on the severity of mitral regurgitation, *Europace* 13:829-838, 2011.

SECTION 9

Device-Based Diagnostics for Heart Failure Monitoring and Remote Monitoring

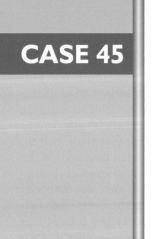

Intrathoracic Impedance (Dietary Incompliance)

Frieder Braunschweig

Age	Gender	Occupation	Working Diagnosis
65 Years	Male	Businessman	OptiVol Alert for Fluid Overload

HISTORY

In August 2008 the patient received a biventricular implantable cardioverter-defibrillator (ICD; Concerto, Medtronic, Minneapolis, Minn.) due to dilated cardiomyopathy with symptomatic heart failure (New York Heart Association [NYHA] class III) despite optimal pharmacologic treatment. Before implantation, his left ventricular ejection fraction (LVEF) was 20%, with a pattern of global hypokinesia. He was in permanent atrial fibrillation, and the surface electrocardiogram (ECG) showed a typical left bundle branch block and QRS duration of 160 ms. After 6 months of cardiac resynchronization therapy (CRT), he had improved to NYHA class II and the LVEF had increased to 35%.

The device collected daily information about intrathoracic impedance and tracked changes in the OptiVol Fluid Index. Intrathoracic impedance can be measured between a right ventricular pacing or defibrillation lead and the device can.[1] Impedance decreases with an increase in blood volume and pulmonary fluid content. The OptiVol fluid index compares the actual patient impedance with a reference impedance derived from a moving average algorithm. When daily impedance falls below the reference, the difference accumulates in the OptiVol Fluid Index. If the OptiVol Fluid Index crosses a certain threshold, an alert can be triggered indicating that the patient is at increased risk for subsequent heart failure decompensation. This may facilitate timely therapeutic interventions. A threshold crossing incident can be indicated to the patient by an audible tone from the device (OptiVol alert) or to the heart failure team by means of remote patient monitoring.

The patient was enrolled in a clinical study. According to the protocol, he was not connected to remote patient monitoring and the OptiVol alert was programmed "on."

Comments

The patient fulfilled essential guideline criteria for implantation of a CRT defibrillator (CRT-D) system. At the time of implantation, the role of CRT in patients with atrial fibrillation was unclear. Nevertheless, implantation of a CRT-D system in a patient such as this reflected common clinical practice.[4] As a result of the beneficial clinical course and improvements in left ventricular function after 6 months, he was considered a responder to CRT treatment.

CURRENT MEDICATIONS

The patient was taking warfarin (INR 2-3), bisoprolol 10 mg daily, enalapril 20 mg daily, spironolactone 25 mg daily, digoxin 0.25 mg daily, and furosemide 40 mg twice daily.

Comments

The medication regimen represents current guideline recommendations. During treatment with bisoprolol and digoxin the spontaneous heart rate was constantly below the basic paced heart rate of 70 bpm (VVIR mode). The proportion of biventricular stimulation was above 98%. Therefore atrioventricular junctional ablation was not deemed necessary.

CURRENT SYMPTOMS

On August 23, 2009, the patient participated in a crayfish party, which is a traditional eating and drinking celebration in the Nordic countries held in late summer during the legal crayfish harvesting period. A crayfish dinner is typically associated with intake of large amounts of salt, and alcohol consumption (with *snaps*, the Swedish for small shots of strong alcohol) may be high. These deviations from essential dietary restrictions prudent for heart failure patients are usually followed by increased water consumption.

During the next several days, a fall in impedance and an increase in the OptiVol Fluid Index was observed. On September 9, the Fluid Index threshold of 60 Ohm*days was crossed and the audible OptiVol alert was activated every morning as long as the Fluid Index remained above threshold values. The patient had been instructed to contact his heart failure clinic in case of an OptiVol alert. Despite this, he waited 12 more days before calling the clinic. Being a well-educated patient, he suspected a causal relationship between the dietary incompliance and the consecutive fluid alert. In fact, he later reported transient symptoms of minor weight increase, dyspnea, and slight ankle swelling for a few days after the dinner. During the last week before contacting the clinic, he took an extra tablet of furosemide 40 mg daily.

On September 10 the patient was seen at the heart failure clinic. At this time, symptoms had disappeared and body weight had normalized. The physical status revealed no sign of overt fluid overload. Information about intrathoracic impedance was read from the device memory. Notably, impedance had increased again for some days and was about to cross the line of the reference impedance. This was consistent with normalization of heart failure signs and symptoms and indicated that the audible alert would soon disappear. It was recommended that the patient continue with his ordinary medical prescription. The patient was reminded about restrictions concerning salt, fluid, and alcohol intake. Flexible use of diuretics in response to subjective signs and symptoms of heart failure was encouraged.

On October 8 a control visit was made. The patient's condition remained unchanged. Device interrogation showed that the OptiVol Fluid Index had normalized soon after the prior visit and impedance had returned to a level indicating normal fluid conditions.

Comments

The patient was asymptomatic at the examination, and the alert could be regarded as a false alert. However, the patient's history indicated transient heart failure deterioration as the most probable explanation. Dietary incompliance can lead to fluid retention[6] and is often involved in heart failure decompensation.[5]

In the present case, the patient had already taken therapeutic action by increasing the dose of diuretics and any additional impact of the clinician encounter cannot be proved. However, during the patient visit the pathophysiologic mechanism of the event was confirmed and important educational advice was provided.

Patient–clinician interaction in a case such as this should rather be established using remote monitoring technology. A phone call together with a remote check of other device diagnostics (i.e., heart rate, heart rate variability, physical activity, ventricular arrhythmia burden, and percentage biventricular pacing, all of which were normal in the present case) would likely be sufficient to resolve this situation without the need for an office visit.

The value of audible alerts has been disputed. In the randomized Diagnostic Outcome Trial in Heart Failure trial, patients in whom the audible alert was activated had a higher incidence of hospitalizations for heart failure.[8] Obviously, audible alerts can trigger patient and physician concerns and thereby lower the threshold for hospitalization. Still, other studies have demonstrated that fluid alerts should direct the attention of clinicians to an increased risk for heart failure–related events.[7,9] Trials evaluating the concept of impedance monitoring in the context of remote patient monitoring are under way.

PHYSICAL EXAMINATION

BP/HR: 110/80 mm Hg/70 bpm (regular)
Height/weight: 192 cm/93 kg
Neck veins: Normal
Lungs/chest: Clear
Heart: Apical systolic murmur (grade 1/6)
Abdomen: Normal status
Extremities: No peripheral edema

COMMENTS

The physical examination on September 10 did not show any sign of heart failure decompensation.

LABORATORY DATA

Hemoglobin: 135 g/dL
Hematocrit: 45%
Mean corpuscular volume: 96 fL
Sodium: 138 mmol/L
Potassium: 4.3 mmol/L
Creatinine: 125 μmol/L

Comments

Findings were normal apart from renal dysfunction.

FOCUSED CLINICAL QUESTIONS AND DISCUSSION POINTS

Question

Why does impedance gradually increase during the first months after implantation?

Discussion

An increase in intrathoracic impedance is commonly observed during the first month after implantation (Figure 45-1, *x*). The typical postoperative impedance pattern is largely explained by the gradual resorption of tissue edema, fluid, and hematoma in the ICD pocket. In the present case, impedance continued to increase for approximately 9 months (see Figure 45-1, *y*) until a plateau was reached. This was likely due to the beneficial long-term effects of CRT with decreasing left ventricular size, blood volume, and pulmonary decongestion.

The typical early impedance increase after surgery may mask a concomitant fluid retention. Therefore the sensitivity of the OptiVol fluid algorithm to detect impending volume overload decompensation is particularly limited during the first few months after device implantation.[2] Similarly, a sudden impedance fall and gradual recovery is observed after a device exchange or other thoracic operations.

Question

What are the possible reasons for an OptiVol fluid alert?

Discussion

Impedance decreases with a consecutive increase of the OptiVol Fluid Index are typically observed in the presence of progressive fluid retention resulting from decompensated heart failure. In the pivotal study by Yu et al (MID-HefFT) study, impedance started to decrease at an average of 18 days before heart failure hospitalization and symptoms first occurred 3 days before hospitalization.[10] Therefore a "true" OptiVol alert can be observed in patients who are asymptomatic or only "mildly" symptomatic. Whether any preventive treatment should be initiated in the latter conditions is currently unclear.

Other reasons for impedance falls include thoracic surgery, pneumonia and bronchitis, and pleural or pericardial effusions. Furthermore, because of the variability

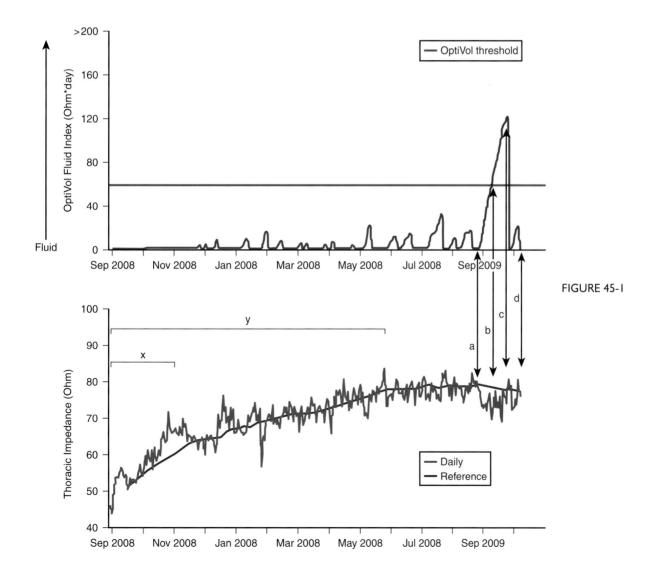

FIGURE 45-1

of thoracic impedance, a false alert with no clinical correlate may occur. A higher specificity can be achieved by increasing the OptiVol threshold.

Question

How should information from impedance monitoring be used in clinical practice?

Discussion

Given the limitations discussed previously, the clinical value of alert features based on impedance is currently unclear, especially if used without concomitant remote patient monitoring. However, it has been shown that information from impedance monitoring alone or in combination with other device-based diagnostics can identify patients who are at higher risk for impending heart failure hospitalization.[9] Therefore regular monitoring of the device diagnostics—for example, in monthly intervals—may improve patient management. Currently, device-based diagnostics appear underused. However, improvements are required for future devices and offline analysis systems to make interpretation of the data more convenient and efficient for the clinicians.[3] This likely requires a multisensor approach.

FINAL DIAGNOSIS

The patient experienced an episode of deteriorating heart failure with fluid retention triggered by dietary incompliance.

PLAN OF ACTION

The patient's medical treatment remained unchanged and he was connected to patient home monitoring.

INTERVENTION

The intervention included recapitulation of dietary restrictions. Self-adjustment of daily diuretics at the lowest possible dose was encouraged.

OUTCOME

The patient remained in NYHA class II with intermittent episodes of congestion that could be handled on an outpatient basis. Remote patient monitoring was initiated and was considered valuable to maintain stable volume conditions.

Selected References

1. Braunschweig F, Ford I, Conraads V, et al: Can monitoring of intrathoracic impedance reduce morbidity and mortality in patients with chronic heart failure? Rationale and design of the Diagnostic Outcome Trial in Heart Failure (DOT-HF), *Eur J Heart Fail* 10:907-916, 2008.
2. Conraads VM, Tavazzi L, Santini M, Oliva F, et al: Sensitivity and positive predictive value of implantable intrathoracic impedance monitoring as a predictor of heart failure hospitalizations: the SENSE-HF trial, *Eur Heart J* 18:2266-2273, 2011.
3. Daubert JC, Saxon L, Adamson PB, et al: 2012 EHRA/HRS expert consensus statement on cardiac resynchronization therapy in heart failure: implant and follow-up recommendations and management, *Europace* 14:1236-1286, 2012.
4. Dickstein K, Bogale N, Priori S, et al: The European cardiac resynchronization therapy survey, *Eur Heart J* 30:2450-2460, 2009.
5. Fonarow GC: The Acute Decompensated Heart Failure National Registry (ADHERE): opportunities to improve care of patients hospitalized with acute decompensated heart failure, *Rev Cardiovasc Med* 4(Suppl 7):S21-S30, 2003.
6. Gudmundsson K, Lynga P, Karlsson H, et al: Midsummer Eve in Sweden: a natural fluid challenge in patients with heart failure, *Eur J Heart Fail* 13:1172-1177, 2011.
7. Tang WH, Warman EN, Johnson JW, et al: Threshold crossing of device-based intrathoracic impedance trends identifies relatively increased mortality risk, *Eur Heart J* 2189-2196, 2012.
8. van Veldhuisen DJ, Braunschweig F, Conraads V, et al: Intrathoracic impedance monitoring, audible patient alerts, and outcome in patients with heart failure, *Circulation* 124:1719-1726, 2011.
9. Whellan DJ, Ousdigian KT, Al-Khatib SM, et al: Combined heart failure device diagnostics identify patients at higher risk of subsequent heart failure hospitalizations: results from PARTNERS HF study, *J Am Coll Cardiol* 55:1803-1810, 2010.
10. Yu CM, Wang L, Chau E, et al: Intrathoracic impedance monitoring in patients with heart failure: correlation with fluid status and feasibility of early warning preceding hospitalization, *Circulation* 112:841-848, 2005.

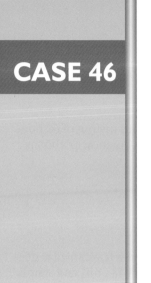

Pulmonary Hypertension and Cardiac Resynchronization Therapy: Evaluation Prior to Implantation and Response to Therapy

Wandy Chan and Richard Troughton

Age	Gender	Occupation	Working Diagnosis
58 Years	Male	Sales Representative	Systolic Heart Failure with Severe Pulmonary Hypertension

HISTORY

The patient was referred from another center for consideration of cardiac resynchronization therapy (CRT) for long-standing ischemic cardiomyopathy and progressive heart failure symptoms. At time of referral he described New York Heart Association (NYHA) class III symptoms despite optimal medical therapy.

The patient's history included ischemic heart disease, first diagnosed at 40 years of age. At that time he also had exertional angina. A 12-lead electrocardiogram (ECG) showed left bundle branch morphology. Echocardiography and left ventriculography demonstrated impaired left ventricular function with a left ventricular ejection fraction of 40%. Coronary angiography demonstrated severe three-vessel coronary artery disease. He underwent coronary bypass grafting at 40 years of age, with left internal mammary grafting to the left anterior descending artery and saphenous vein grafts to the lateral circumflex and posterior descending arteries. He then remained asymptomatic until ventricular fibrillation arrest occurred while driving in a car race at 50 years of age. Coronary bypass grafts were intact, with no new native coronary lesions suitable for percutaneous intervention. Left ventricular function remained mildly impaired. Treatment with amiodarone was initiated, and he underwent implantation of an implantable cardioverter-defibrillator at that time. He had no further ventricular arrhythmias or device therapies delivered, but over the ensuing 8 years he developed progressive symptoms of heart failure accompanied by a decline in left ventricular systolic function. At the time of referral

for CRT, he had no symptoms of ischemic heart disease and coronary angiography demonstrated patent grafts but diffuse native coronary disease.

Apart from hyperlipidemia, the patient had no history of other significant medical conditions.

CURRENT MEDICATIONS

The patient was taking spironolactone 25 mg daily, furosemide 120 mg daily, atorvastatin 20 mg daily, carvedilol 12.5 mg twice daily, enalapril 5 mg twice daily, amiodarone 200 mg daily, and enteric coated aspirin 100 mg daily.

Comments

Although the patient practiced good adherence to guideline–based heart failure medications, maximal doses of carvedilol and enalapril were not tolerated because of hypotension and azotemia. Occasional additional midday furosemide doses were self-administered by the patient according to an action plan based on weight and symptoms.

CURRENT SYMPTOMS

The patient experienced NYHA class III symptoms of shortness of breath and fatigue and occasional orthopnea and paroxysmal nocturnal dyspnea. He had no syncope, palpitations, or anginal symptoms.

PHYSICAL EXAMINATION

BP/HR: 105/60 mm Hg/60 bpm
Height/weight: 171 cm/77 kg
Neck veins: +4 cm, hepatojugular reflux positive
Lungs/chest: Resonant to percussion, vesicular breath sounds with bibasal fine, late-inspiratory crackles
Heart: Laterally displaced, diffuse apex beat impulse, first heart sound (S_1) + second heart sound (S_2) + third heart sound (S_3); grade 3 apical pan-systolic murmur radiating to the axilla
Abdomen: No abnormality
Extremities: No edema, normal volume pulses

Comments

Physical examination elicited signs consistent with left ventricular dysfunction and mild volume overload.

LABORATORY DATA

Hemoglobin: 12.6 mg/dL
Hematocrit/packed cell volume: 39%
Mean corpuscular volume: 91 fL
Platelet count: $272 \times 10^3/\mu L$
Sodium: 136 mmol/L
Potassium: 4.3 mmol/L
Creatinine: 1.58 mg/dL
Blood urea nitrogen: 82 mg/dL

Comments

Hematologic investigations were within normal limits. Biochemical testing revealed mild renal dysfunction consistent with prerenal azotemia, with no evidence of intrinsic renal disease on subsequent testing.

ELECTROCARDIOGRAM

Findings

The ECG in Figure 46-1 shows a sinus rhythm of 60 bpm, left bundle branch block, and QRS duration of 190 ms.

ECHOCARDIOGRAM

Findings

The echocardiogram showed severe left ventricular dilation with an end-diastolic volume of 484 mL, end-systolic volume of 380 mL, with severe global systolic dysfunction and calculated ejection fraction of 21% (Figure 46-2).

Comments

In addition to severe systolic dysfunction, evidence of mechanical dyssynchrony with a prolonged left ventricular preejection time of 190 ms was noted (Figure 46-3).

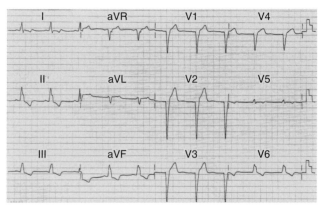

FIGURE 46-1   Resting electrocardiogram.

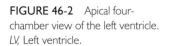

FIGURE 46-2   Apical four-chamber view of the left ventricle. *LV,* Left ventricle.

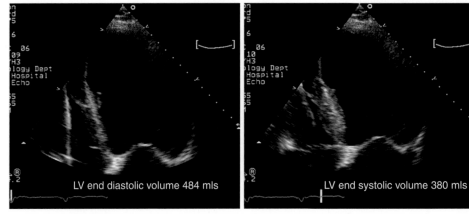

Findings

The echocardiogram also showed normal mitral valve leaflets, tenting of leaflets resulting from left ventricular dilation, severe functional mitral regurgitation, effective regurgitant orifice 0.5 cm², and the regurgitant volume of 72 mL by the proximal isovelocity surface area method.

Comments

The findings on echocardiography were consistent with those of severe functional mitral regurgitation as a consequence of ischemic cardiomyopathy with severe ventricular dilation (Figure 46-4).

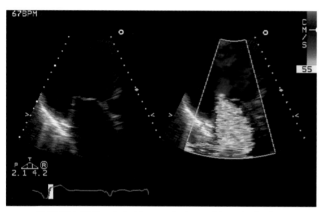

FIGURE 46-3 Apical long axis view of the mitral valve.

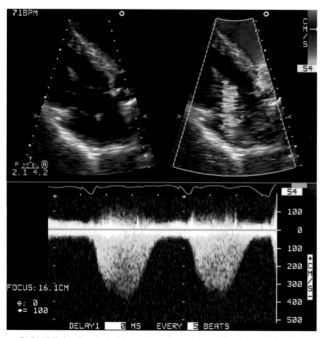

FIGURE 46-4 Apical four-chamber view of the tricuspid valve.

Findings

Moderately severe functional tricuspid regurgitation, with peak velocity of 3.8 ms, consistent with estimated right ventricular systolic pressure of 58 mm Hg above right atrial pressure.

PHYSIOLOGIC TRACINGS

Findings

The initial hemodynamic recordings demonstrated elevated pulmonary artery pressures (Figures 46-5 through 46-8). The pulmonary capillary wedge pressure was elevated, and the waveform demonstrated large c-V waves consistent with mitral regurgitation. The transpulmonary gradient was 9 mm Hg, and the calculated pulmonary vascular resistance was 2.5 Wood units. After administration of intravenous nitroglycerin, a significant fall in pulmonary artery and pulmonary capillary wedge pressure occurred. Abolition of the prominent c-V wave was also seen on the pulmonary capillary wedge tracing.

CATHETERIZATION

Right heart catheterization was performed to evaluate pulmonary hypertension.

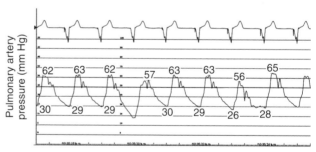

FIGURE 46-5 Pulmonary artery pressure trace at baseline before cardiac resynchronization therapy.

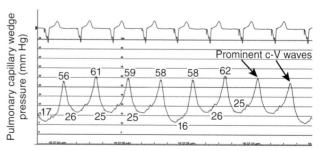

FIGURE 46-6 Pulmonary capillary wedge pressure trace at baseline before cardiac resynchronization therapy.

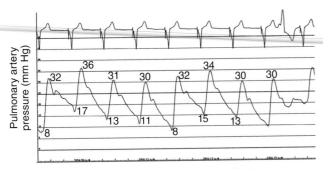

FIGURE 46-7 Pulmonary artery pressure trace after intravenous nitroglycerin 300 mcg demonstrating a significant fall in mean pulmonary artery pressure.

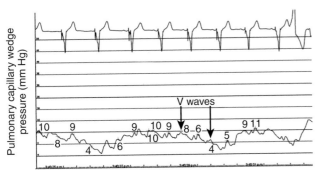

FIGURE 46-8 Pulmonary capillary wedge pressure trace after intravenous nitroglycerin 300 mcg demonstrating a significant fall in mean capillary wedge pressure.

Hemodynamics

Baseline

HR/BP: 102/61 mm Hg, mean 82 mm Hg/60 bpm
Right atrial pressure: Mean 11 mm Hg
Right ventricular pressure: 59/7 mm Hg, end-diastolic pressure 11 mm Hg
Pulmonary artery pressure: 61/28 mm Hg, mean 41 mm Hg
Pulmonary capillary wedge pressure: Mean 32 mm Hg
Cardiac output: 3.6 L/min
Pulmonary vascular resistance: 198 dynes*s/cm⁵ (2.5 Wood units)

After Intravenous Nitroglycerin 300 mcg

HR/BP: 88/61 mm Hg, mean 68 mm Hg/60 bpm
Pulmonary artery pressure: 32/8 mm Hg, mean 16 mm Hg
Pulmonary capillary wedge pressure: Mean 8 mm Hg
Cardiac output: 3.4 L/min
Pulmonary vascular: 188 dynes*s/cm⁵ (2.4 Wood units)

FOCUSED CLINICAL QUESTIONS AND DISCUSSION POINTS

Question

Is pulmonary hypertension a contraindication to CRT?

Discussion

Pulmonary hypertension in the setting of heart failure is associated with increased risk for adverse outcome and death,[2,4] particularly if pulmonary hypertension persists on serial measurement once medical therapy has been optimized.[3] The risk is highest in subjects with "precapillary" or "reactive" pulmonary hypertension that reflects pulmonary vascular remodeling either as a consequence of sustained elevation of pulmonary pressures in the context of left heart disease or as a result of collagen vascular disease or other causes.[1,4]

Pulmonary hypertension has been associated with a worse prognosis after CRT.[8,9] However, reductions in pulmonary artery pressures occur frequently after CRT and are associated with improved clinical outcome.[7]

Pulmonary hypertension was not an exclusion criterion in landmark CRT trials and is not currently considered a contraindication to CRT. However, patients with pulmonary hypertension warrant careful evaluation to confirm the severity of pulmonary artery pressure elevation and response to vasodilator challenge.[4] When precapillary or reactive pulmonary hypertension is identified, the risk for implantation and the potential role of alternative therapies such as pulmonary vasodilator agents (e.g., sildenafil) should be carefully considered.[4]

Question

What is the best way to assess pulmonary hypertension in preparation for CRT?

Discussion

Echocardiography is the best screening test for evaluation of pulmonary hypertension in the setting of left heart disease, but it has limitations.[4] Although right ventricular systolic pressure as a surrogate for pulmonary artery systolic pressure can be estimated from Doppler velocity of the tricuspid regurgitation jet, these estimates may be inaccurate in the setting of a suboptimal acoustic window or incomplete tricuspid regurgitation Doppler trace.[6] Echocardiography does not allow accurate measurement of the transpulmonary pressure gradient or pulmonary vascular resistance.[6]

Right heart catheterization is the gold standard for evaluation of pulmonary vascular hemodynamics and can be performed with minimal risk.[4,6] Direct measurement of pulmonary artery pressure, pulmonary capillary wedge pressure, and cardiac output (by thermodilution or Fick method) allows the most accurate calculation of transpulmonary gradient and pulmonary vascular resistance.[4] When pulmonary capillary wedge pressure is greater than 15 mm Hg and the transpulmonary gradient is less than 15 to 20 mm Hg or the pulmonary vascular resistance less than 3 Wood units, pulmonary hypertension is consistent with left atrial pressure elevation[4] and is likely to improve if left atrial pressure falls after CRT.[7] A fall in pulmonary artery pressures after challenge with a vasodilator, such as nitroprusside, also identifies patients in whom pulmonary hypertension is likely to improve if left atrial pressures fall after intervention with CRT. Reactive or precapillary pulmonary hypertension can be identified when the transpulmonary gradient is greater than 20 or pulmonary vascular resistance is greater than 3. A reduction in pulmonary artery pressures after CRT intervention is less likely in this setting and is also unclear for patients in whom pulmonary artery pressures do not fall after an acute vasodilator challenge.

Question

Should all patients who are being considered for CRT undergo right heart catheterization if evidence is present of pulmonary hypertension at the time of echocardiography?

Discussion

Right heart catheterization is not indicated in all patients undergoing CRT, but may be appropriate in patients with more severe elevation of pulmonary artery pressures (mean pulmonary artery pressure >40 mm Hg), patients with suspected reactive pulmonary hypertension who may be less likely to improve with CRT, and those in whom elevation of pulmonary artery pressure appears disproportionate to the severity of left ventricular or valvular dyfunction and in whom an alternative cause for pulmonary hypertension may be present.[4,6]

Question

Can all patients with pulmonary hypertension secondary to left ventricular dysfunction or functional mitral regurgitation expect to improve after CRT?

Discussion

A reduction in pulmonary artery pressures occurs in many patients after CRT through a variety of mechanisms and is associated with improved clinical outcomes.[7,5] A reduction in mitral regurgitation is seen in a large proportion of subjects receiving CRT and is

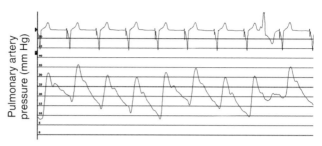

FIGURE 46-9 Pulmonary artery pressure trace 3 months after cardiac resynchronization therapy.

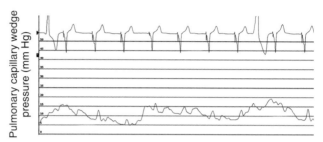

FIGURE 46-10 Pulmonary capillary wedge pressure trace 3 months after cardiac resynchronization therapy.

associated with reductions in pulmonary artery pressures (Figures 46-9 and 46-10).[5,10]

Reductions in pulmonary artery pressure are less likely to occur in CRT nonresponders, as a consequence of persisting elevation in left atrial pressures or persisting mitral regurgitation. Correction of elevated pulmonary artery pressures after CRT is also less likely in the context of reactive pulmonary hypertension, in which pulmonary vascular remodeling contributes to persisting pulmonary hypertension.

FINAL DIAGNOSIS

This patient had severe ischemic cardiomyopathy with severe functional mitral regurgitation and secondary pulmonary hypertension, with normal pulmonary vascular resistance.

PLAN OF ACTION

The plan for this patient was cardiac resynchronization with consideration of subsequent mitral valve repair, with left ventricular assist device back-up.

INTERVENTION

Cardiac resynchronization therapy with CRT-D was performed.

OUTCOME

The CRT-D was successfully implanted.

Findings

The patient had a clinical response with improvement to class II. Brain natriuretic peptide improved from 1414 pg/mL to 574 pg/mL. Left ventricular volumes fell to 341/255 mL. Improvement in left ventricular ejection fraction to 25% also was noted. Mitral regurgitation reduced to moderately severe, with an effective regurgitant orifice area of 0.39 cm^2 and regurgitant volume of 44 mL using the proximal isovelocity area method.

Improvement was seen at follow-up right heart catheterization performed 3 months after CRT-D, with pulmonary artery pressures of 35/12 mm Hg, mean 24 mm Hg, and pulmonary capillary wedge mean of 12 mm Hg with relatively normal V waves, giving a transpulmonary gradient of 12 mm Hg and calculated pulmonary vascular resistance of less than 3 Wood units.

Comments

CRT-D implantation was associated with beneficial reverse left ventricular remodeling, a reduction in mitral regurgitation, and a reduction in pulmonary artery pressures. Right heart catheterization before CRT-D implantation indicated that pulmonary hypertension was secondary to elevated left atrial pressure as a consequence of severe functional mitral regurgitation. Findings indicated normal pulmonary vascular resistance and reversibility of pulmonary hypertension when left atrial pressure was lowered with acute vasodilator therapy. Follow-up right heart catheterization after implantation confirmed the finding that pulmonary hypertension was reversible and normalized once left atrial pressures fell after implantation.

Selected References

1. Aronson D, Eitan A, Dragu R, et al: Relationship between reactive pulmonary hypertension and mortality in patients with acute decompensated heart failure, *Circ Heart Fail.* 4:644-650, 2011.
2. Chatterjee NA, Lewis GD: What is the prognostic significance of pulmonary hypertension in heart failure? *Circ Heart Fail.* 4:541-545, 2011.
3. Grigioni F, Potena L, Galie N, et al: Prognostic implications of serial assessments of pulmonary hypertension in severe chronic heart failure, *J Heart Lung Transplant* 25:1241-1246, 2006.
4. Guazzi M, Borlaug BA: Pulmonary hypertension due to left heart disease, *Circulation* 126:975-990, 2012.
5. Liang YJ, Zhang Q, Fung JW, et al: Different determinants of improvement of early and late systolic mitral regurgitation contributed after cardiac resynchronization therapy, *J Am Soc Echocardiogr* 23:1160-1167, 2010.
6. McLaughlin VV, Archer SL, Badesch DB, Barst RJ, Farber HW, Writing Committee, American College of Cardiology Foundation Task Force on Expert Consensus Documents, American Heart Association, American College of Chest Physicians, American Thoracic Society, Pulmonary Hypertension Association, et al: ACCF/AHA 2009 expert consensus document on pulmonary hypertension, *Circulation* 119:2250-2294, 2009.
7. Shalaby A, Voigt A, El-Saed A, et al: Usefulness of pulmonary artery pressure by echocardiography to predict outcome in patients receiving cardiac resynchronization therapy heart failure, *Am J Cardiolo* 101:238-241, 2008.
8. Stern J, Heist EK, Murray L, et al: Elevated estimated pulmonary artery systolic pressure is associated with an adverse clinical outcome in patients receiving cardiac resynchronization therapy, *Pacing Clin Electrophysiol* 30:603-607, 2007.
9. Tedrow UB, Kramer DB, Stevenson LW, et al: Relation of right ventricular peak systolic pressure to major adverse events in patients undergoing cardiac resynchronization therapy, *Am J Cardiol* 97:1737-1740, 2006.
10. van Bommel RJ, Marsan NA, Delgado V, et al: Cardiac resynchronization therapy as a therapeutic option in patients with moderate-severe functional mitral regurgitation and high operative risk, *Circulation* 124:912-919, 2011.

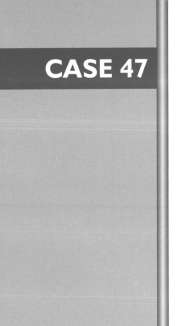

CASE 47

Role of Left Atrial Pressure Monitoring in the Management of Heart Failure

Kimberly A. Parks and Jagmeet P. Singh

Age	Gender	Occupation	Working Diagnosis
60 Years	Male	Teacher	Congestive Heart Failure, Stage C, New York Heart Association Class III

HISTORY

This 60-year-old man had coronary atherosclerosis, left bundle branch block (LBBB) with a QRS duration of 154 ms, peripheral vascular disease, and cardiomyopathy. He sought an opinion regarding management of his cardiomyopathy, which was diagnosed 10 years previously after he went to a local emergency department with chest tightness and shortness of breath. A coronary angiogram was performed that showed total occlusion of his right coronary artery, with no other significant coronary disease. His left ventricular ejection fraction (LVEF) at that time was 40%. He was managed medically, his symptoms improved markedly, and he returned to his baseline functional capacity. He was riding his bicycle regularly, working full time as a high school teacher, and doing heavy housework without difficulty. Approximately 2 years earlier, he noticed a decline in his exercise tolerance and developed intermittent dyspnea on exertion. His medical regimen was optimized, but he had no improvement in his symptoms. His LVEF was noted to have declined to 32%. A workup for ischemia was negative, and given his underlying LBBB and New York Heart Association (NYHA) class III symptoms, he was then referred for a biventricular pacemaker and treated with cardiac resynchronization therapy (CRT). Despite an optimal medical regimen and CRT, he had progressive dyspnea on exertion and worsening functional capacity. He reported development of lower extremity edema over the past 6 months and had frequent episodes of congestion. He required hospitalization five times in the previous 6 months for treatment of acute decompensated heart failure. His most recent two-dimensional echocardiogram revealed an LVEF of 29%, mild right ventricular dysfunction, and a moderately dilated left ventricle with mild mitral regurgitation. He has orthopnea that requires four pillows and frequently sleeps in a recliner. After his most recent hospitalization, he was enrolled in a home telemonitoring program, but did not experience improvement in his symptoms. He is obese and was recently diagnosed with sleep apnea, for which he uses continuous positive airway pressure at night.

Comments

The patient had chronic heart failure with progressive worsening in symptoms despite an optimized medical regimen. His volume status was difficult to manage over the past year, even with the addition of home telemonitoring. He should be counseled about the importance of sodium restriction, medication, and dietary compliance. Given his obesity, his volume status might be difficult to assess, and evaluation of his hemodynamics by right catheterization would be helpful in establishing his true volume status. He might require advanced therapies for heart failure in the near future, including heart transplantation or a left ventricular assist device, and consideration should be given for other novel therapies that might assist in symptom management. Controlling volume status will help delay disease progression.

CURRENT MEDICATIONS

The patient was taking carvedilol 25 mg twice daily, lisinopril 40 mg daily, torsemide 80 mg twice daily, metolazone 2.5 mg as needed for weight gain of more than 5 lb in 48 hours, spironolactone 25 mg daily, digoxin 0.125 mg daily, atorvastatin 20 mg daily, and aspirin 81 mg daily.

Comments

He was on a standard medication regimen to promote neurohormonal blockade and manage heart failure.

CURRENT SYMPTOMS

The patient reported orthopnea for the previous 2 weeks and noted chronic lower extremity edema over the past 6 to 7 months. He was unable to walk more than 20 feet without significant dyspnea.

PHYSICAL EXAMINATION

BP/HR: 98/54 mm Hg/60 bpm
Height/weight: 177.8 cm/131 kg
Neck veins: Difficult to assess secondary to body habitus, short neck
Lungs/chest: Clear to auscultation and percussion
Heart: Point of maximal impulse is lateral to the left midclavicular line, no right ventricular or left ventricular heave, distant heart sounds, normal first heart sound (S_1) and second heart sound (S_2) and a faint (S_3) gallop, 1 to 2/6 holosystolic murmur at the left sternal border that increases in intensity with inspiration
Abdomen: Soft, obese, nontender, and nondistended, no ascites; liver palpable 1 cm below the costal margin; no abdominal bruits
Extremities: Warm and well perfused with 2+ pulses bilaterally, 2+ pitting edema to the midcalf, and skin changes consistent with chronic venous stasis

Comments

The patient's body habitus limited the sensitivity of the examination. The combination of the presence of an S_3 gallop, a murmur of tricuspid regurgitation, and lower extremity edema suggested he was volume overloaded and likely had a component of both left and right heart failure.

LABORATORY DATA

Hemoglobin: 14 mg/dL
Hematocrit/packed cell volume: 39%
Platelet count: 204 × 10^3/µL
Sodium: 129 mmol/L
Potassium: 4.2 mmol/L
Creatinine: 1.5 mg/dL
Blood urea nitrogen: 54 mg/dL

Comments

The patient has hyponatremia and renal insufficiency, both of which can be attributable to high filling pressures and volume overload.

ELECTROCARDIOGRAM

Findings

The electrocardiogram shows an atrial paced, biventricular paced rhythm.

FOCUSED CLINICAL QUESTIONS AND DISCUSSION POINTS

Question

What implantable monitors are available for this patient that may assist in management of his condition?

Discussion

Many available implantable cardioverter-defibrillators have the ability to measure impedance, which may be a marker of pulmonary edema,[8] as well as other indicators of impending heart failure such as heart rate variability[2] and activity level. Several investigational implantable sensors have been tested, including a pulmonary artery sensor and a left atrial pressure sensor. These devices remain investigational as of this publication and are available only in clinical trials. Other sensors have been tested as part of pacemaker or defibrillator leads and can measure hemodynamics. The Chronicle Offers Management to Patients with Advanced Signs and Symptoms of Heart Failure (COMPASS HF) trial assessed the efficacy of using a right ventricular pressure sensor to aid physician-guided management in patients with NYHA class III to IV heart failure symptoms.[5] This study reached its safety end points, but did not reach its primary end point of reducing the rate of heart failure–related events. A separate analysis demonstrated a reduction in time to first heart failure rehospitalization. The Reducing Decompensation Events Utilizing Intracardiac Pressures in Patients with Chronic Heart Failure (REDUCE hf) trial assessed the use of continuous hemodynamic monitoring using right ventricular pressures in patients with NYHA class II to III heart failure symptoms; however, the study was terminated early because of lead failures and thus clinical efficacy was unable to be assessed.[3] A pulmonary artery sensor was tested in the CardioMEMS Heart Sensor Allows Monitoring of Pressure to Improve Outcomes in NYHA Class III Patients (CHAMPION) trial, in which qualifying patients received a pulmonary artery sensor that was embolized into a branch of the right or left pulmonary artery using catheters. A total of 550 patients were enrolled; patients were randomized in a 1:1 fashion with the control group receiving standard medical therapy for heart failure and the treatment group receiving the pulmonary sensor. Those in the treatment group received medical therapy tailored to pulmonary artery pressure goals. Results of the study revealed a significant reduction in hospitalization for heart failure at 6 months (30% reduction, p = 0.022), a reduction in mean pulmonary artery pressure at 6 months, and improvement in quality of life.[1] This device is not currently available and has not received U.S. Food and Drug Administration approval. The second device now available in clinical trials is a left atrial pressure sensor. This device was tested in a feasibility study, the Home Self-Therapy in Severe Heart Failure Patients (HOMEOSTASIS) trial,[7] which suggested that direct left atrial sensing, in combination with physician-directed patient self-management, had the potential to improve outcomes in patients with advanced heart failure. It demonstrated a reduction in mean left atrial pressure of 3.6 mm Hg at 12 months. The left atrial pressure sensor is currently available as part of a large, randomized controlled trial called the Left Atrial Pressure Monitoring to Optimize Heart Failure Therapy Study (LAPTOP-HF) and is limited to investigational use only.

Question

Is this patient a good candidate for the use of implantable sensors?

Discussion

This patient was an ideal candidate for implantable sensor technology. His symptoms were difficult to manage, and his physical examination was unreliable in assessing his volume status. Most hospitalizations for heart failure are related to worsening volume status and congestion. Filling pressures have been shown to increase 5 to 7 days before the development of symptoms severe enough to warrant hospitalization[4]; therefore knowledge of his true filling pressures will allow tight control of volume status and potentially reduce heart failure symptoms and need for hospitalization.

Question

What is the appropriate medical regimen for patients with systolic heart failure?

Discussion

Major society guidelines, based on evidence-based practice, recommend the use of an angiotensin-converting enzyme (ACE) inhibitor and beta blockers in patients with reduced LVEF (≤0.40) with or without symptoms of heart failure. Three beta blockers have proved beneficial in patients with heart failure with reduced LVEF: carvedilol, metoprolol succinate, and bisoprolol. Angiotensin-receptor blockers (ARBs) should be used in patients who are intolerant of ACE inhibitors. ARBs are recommended as additive therapy in patients who have moderately severe to severe heart failure symptoms and can be monitored for hyperkalemia and or worsening renal function.[6]

FINAL DIAGNOSIS

This patient had advanced heart failure with a reduced LVEF. He was placed on an optimal medical regimen and treated with CRT. Despite this, he remained unresponsive to these therapies and had persistent heart failure symptoms.

PLAN OF ACTION

After discussion, the patient was given a left atrial pressure sensor.

INTERVENTION

The patient was taken to the electrophysiology laboratory, where he was placed under general anesthesia and prepared and draped using standard sterile precautions. The left atrium was inspected using intracardiac echocardiography. After the right atrium was accessed by an inferior approach from the right femoral vein, the left atrium was inspected and found to be free of thrombus and then accessed by a transseptal approach. The left atrial pressure sensor was anchored into the intraatrial septum and pressure measurements obtained. The left atrial pressure was 20 mm Hg. Placement was confirmed using intracardiac echocardiography (Figure 47-1), followed by obtaining pulmonary and lateral chest radiographs (Figure 47-2).

OUTCOME

The patient was given instructions on how to measure left atrial pressure twice daily using a handheld device. This device—the patient advisory module—had a physician-directed algorithm built in that directed his medication regimen based on direct left atrial pressure measurement beginning at 3 months after implantation. After treatment, he experienced significant improvement in heart failure symptoms, with a reduction in NYHA class to NYHA II. Additionally, he remained free of hospitalization for heart failure for the subsequent year. His mean left atrial pressure fell from 32 mm Hg at 3 months to 9.8 mm Hg at 1 year after implantation (Figure 47-3).

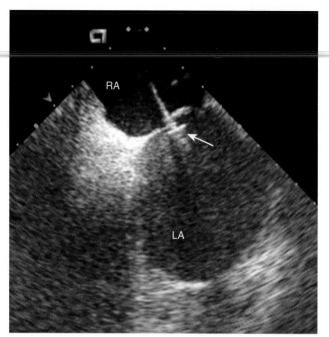

FIGURE 47-1   Intracardiac echocardiogram showing the left atrial pressure sensor in situ, anchored across the intraatrial septum from the right atrium. *Caution:* This is an investigational device, restricted by U.S. law to investigational use. *LA,* Left atrium; *RA,* right atrium.

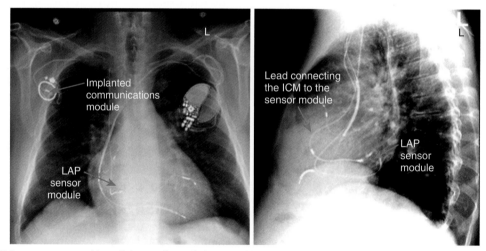

FIGURE 47-2   Pulmonary artery and lateral chest radiograph demonstrating proper placement of the left atrial pressure *(LAP)* monitoring system. The implanted communications module is used to transmit the pressure readings from the sensor module. The patient also has a cardiac resynchronization therapy device with an implantable cardioverter-defibrillator. *Caution:* This is an investigational device, restricted by U.S. law to investigational use. *ICM,* Implanted Communications Module.

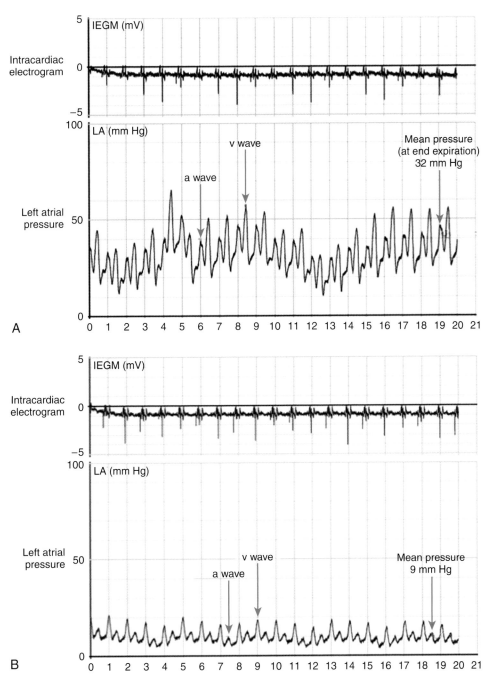

FIGURE 47-3 **A,** Left atrial pressure tracing obtained 3 months after implantation of the left atrial pressure (LAP) sensor, before initiation of a tailored regimen based on pressure readings. The waveform can be correlated with the atrial electrocardiogram and demonstrates significantly elevated pressure. **B,** LAP tracing obtained 12 months after implantation of the LAP sensor, after treatment was tailored using pressure readings. The waveform demonstrates a significant reduction in LAP in contrast to 9 months previously CAUTION: This is an investigational device, restricted by U.S. law to investigational use. *IEGM,* Intracardiac electrogram.

Selected References

1. Abraham W, Adamson P, Bourge R, et al: Wireless pulmonary artery haemodynamic monitoring in chronic heart failure: a randomised controlled trial, *Lancet* 377:658-666, 2011.
2. Adamson PB: Continuous heart rate variability from an implanted device: a practical guide for clinical use, *Congest Heart Fail* 11:327-330, 2005.
3. Adamson PB, Gold MR, Bennett T, et al: Continuous hemodynamic monitoring in patients with mild to moderate heart failure: results of The Reducing Decompensation Events Utilizing Intracardiac Pressures in Patients, *Congest Heart Fail* 17:248-254, 2011.
4. Adamson PB, Magalski A, Braunschweig F, et al: Ongoing right ventricular hemodynamics in heart failure: clinical value of measurements derived from an implantable monitoring system, *J Am Coll Cardiol* 41:565-571, 2003.
5. Bourge RC, Abraham WT, Adamson PB, et al: Randomized controlled trial of an implantable continuous hemodynamic monitor in patients with advanced heart failure: the COMPASS-HF study, *J Am Coll Cardiol* 51:1073-1079, 2008.
6. Hunt SA, Abraham WT, Chin MH, et al: 2009 focused update incorporated into the ACC/AHA 2005 Guidelines for the Diagnosis and Management of Heart Failure in Adults: a report of the American College of Cardiology Foundation/American Heart Association Task Force on Practice Guidelines: developed in collaboration with the International Society for Heart and Lung Transplantation, *Circulation* 119, 2009, e391.
7. Ritzema J, Troughton R, Melton I, et al: Physician-directed patient self-management of left atrial pressure in advanced chronic heart failure, *Circulation* 121:1086-1095, 2010.
8. Yu CM, Wang L, Chau E, et al: Intrathoracic impedance monitoring in patients with heart failure: correlation with fluid status and feasibility of early warning preceding hospitalization, *Circulation* 112:841-848, 2005.

Role of Remote Monitoring in Managing a Patient on Cardiac Resynchronization Therapy: Medical Therapy and Device Optimization

Mary P. Orencole and Jagmeet P. Singh

Age	Gender	Occupation	Working Diagnosis
54 Years	Male	Business Entrepreneur	Non-ischemic idiopathic cardiomyopathy

HISTORY

This 54-year-old man first sought treatment in 2005 with symptoms of progressive dyspnea on exertion, pedal edema accompanied by paroxysmal nocturnal dyspnea, and orthopnea. He had initially been treated in the community for upper respiratory tract infection with oral antibiotics but then developed symptoms of shortness of breath and fatigue. On further medical testing, he was diagnosed with dilated cardiomyopathy. His initial echocardiogram showed dilated cardiomyopathy with left ventricular internal diameter at end-diastole of 64 mm Hg, left ventricular ejection fraction (LVEF) of 18% with diffuse hypokinesis, moderate mitral regurgitation, left atrial enlargement, and moderate-to-severe tricuspid regurgitation.

The patient's risk factors included active cigarette smoking, with a 25 pack-year history, and hyperlipidemia. He underwent cardiac catheterization, which showed mild obstructive coronary artery disease; however, this was unlikely to explain the severity of his cardiomyopathy and symptoms.

A single-lead implantable cardioverter-defibrillator (ICD) was originally placed in March 2010 for New York Heart Association (NYHA) class II symptoms with a QRS duration of 110 ms. Progressive worsening and widening of his QRS duration resulted in an upgrade to a cardiac resynchronization therapy defibrillator (CRT-D) with the addition of atrial and left ventricular leads. His NYHA classification had worsened to NYHA class III with hospitalizations for heart failure. Because of his relatively narrow QRS duration (126 ms), he also underwent a dyssynchrony echocardiographic study to ascertain the potential value of an upgrade of his ICD.

After the upgrade he came to our clinic for an unscheduled visit after being "bothered" by an audible tone from his device occurring every morning over several consecutive days. He described it as "an annoying occurrence" during his morning business meetings. His device interrogation was notable for inappropriate ICD therapy having occurred while he was asleep 7 days previously. The intracardiac electrograms documented atrial fibrillation with rapid ventricular response, which converted to sinus rhythm after he received one 34-J shock. After this initial shock he connected and established himself on our remote monitoring system.

He proceeded over the next several months to have several episodes of paroxysmal atrial fibrillation, which were detected accurately by his remote monitoring intracardiac electrograms, as exemplified in Table 48-1. Amiodarone therapy was started, but poorly tolerated secondary to neurologic effects of increased somnolence and fatigue, which led to the patient discontinuing the medication. On the amiodarone, his activity level decreased significantly, as seen on remote monitoring, although his biventricular pacing quantities went up significantly, as highlighted and circled in Figure 48-1.

The choices for alert alarms are audible and/or system monitor alerts that can range from 3 to 24 hours, including settings for the accompanying ventricular rates. For patients with heart failure, it is beneficial to set these parameters conservatively because the onset of atrial fibrillation could exacerbate their heart failure.

As a result of increasing heart failure symptoms, a month-long trial of turning off the left ventricular lead was done, but his heart failure symptoms worsened over the following weeks. As indicated earlier, his baseline

TABLE 48-1   Remote Arrhythmia Episode List

Type	ATP Seq	Shocks	Success	ID no.	Date	Time hh:mm	Duration hh:mm:ss	Average BPM A/V
AT/AF				102	17-Sep-2012	04:32	(Episode in progress)	
AT/AF				101	17-Sep-2012	03:48	:44:22	178/98
AT/AF				100	17-Sep-2012	00:16	03:31:53	180/90
AT/AF				99	16-Sep-2012	02:17	21:58:27	180/91
AT/AF				98	15-Sep-2012	23:20	02:57:42	178/89
AT/AF				97	15-Sep-2012	01:10	22:09:17	180/90
AT/AF				96	15-Sep-2012	00:06	01:04:13	175/87
AT/AF				95	14-Sep-2012	14:10	09:56:19	178/88
AT/AF				94	14-Sep-2012	13:59	:10:43	176/88
AT/AF				93	14-Sep-2012	08:20	05:38:34	176/88
AT/AF				92	14-Sep-2012	05:22	02:57:52	176/86
AT/AF				91	13-Sep-2012	19:38	09:44:24	169/83

AF, Atrial fibrillation; *AT,* atrial tachycardia; *ATP Seq,* anti-tachycardial pacing sequence; *A/V,* atrioventricular; *BPM,* beats per minute; *hh,* hours; *ID,* identification; *mm,* minutes; *ss;* seconds.

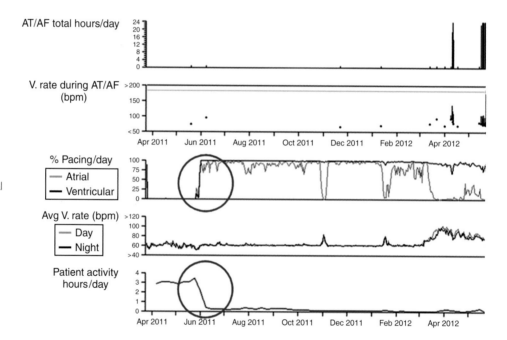

FIGURE 48-1 Decreased quantities of biventricular pacing present along with activity level trends. *AF,* Atrial fibrillation; *AT,* atrial tachycardia; *V,* ventricular.

QRS duration was fairly narrow, at 126 ms, which can be a substrate for nonresponse to CRT.

As his heart failure progressed, he developed multiple episodes of nonsustained ventricular tachycardia, some of which occurred at ventricular rates as low as 131 bpm. These ventricular arrhythmias were preceded by elevations in his intrathoracic lead impedance fluid index trends measured in Ohms and identified as OptiVol in Medtronic (Medtronic, Minneapolis, Minn.) devices. His impedance measurements became important to monitor on a regular basis, because they were an accurate predictor of his heart failure exacerbations.

Remote monitoring trends of these episodes are viewed in Figure 48-2.

The patient's clinical trajectory went further downhill as he developed persistent atrial fibrillation, with rapid ventricular rates and decreased percentages of biventricular pacing ultimately requiring cardioversion. Because of the size of his left atrium, the occurrence of atrial fibrillation was not unexpected. He had not been on anticoagulation therapy and was started on dabigatran when his lifestyle proved that he would not be compliant for frequent blood level international normalized ratio blood sample checks on warfarin.

CURRENT MEDICATIONS

The patient was taking captopril 6.25 mg three times daily, carvedilol 6.25 mg twice daily, furosemide 40 mg twice daily, spironolactone 25 mg daily, digoxin 0.125 mg daily, atorvastatin 80 mg daily, and aspirin 81 mg daily. Carvedilol was discontinued when his blood pressure was no longer high enough, and metoprolol was resumed. His diuretic medications included torsemide 80 mg twice daily, with an additional 80 mg as needed based on daily weight. Metolazone 2.5 mg was then added on an as-needed basis. His intolerance of amiodarone and ongoing ventricular arrhythmias necessitated the initiation of low-dose sotalol, which was eventually

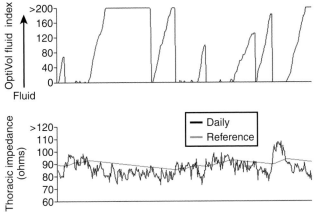

FIGURE 48-2 Intrathoracic impedance trends.

titrated up to 120 mg twice daily for treatment of ventricular arrhythmias as documented by his remote transmission (Figure 48-3) that required ICD therapies.

Comments

The remote monitoring of cardiac implantable devices is rapidly growing throughout most of our clinical practices. Remote transmissions are being used to replace in-office device checks and provide a method of surveillance for recalled leads. For patients with CRT devices, programmed device alerts are frequently indicative of a clinical change requiring intervention. Previous work reported that 86% of remote monitoring events done on daily transmissions were due to medical conditions, including detection of supraventricular or ventricular arrhythmias, ICD therapy, or paroxysmal atrial fibrillation, as opposed to lead or technical problems.[5] Early detection of these electrophysiologic issues or clinical trends can result in earlier intervention and decreased mortality. In this case study, close monitoring of the patient alerts through the remote system prevented several potential admissions and ICD therapies because his medications were adjusted while he remained at home. In this single case study the audible alert actually prompted the patient's first clinic visit. He sought health care only because of the bothersome audible tone coming from his device. This may serve as a useful feature to keep programmed on in patients with issues of compliance. The Diagnostic Outcome Trial in Heart Failure

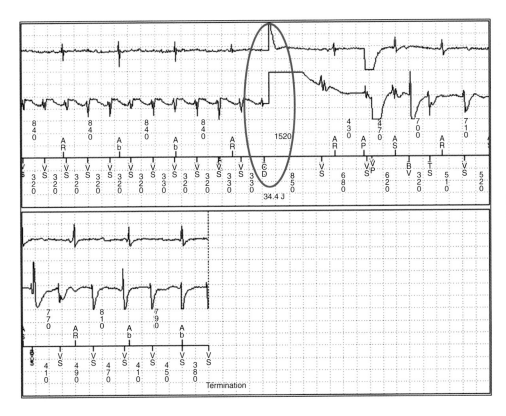

FIGURE 48-3 Ventricular tachycardia with a 35-J shock.

(DOT-HF) study demonstrated that audible alerts may increase hospital admissions. This is because OptiVol measures as a predictor of heart failure exacerbations lack specificity and may result in patients and physicians overreacting to a false-positive alert.

PHYSICAL EXAMINATION

BP/HR: 120/70 mm Hg/80 bpm
Height/weight: 97.5 kg/182.9 cm
Body mass index: 29.2
Head, ears, eyes, nose, throat: Unremarkable
Neck: Supple; positive jugular venous distention up to 9 cm without carotid bruits
Lungs: Scattered crackles were present bilaterally
Heart: Regular rate and rhythm, normal first heart sound (S_1) and second heart sound (S_2), no murmurs or gallops
Abdomen: Soft, nontender, with no organomegaly
Extremities: Trace edema present laterally, with 2+ distal pulses

LABORATORY DATA

Hemaglobin: 9.3 g/dL
Hematocrit/packed cell volume: 29.3%
Platelet count: 195 × 10^3/μL
Sodium: 122 mmol/L
Potassium: 4.3 mmol/L
Creatinine: 3.2-4.8 mmol/L
Blood urea nitrogen: 39-72 mg/dL

ELECTROCARDIOGRAM

The electrocardiogram showed sinus rhythm at 67 bpm, first-degree atrioventricular block with a PR interval of 228 ms, QRS duration 126 ms, left axis deviation consistent with a left anterior fascicular hemiblock, poor R-wave progression across the precordium, and Q-waves in the inferior leads.

CHEST RADIOGRAPH

On chest radiography the cardiomyopathy was shown to be stable. Both lungs were inflated and clear (Figure 48-4).

EXERCISE TESTING

In the myocardial imaging (Regadenoson) stress test, the patient's heart rate reached 37% of predicted rate, achieving the metabolic equivalent of task of 1. No evidence of ischemia was found, and the LVEF was 33%. Moderate right and left ventricular dilation were present.

DYSSYNCHRONY ECHOCARDIOGRAM

The dyssynchrony echocardiogram revealed a left atrial pressure of 53 mm, left ventricular internal diameter at end-diastole of 63 mm, left ventricular internal diameter at end-systole of 54 mm, right ventricular systolic pressure of 35, and LVEF of 26%. For interventricular mechanical delay, the difference between left ventricular and right ventricular preejection intervals, the patient's value was –37 ms. The left ventricular preejection interval was 174 ms. The left ventricular filling ratio, the ratio of left ventricular filling time to cardiac cycle length, was 29%. The opposing wall delay between the peak longitudinal systolic velocities in the basal septal and lateral walls was 185 ms, the maximum difference in time to peak longitudinal systole was 202 ms, and the standard deviation in time to peak longitudinal systolic velocity among 10 left ventricular segments (midanterior and posterior segments were excluded) was 76 ms. Mechanical dyssynchrony was present, with the lateral segments demonstrating the most delayed systolic motion.

CARDIAC CATHETERIZATION

The patient's cardiac output is 3.68 L/min, cardiac index is 1.8 L/min/m², peripheral vascular resistance was

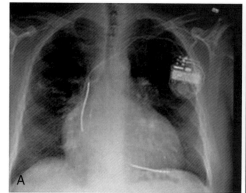
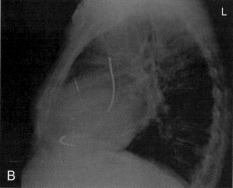

FIGURE 48-4 Chest radiographs. **A,** Posterior anterior view. **B,** Lateral view.

109 dyn*s/cm5, and systemic vascular resistance was 1475, with a ratio of 0.075. The right atrium was 30/20 (v/m), right ventricle was 40/9 s/edp, wedge was 37/32, pulmonary artery was 45/32/37, and left ventricle was 97/37. His left main coronary artery was normal; 40% focal stenosis was found in the proximal third of the mid–left anterior descending artery. The left circumflex and right coronary arteries were normal. Combined systolic and diastolic heart failure also was present.

PULMONARY FUNCTION TESTING

The patient's forced expiratory volume in 1 second measured 2.94 L/second, which is 75% of predicted value. His forced vital capacity measured 4.13 L, which was 83% of predicted value, with forced expiratory flow measuring 2.94 L/second, or 52% of predicted capacity. The findings demonstrated a mild obstructive ventilatory defect.

OUTCOME

As the patient's heart failure and arrhythmias worsened, his remote alerts became more frequent and the management of his care on an outpatient basis was facilitated by these alerts. He went into atrial flutter with ventricular sensed response pacing. Examination of his remote internal electrograms demonstrated the presence of ventricular trigger pacing (Figure 48-5).

FINAL DIAGNOSIS

This patient had dilated cardiomyopathy, with both paroxysmal atrial fibrillation and ventricular arrhythmias.

Comments

Remote monitoring of this patient's device led to multiple interventions, some of which prevented hospitalizations

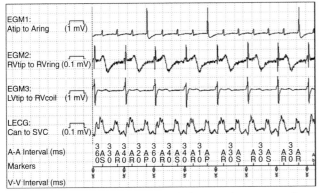

FIGURE 48-5 Atrial flutter with ventricular sensed response pacing and loss of true biventricular pacing. *EGM*, Electrogram; *LV*, left ventricle; *RV*, right ventricle; *SVC*, superior vena cava; *VS*, ventricular sensing.

and led to earlier detection of both atrial and ventricular arrhythmias. The importance of examining and monitoring the quantity of biventricular pacing and differentiating the degree of trigger or ventricular assisted pacing is essential in this fragile population. At time of publication, biventricular pacing alerts are not available on all device platforms, but support for their value has been demonstrated.[3,4] Ultimately, with the assistance of these last remote alerts, it was determined that the patient was nearing the end of life. He had declined the option of heart transplantation. The decision was made to not proceed with synchronized electrical cardioversion for his last episode of atrial flutter and to turn off his defibrillator. The focus then became quality at the end of life; he was then admitted to hospice, where he died within 48 hours.

FOCUSED CLINICAL QUESTIONS AND DISCUSSION POINTS

Question

Does the usage of remote monitoring decrease health care usage?

Discussion

Although the mortality and hospitalization benefits of remote monitoring have been demonstrated,[5,7] it appears that other potential cost savings have not consistently been supported, possibly because of nonstandardization of monitoring protocols, procedures, and equipment. A significant amount of variability exists among alert settings, which can lead to increased health care costs. In the intrathoracic impedance monitoring study DOT-HF,[9] which examined whether heart failure patient management using measurements of intrathoracic impedances with an implanted device as a means of detecting increases in pulmonary fluid would lead to a reduction in the combined end point of all-cause mortality or heart failure hospitalizations, results included an increase in heart failure admissions and outpatient visits because of patients receiving audible alerts for daily fluctuations in impedance that were not clinically significant.

Audible patient tone alerts can create increased anxiety for patients and cannot be cleared without a visit to a device clinic or emergency room. This can be burdensome to patients who do not have easy access to a device clinic or especially if these alerts occur during nonclinic hours. At this juncture the use of these alerts should be individualized, based on the patient's clinical condition and some prior information on the correlation of these alerts with cardiac decompensation.

Having an audible alert was very important for this patient, who had not set up his remote system. Clearly if the audible alert had not gone off, he would not have gone to the clinic. On some devices, certain alerts can be evaluated and then cleared remotely. This alleviates undue anxiety for both patients and their household members or associates. In addition, with newer device implants, unfamiliarity and lack of education about these vibratory tones can be confused with antitachycardia pacing therapy or diaphragmatic stimulation.

Question

Does remote monitoring decrease mortality?

Discussion

The work done in the Altitude Survival Study that followed patients on the Boston Scientific Corporation (Natick, Mass.) remote monitoring system LATITUDE demonstrated a 50% relative reduction in the risk for death in contrast to that of patients followed in-clinic only.[7] Patients who transmitted weight and blood pressure data via the LATITUDE system experienced an additional 10% reduction in the risk for death in contrast to other networked CRT-D patients followed on LATITUDE. Patients who transmitted regular weight and blood pressure data in addition to their ICD parameters experienced an additional 10% mortality reduction in contrast to others who had only ICD parameters monitored on LATITUDE.

Question

Should we standardize remote alert settings according to diagnosis or device clinic practices?

Discussion

A great deal of variation remains among clinical practices regarding the manner in which remote monitoring is used. In a study of remote alerts, the remote alert settings appeared to be a crucial parameter in the efficacy of remote monitoring. This study found that more attention was paid to critical technical data such as battery exhaustion, impedances, sensing, and threshold measurements than to patients' clinical profiles, including heart rate monitoring and supraventricular arrhythmias.[2]

In addition, the time intervals between device checks and the level of personnel monitoring the transmission of this information have no clear standardization. Some practices continuously use it, in addition to routine scheduled device follow-up, and actively evaluate clinical parameters between visits. The actual practice standard of usage was 62% of CRT-D in patients managed by physicians with remote monitoring in addition to routine office follow-up.[7] No homogeneous standard of practice exists for evaluations, with times ranging from 3 months to only once annually.[6] Other clinical parameters that can be used to monitor heart failure include heart rate variability, lower

daily activity, weights, and abnormal heart rates, all of which provide ongoing trends between scheduled visits. These parameters will not be used to their fullest capacity until consensus can be reached regarding convenience and efficient usage for clinicians.[1] Preventing heart failure hospitalization necessitates thinking about remote monitoring differently and understanding that parameters that may help predict heart failure exacerbation must be monitored more carefully. Some of the parameters shown to be predictive of increased mortality include mean heart rate, heart rate variability, and physical activity.[8] The Program to Access and Review Trending Information and Evaluate Correlation to Symptoms in Patients With Heart Failure (PARTNERS HF) study evaluated variables to predict heart failure. Patients were observed to have a higher hospitalization rate if they had two of the following abnormal criteria during a 1-month period: long atrial fibrillation duration, rapid ventricular rate during atrial fibrillation, high (≥60) fluid index, low patient activity, abnormal autonomics (high night heart rate or low heart rate variability), or notable device therapy (low CRT pacing or ICD shocks) or if they only had a very high (≥100) fluid index.[10]

An international variability also remains in the usage of remote monitoring, which is affected by variables outside of clinician control such as the type of telecommunications equipment in patient homes, reimbursement for remote follow-up visits, and geographic distance between clinics and patient homes. The legal ramifications for identification and intervention of remote alerts in clinical settings with varied resources on a timely basis also need to be clarified.

Question

Is the percentage of biventricular pacing present an important parameter to monitor remotely?

Discussion

The percentage of biventricular pacing that matters, as discussed earlier, is not a parameter standardized as an alert on all CRT device remote alert systems. In a cohort study of 36,935 patients followed on the LATITUDE management system, mortality was inversely associated with the percentage of biventricular pacing both in the presence of sinus rhythm and when atrial pacing or atrial fibrillation was present. The greatest magnitude of reduction of mortality was observed with a biventricular pacing cutoff in excess of 98%.[3]

Selected References

1. Daubert JC, Saxon L, Adamson PB, et al: 2012 EHRA/HRS expert consensus statement on cardiac resynchronization therapy in heart failure: implant and follow-up recommendations and management, *Heart Rhythm* 9:1524-1576, 2012.

2. Folino AF, Chiusso F, Zanotto G, et al: Management of alert messages in the remote monitoring of implantable cardioverter defibrillators and pacemakers: an Italian single-region study, *Europace* 13:1281-1291, 2011.

3. Hayes DL, Boehmer JP, Day JD, et al: Cardiac resynchronization therapy and the relationship of percent biventricular pacing to symptoms and survival, *Heart Rhythm* 8:1469-1475, 2011.

4. Koplan BA, Kaplan AJ, Weiner S, et al: Heart failure decompensation and all-cause mortality in relation to percent biventricular pacing in patients with heart failure: is a goal of 100% biventricular pacing necessary? *J Am Coll Cardiol* 53:355-360, 2009.

5. Lazarus A: Remote, wireless, ambulatory monitoring of implantable pacemakers, cardioverter defibrillators, and cardiac resynchronization therapy systems: analysis of a worldwide database, *Pacing Clin Electrophysiol* 30(Suppl 1):S2-S12, 2007.

6. Marinskis G, van Erven L, Bongiorni MG, et al: Practices of cardiac implantable electronic device follow-up: results of the European Heart Rhythm Association survey, *Europace* 14: 423-425, 2012.

7. Saxon LA, Hayes DL, Gilliam FR, et al: Long-term outcome after ICD and CRT implantation and influence of remote device follow-up: the ALTITUDE survival study, *Circulation* 122:2359-2367, 2010.

8. Singh JP, Rosenthal LS, Hranitzky PM, et al: Device diagnostics and long-term clinical outcome in patients receiving cardiac resynchronization therapy, *Europace* 11:1647-1653, 2009.

9. van Veldhuisen DJ, Braunschweig F, Conraads V, et al: Intrathoracic impedance monitoring, audible patient alerts, and outcome in patients with heart failure, *Circulation* 124:1719-1726, 2011.

10. Whellan DJ, Ousdigian KT, Al-Khatib SM, et al: Combined heart failure device diagnostics identify patients at higher risk of subsequent heart failure hospitalizations: results from PARTNERS HF (Program to Access and Review Trending Information and Evaluate Correlation to Symptoms in Patients With Heart Failure) study, *J Am Coll Cardiol* 55:1803-1810, 2010.

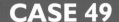

CASE 49

Role of Remote Monitoring in Managing a Patient on Cardiac Resynchronization Therapy: Atrial Fibrillation

Niraj Varma

Age	Gender	Occupation	Working Diagnosis
69 Years	Male	Retired Accountant	Persistent Atrial Fibrillation After Cardiac Surgery

HISTORY

In March 2012 this 68-year-old male patient sought treatment for chest pain. Non–ST segment elevation myocardial infarction (NSTEMI) was diagnosed, and, on catheterization, the patient was found to have severe three-vessel disease. This was unsuitable for percutaneous coronary intervention. He was therefore treated with bypass grafting and mitral valve repair.

The patient also had multiple myeloma (immunoglobulin G kappa), which was being treated with bortezimib and decadron; recurrent anemia resulting from myeloma and chemotherapy and requiring periodic blood transfusions; and thrombocytopenia. He was recommended to have platelet transfusions whenever his platelet concentration dropped below 20,000/μL or signs of bleeding occurred.

He had been previously diagnosed with mixed non-ischemic and ischemic cardiomyopathy. He had a history of adriamycin exposure and thoracic radiation for myeloma. Magnetic resonance imaging 3 months previously revealed a severely dilated left ventricle (left ventricular ejection fraction [LVEF], 28%) with an akinetic inferior wall and left ventricular scar area of 9%. There was no evidence of infiltrative disease, for example, amyloidosis.

The patient had previously experienced frequent premature ventricular contractions, possibly contributing to left ventricular dysfunction. Their origin was the inferior scar margin, and they had been successfully ablated 3 months previously (December 2011). Programmed electrical stimulation at that time induced a sustained monomorphic ventricular tachycardia. In view of this,

and baseline prolonged QRS duration with a left bundle branch block configuration, he received a cardiac resynchronization therapy defibrillator (CRT-D) implant (February 2012) with automatic remote monitoring capability. The implant was complicated by a significant anterior chest wall hematoma, but did not require evacuation. He had no prior history of atrial fibrillation.

The patient's other significant comorbidities were chronic renal dysfunction, with a creatinine value normally approximately 2.0, and carotid artery disease, for which he had undergone left carotid endarterectomy in 2009.

PHYSICAL EXAMINATION

Thirty-six hours after cardiac surgery, the patient developed atrial fibrillation with a rapid ventricular response.

BP/HR: 100/60 mm Hg/156 bpm
Neck: No jugular venous distention
Lungs: Bilaterally diminished breath sounds
Heart: Irregular pulse, short mitral systolic murmur
Abdomen: Soft, nontender
Extremities: Intact pulses, no edema

LABORATORY DATA

Hemoglobin: 10.6 mg/dL
Hematocrit/packed cell volume: 31.3%
Platelet count: 37×10^3/μL
Creatinine: 2.1 mg/dL

POSTOPERATIVE ECHOCARDIOGRAM

On the echocardiogram a moderate pericardial effusion was seen adjacent to the right ventricle and right atrium measuring 2.3 cm and a small circumferential pericardial effusion adjacent to the left ventricle. Pleural effusions were noted bilaterally. The LVEF was 15 ±5%. The mitral valve ring had moderate (2+) mitral valve regurgitation.

Comments

An attempt was made to restore normal rhythm. Unusually, this case of postoperative atrial fibrillation was resistant to amiodarone therapy and electrical cardioversion. Sinus rhythm could not be maintained for even a few minutes.

Ideally, this patient should have been placed on anticoagulation therapy. However, this would have risked expansion of postoperative pericardial and pleural effusions in the setting of thrombocytopenia and predilection for occult bleeding. In view of this hematologic disorder, anemia, and general postoperative debilitation risking falls (requiring wheelchair), the risk to benefit balance favored postponing anticoagulation. This strategy nevertheless risked both thromboembolism and heart failure precipitated by reduction of CRT pacing level. However,

because the patient had a device with remote monitoring, his condition could potentially be monitored closely without requirement for hospital visits. In particular, rate control could be optimized. The patient preferred this approach. He was discharged to a rehabilitation facility.

FOLLOW-UP

Postoperative 2 Weeks

The patient was readmitted with decompensated systolic heart failure and continued atrial fibrillation, with ventricular rates exceeding 110 bpm (CRT pacing level <60%). He underwent thoracentesis. He was placed on diuretic therapy, and his heart failure medications were slowly optimized. This was a difficult balance in view of his systolic blood pressure of approximately 100 mm Hg. A sternal wound infection was discovered and treated with antibiotics. Tremor related to amiodarone exposure was noted.

Postoperative 4 Weeks

The patient was admitted with a chest infection, which was treated with antibiotics. He was anemic (hemoglobin 8.8 mg/dL and hematocrit 26%) and received transfusion.

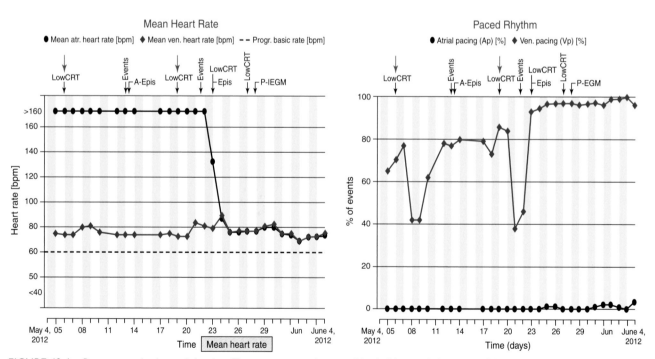

FIGURE 49-1   Remote monitoring website data. Two separate panels across identical 1-month time spans (May 4 to June 4) show separate graphic parameter trends. Low cardiac resynchronization therapy (CRT) events along the top of the panels represent alert notifications automatically delivered by the remote monitoring technology. *Left panel*, Persistent atrial fibrillation spontaneously terminates (May 23). *Right panel*, Episodic dips in CRT pacing percentage are noted, from baseline levels of approximately 80%. Atrial fibrillation terminates (May 23) and then CRT pacing percentage stabilizes at approximately 98%. Atrial pacing percentage remains negligible.

Postoperative 6 Weeks

The patient received remote follow-up. This showed that he was still in atrial fibrillation, with ventricular rates at 110 bpm reducing CRT pacing to less than 60%. He was contacted, and beta blockade was increased and digoxin added for rate control.

Postoperative 8 Weeks

Figure 49-1 shows the most recent remote trends from May 2012 onward. Periods of loss of CRT pacing (see Figure 49-1, *top right*) were notified within 24 hours of occurrence *(red arrows)*. These were treated promptly, resulting in resolution and gradual increase in the overall trend of the CRT pacing level over several weeks. These events were clinically silent but detected and signaled automatically by the device without patient participation and occurred irrespective of his location—his postoperative convalescence was spent alternately in skilled nursing facilities and home. Treatment could be implemented early and prevent future heart failure decompensation.

Spontaneous reversion to normal sinus rhythm occurred on May 24. The event was notified together with confirmatory electrograms (Figure 49-2, *bottom*). The CRT pacing level was maintained at 100% thereafter.

FOCUSED CLINICAL QUESTIONS AND DISCUSSION POINTS

Question

Is it important to monitor atrial fibrillation in patients with CRT devices?

Discussion

Atrial fibrillation in a patient treated with CRT worsens prognosis.[7] Device-detected persistent atrial tachycardia or atrial fibrillation was strongly associated with a two-fold increase in the composite death or heart failure hospitalization end point. Causes involve increased thromboembolic risk (even with a duration of a few minutes) hemodynamic deterioration and heart failure, and facilitation of ventricular arrhythmias. Periods of rapid atrioventricular conduction result in withdrawal of ventricular pacing and neutralize the beneficial effect of CRT. Thus reduction in CRT pacing to less than 92% increased mortality.[5] The detection and treatment of

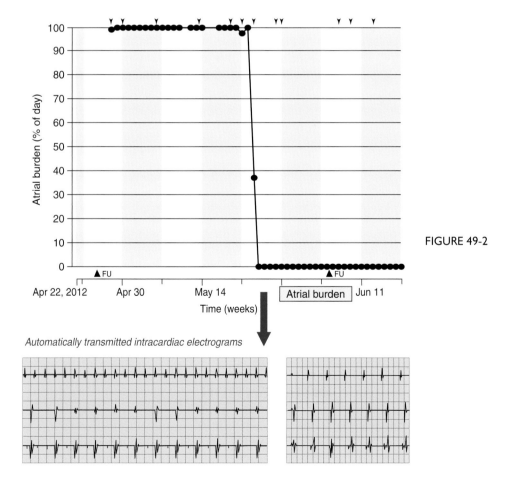

FIGURE 49-2

atrial fibrillation in patients on CRT is therefore important.

Question

How is monitoring performed for atrial fibrillation, treatment, and recurrence?

Discussion

The challenges in monitoring are in diagnosis of a silent, episodic problem, and measurement of its burden; treatment, which requires assessment of the risk to benefit ratio for appropriate anticoagulant therapy and attention to rapid ventricular responses; and monitoring to evaluate response, because patient symptoms are inaccurate and do not provide a suitable guide. Potential solutions are to schedule frequent in-clinic evaluations, which are burdensome and miss interim problems, and external monitoring, but this can be used only for short periods. However, implanted devices collect and quantify data and those embedded with remote monitoring technology enable early discovery, thus overcoming many of these barriers.[4,8] In regard to atrial fibrillation, delivery of intracardiac electrograms permits confirmation of device diagnosis (mode switch data in isolation may be vulnerable to false-positive results). Continuous monitoring with daily updating of parameter trends enables accurate measurements, and automatic notification of changes facilitates early clinical management.[9]

Question

Should the patient receive anticoagulation therapy?

Discussion

Generally, early discovery enables early anticoagulation prescription decisions, if necessary. This may reduce thromboembolic risk.[1] However, the decision to treat requires careful adjudication in each individual case. This is complicated given the different choices of measures for assessing risk from either the arrhythmia (e.g., CHADS versus CHADS VASC) or, importantly, the treatment itself (HAS-BLED versus HEMORRHAGES) cited in guidelines issued by various professional societies.[2] Selection of anticoagulant becomes complicated with the recent availability of three new anticoagulants, none of which have been compared head-to-head in similar populations. Additionally, the inclusion of patient perspective on the decision is vital. A risk prediction model incorporating the several aspects of clinical decision making may permit tailored prescription of novel agents on an individual basis to achieve desired risk reductions.

Question

Is it important to monitor for rate control?

Discussion

High ventricular rates in patients on CRT are particularly important because they result in withdrawal of CRT, which removes its beneficial effect in heart failure. Even a less than 10% loss of pacing may reduce mortality by 25% to 30%. Thus, in this case, the patient had acute heart failure decompensation 2 weeks after discharge that required readmission (however, subsequent loss of CRT was rapidly rectified with the use of remote monitoring).

Several mechanisms are employed by manufacturers to promote continuous CRT delivery during atrial fibrillation. For example, each right ventricular sensed event may trigger a paced response immediately (within 10 ms) in one or both ventricles depending on how ventricular pacing is programmed.[3] However, these most likely generate partially resynchronized complexes, and their efficacy is likely limited. It is therefore important to commit to pacing. This may be accomplished by restoring normal sinus rhythm if possible. For persistent atrial fibrillation, atrioventricular nodal ablation restores consistent 100% ventricular capture and has shown mortality and functional benefits.[6]

FINAL DIAGNOSIS

The diagnosis in this patient was persistent atrial fibrillation with rapid ventricular rates in the presence of heart failure, a CRT device, and balance of risk to benefit considerations for anticoagulation that favored withholding therapy at the time of initial consultation.

PLAN OF ACTION

Immediate restoration of normal rhythm and accompanying anticoagulation were not possible; therefore a strategy of rate control was implemented with the aim of preventing rapid conducted rates and loss of CRT pacing. If medical measures were unsuccessful, atrioventricular nodal ablation would be indicated. These objectives would be followed with extended remote monitoring. If the balance of comorbidities changed in the future, anticoagulation could be reconsidered. This management strategy depended on continuous monitoring.

INTERVENTION

Accelerated ventricular rates sporadically caused loss of CRT pacing level (see Figure 49-1). Such events are typically unsuspected by both patients and physicians,

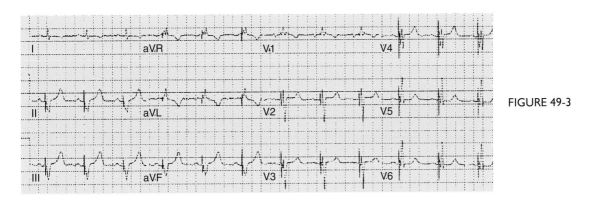

FIGURE 49-3

until they lead to symptomatic deterioration. Remote monitoring–derived trends revealed that the ventricular rate was usually controlled, but prone to periods of acceleration during which CRT pacing loss was further aggravated. However, these events were treated effectively. Atrioventricular nodal ablation would have been indicated if atrial fibrillation had persisted and ventricular rate accelerations had become more prolonged.

The case illustrates how remote monitoring–derived arrhythmia and pacing trends guided clinical decision making over a period of several months of a difficult convalescence phase with changing status of comorbidities. Parameter trending permitted close monitoring. Parameter deviations (e.g., for loss of CRT pacing level) were self-declared by the device and enabled clinical action to optimize medications within 24 hours. This preemptive care (rather than reactive to clinical decompensation) over the course of several months resulted in gradual improvement and likely avoided further heart failure decompensation and inpatient admissions. Event notification for atrial fibrillation termination with confirmatory electrograms resolved a persistent anxiety and permitted patient reassurance, stabilization of medical therapy, and correlation with clinical recovery.

Remote monitoring was continued to provide early (<24-hour) notification of atrioventricular recurrence and enable prompt cardioversion if necessary.

OUTCOME

Postoperative atrial fibrillation is usually reversible and self-limited, but in this case persisted for almost 3 months. Unusually, it was recalcitrant to therapy, including amiodarone (which resulted in adverse effects) and electrical cardioversion. In view of renal dysfunction and coronary artery disease, other antiarrythmics were contraindicated. Although conducted ventricular rates were eventually maintained at fewer than 90 bpm (see Figure 49-1), these occasionally were accompanied by loss of CRT pacing level. Spontaneous termination of atrial fibrillation resolved the dilemma about the necessity for atrioventricular nodal ablation and chronic anticoagulation.

Findings

No atrial fibrillation recurred, and CRT pacing has been sustained at 100% (Figure 49-3). The patient has been managed without anticoagulation and recovered well. He has resumed a physically active lifestyle.

Comments

In summary, in recipients of CRT devices, remote monitoring technology provides a high-definition image of patterns of atrial fibrillation occurrence, measurement of its daily burden, and associated ventricular rate and interaction with pacing. These data may guide clinical decision processes regarding anticoagulation and efficacy of antiarrhythmic measures undertaken, including drug therapy, ablation, and pacing systems. This ability for close monitoring is important in patients with multiple medical conditions, prone to episodic decompensations and presenting difficult management decisions.

Selected References

1. Boriani G, Santini M, Lunati M, et al: Improving thromboprophylaxis using atrial fibrillation diagnostic capabilities in implantable cardioverter-defibrillators: the multicentre Italian ANGELS of AF Project, *Circ Cardiovasc Qual Outcomes* 5:182-188, 2012.
2. Camm AJ, Kirchhof P, Lip GY, et al: Guidelines for the management of atrial fibrillation: the Task Force for the Management of Atrial Fibrillation of the European Society of Cardiology (ESC), *Eur Heart J* 31:2369-2429, 2010.
3. Ganesan AN, Brooks AG, Roberts-Thomson KC, et al: Role of AV nodal ablation in cardiac resynchronization in patients with coexistent atrial fibrillation and heart failure: a systematic review, *J Am Coll Cardiol* 59:719-726, 2012.
4. Healey JS, Israel CW, Connolly SJ, et al: Relevance of electrical remodeling in human atrial fibrillation: results of the asymptomatic atrial fibrillation and stroke evaluation in pacemaker patients and the atrial fibrillation reduction atrial pacing trial mechanisms of atrial fibrillation study, *Circ Arrhythm Electrophysiol* 5:626-631, 2012.
5. Koplan BA, Kaplan AJ, Weiner S, et al: Heart failure decompensation and all-cause mortality in relation to percent biventricular pacing in patients with heart failure: is a goal of 100% biventricular pacing necessary? *J Am Coll Cardiol* 53:355-360, 2009.

6. Varma N, Wilkoff B: Device features for managing patients with heart failure, *Heart Fail Clin* 7:215-225, 2011. viii.

7. Santini M, Gasparini M, Landolina M, et al: Device-detected atrial tachyarrhythmias predict adverse outcome in real-world patients with implantable biventricular defibrillators, *J Am Coll Cardiol* 57:167-172, 2011.

8. Varma N, Stambler B, Chun S: Detection of atrial fibrillation by implanted devices with wireless data transmission capability, *Pacing Clin Electrophysiol* 28(Suppl 1):S133-S136, 2005.

9. Varma N, Epstein A, Irimpen A, et al: TRUST Investigators. Efficacy and safety of automatic remote monitoring for ICD follow-up: the TRUST trial, *Circulation* 122:325-332, 2010.

Index